50 HEALTH SCARES THAT FIZZLED

50 HEALTH SCARES THAT FIZZLED

JOAN R. CALLAHAN

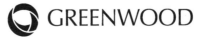 GREENWOOD

AN IMPRINT OF ABC-CLIO, LLC
Santa Barbara, California • Denver, Colorado • Oxford, England

Library of Congress Cataloging-in-Publication Data

Callahan, Joan R.
  50 health scares that fizzled / Joan R. Callahan.
    p. cm.
  Fifty health scares that fizzled
  Includes bibliographical references and index.
    ISBN 978–0–313–38538–4 (hard copy : alk. paper) — ISBN 978–0–313–38539–1 (ebook)
1. Medical misconceptions. 2. Health risk assessment. I. Title. II. Title: Fifty health scares that fizzled.
    [DNLM: 1. Health Education. 2. Mass Media. 3. Fear—psychology. 4. Fraud—psychology.
5. Health Behavior. WA 590]
R729.9.C35 2011
613—dc22   2010046067

ISBN: 978–0–313–38538–4
EISBN: 978–0–313–38539–1

15 14 13 12 11   1 2 3 4 5

This book is also available on the World Wide Web as an eBook.
Visit www.abc-clio.com for details.

Greenwood
An Imprint of ABC-CLIO, LLC

ABC-CLIO, LLC
130 Cremona Drive, P.O. Box 1911
Santa Barbara, California 93116-1911

This book is printed on acid-free paper ∞

Manufactured in the United States of America

CONTENTS

INTRODUCTION

It's much easier to scare people than to unscare them.

—Dr. Paul Offit (*Autism's False Prophets*, 2008)

As the title suggests, this book is about media events known as health scares that have ended (or mostly ended) not with a bang but a whimper. To "fizzle" means to end in a way that someone finds unsatisfactory. It often refers to an event or trend that holds the promise of a dramatic conclusion and then goes nowhere. A party might be said to fizzle if the guests fall asleep or go home early. The Ford Edsel is a famous example of a car that fizzled, only to be reborn as a classic. Many a child actor's career has fizzled at puberty.

In the case of a health scare, however, fizzling is more often a cause for celebration. If the latest disease outbreak or toxic exposure du jour turns out to be less dangerous than expected—or if the public and the news media simply lose interest, irrespective of actual risk—then the scare fizzles. But even a false alarm may cause a great deal of fuss and expense that often requires a scapegoat, such as a government agency that acted on the best information available at the time, or the scientists who reported preliminary study findings and lived to eat them.

The English word *fizzle* was in use by about 1600, when it meant to break wind. By the nineteenth century, however, fizzle referred to a comparable hissing or fizzing noise produced by wet blasting powder when it burned briefly and then went out instead of exploding. Again, whether this outcome was good or bad depended on the narrator's perspective. As a result of this phenomenon, "keeping one's powder dry" has become a metaphor for maintaining a constant state of readiness for something.

WHAT IS A HEALTH SCARE?

A health scare is a highly publicized threat (or perceived threat) to human health. These scares come in all shapes and sizes, ranging from the fear of high-voltage power lines to the fear of contaminated watercress. Yet the fact that we call something a health "scare" does not necessarily imply that the scare is unfounded, or that people are gullible. A health scare often starts with a valid discovery or hypothesis that somehow fires the public imagination. The scare typically undergoes a period of growth, sometimes budding off new scares in the process, and then fizzles or otherwise ends for a variety of reasons, such as the discovery of a cure, the banning of a toxic chemical, the debunking of an urban legend, or the arrival of a newer, more photogenic health scare. Some scares repeatedly fizzle, only to be reborn in new shapes.

The public often attributes health scares to conspiracies—by the pharmaceutical industry, the government, or the environmental left—but more often these scares seem to result from the absence of conspiracy. That is, the word "conspiracy" implies that people work together in a coordinated fashion to achieve an outcome that is detrimental to someone else's interests. But when people fail to work together at all, the results can be even worse, with independent agencies and experts and quacks all going off half-cocked. The contradictory news reporting that immediately followed the 1979 accident at Three Mile Island (Chapter 36) is a good example; early coverage of the 2009 swine flu pandemic (Chapter 8) is another. We all seem to want clear answers from closed ranks of unimpeachable experts, but instead we get exactly what the Bill of Rights guarantees: freedom of speech, and lots of it. The Internet provides immediate access to so many opinions on every issue that it is sometimes hard to take anyone seriously.

HOW A HEALTH SCARE STARTS

A health scare does not necessarily require any precipitating event. In the 1890s, for example, famed physician and Atlantean theorist Dr. Joseph P. Widney (1841–1938) wanted to create an inland sea in California's Salton Basin. He immediately encountered opposition from area residents and journalists who claimed—among other things—that the project would encourage boa constrictors and alligators to take up residence in southern California, thus endangering women and children.

Although the danger probably seemed real at the time, its proponents did not explain how these reptiles would travel from the Gulf Coast states to the Salton Basin, or why they would not also eat men. In 1905, the matter was resolved when the Colorado River jumped its banks (not for the first time in history) and filled the Salton Basin anyway. More than a century later, it is probably fair to say that boa constrictors and alligators are among the few health hazards that have *not* attended the aging of the Salton Sea.

More often, a health scare starts because of something that has actually happened. The news media frequently report that a new infectious disease is spreading somewhere in the world, or that exposure to an industrial chemical is endangering our lives, or that a widely used food, drug, appliance, or lifestyle choice causes cancer or heart disease or diabetes. All these are examples of health scares. Responsible journalists do not invent these stories out of thin air; typical sources include medical journal articles, comments by public figures, and agency press releases. When sources disagree on the level of threat, or fail to explain the problem clearly, reporters must interpret the available information as best they can.

A health scare may result from various combinations of circumstances, as summarized in Table I.1. What all these combinations have in common is that the news media report high risk. This media response appears to be a necessary condition for a major health scare, but not always sufficient to keep it going for long. Sometimes news reporting is truly scary, but the public doesn't buy it, as in the case of the 2009 H1N1 swine flu, when the health scare largely fizzled before the real pandemic had even ended (Chapter 8). To be

Table I.1 Health Scare Conditions and Outcomes

Actual Risk	Study Findings	Media Response	Outcome	Examples
High	High	High	Scare	Tobacco
High	Mixed	High	Scare	Hormone replacement therapy
Low	Mixed	High	Scare	Toxic mold
Low	Low	High	Scare	Return of smallpox
High	High	Low	No scare	Isotretoin
High	Mixed	Low	No scare	Dengue
Low	Mixed	Low	No scare	New World arenaviruses
Low	Low	Low	No scare	Clams at Torbay beach (see text)

effective, the media must often report what the public is already thinking; and in 2009, most people were probably thinking about the economic recession and terrorism and the healthcare crisis, not about the possibility of catching something as familiar as the flu.

In Table I.1 and throughout this book, the assessment of risk as high does not mean that a thing is "bad," but simply that its use or presence involves the potential for harm that may outweigh the benefits (if any). This is a highly subjective decision in many cases. Also, note that some possible combinations of circumstances are missing from Table I.1, because they would make no sense. For example, we can't list "actual risk" as high and "study findings" as low, or vice versa, because that would mean all the studies were wrong, and we would have nothing on which to base the assessment.

HOW A HEALTH SCARE KEEPS GOING

Some health scares, such as lead poisoning, have been with us for thousands of years and show no signs of ever ending. There are recent disturbing reports of lead-contaminated candy, toys, and other products exported from Mexico and China. A valid health scare such as this one cannot fizzle (or otherwise end) until the source is somehow brought under control, because newsworthy events continually return it to public scrutiny.

By contrast, many lesser health scares—including some that never made sense in the first place—keep going for years or centuries because of the so-called Bellman's Fallacy. We owe this happy phrase to Dr. Harry A. Waldron and to an 1874 poem called "The Hunting of the Snark," by Lewis Carroll, better known as the author of *Alice in Wonderland*. In the poem, a character called the Bellman states: "What I say three times is true." Indeed, whatever stories or statements we hear often enough may take on the outward appearance of truth. Many health scares resemble urban legends, in that everyone has heard someone else speak of the scare as fact, but nobody quite remembers the original source. For example, everybody knows that poinsettia leaves are poisonous, but they aren't. Everybody knows that camels carry syphilis, but they don't.[1] And everybody knows that 90,000 Chicagoans died from a waterborne disease epidemic in 1885, but they didn't.[2]

Yet other scary incidents never become health scares at all. The Bellman does not repeat these stories three times, or even once. In the summer of 1998, for example, the wire services reported that more than 130 people wading in the ocean near the English town of Torbay suddenly began screaming and ran from the surf with severely lacerated feet. Was it a great white shark, a sea serpent, an aquatic Jack the Ripper, or a secret weapon that a military agency was testing offshore?

The British Coast Guard and police evacuated the beach, posted warning signs, summoned air ambulances to transport the victims, and set out grimly in search of a would-be killer. And there the story ended, for the officers soon identified the menace as ordinary razor clams buried in the sand. The combination of a low tide and a hot day had prompted bathers to wade out farther than usual, and they had simply stepped on broken clamshells. The wire services bleeped once, and the incident was forgotten. Yet this story would appear to be newsworthy by the usual criteria. Although nobody died, there was a show of blood, and screaming children were involved. The injuries were sudden, mysterious, and unprecedented. But either the local authorities handled the media exceptionally well, or else the general public simply did not find the story that interesting.

Health scares that involve death may persist longer than others, but not even that rule is absolute. In 1999 and 2000, three women in California died from a previously unknown arenavirus infection, which turned out to be closely related to a dreaded African hemorrhagic fever called Lassa fever and an equally deadly South American disease called Machupo. The wild rodents that serve as a reservoir for arenaviruses in California are common, and the mode of transmission to those three unrelated victims was never determined, or at least never publicized. Yet that health scare, too, fizzled almost immediately. In other words, as a general rule, there is no general rule.

HOW A HEALTH SCARE ENDS

Most health scares eventually end, but not always by fizzling. For example, the 2003 outbreak of severe acute respiratory syndrome (SARS) in Asia caused a well-deserved worldwide health scare. The outbreak ended in 2004, with nearly 10 percent of its victims dead; but although the disease appears to be gone, a reservoir of infected animals may still exist. The outbreak probably ended because an intensive and well-coordinated public health response brought it under control, but there is no way to be certain of its present status until or unless it strikes again.

The 2001 anthrax mailing was another major health scare that ended quickly but did not fizzle. It ended because the perpetrator(s) apparently achieved the intended objective and decided to stop. Inhalation anthrax and domestic terrorism both remain as dangerous as ever, given the opportunity for exposure. A third example of a health scare that ended abruptly involves the drug thalidomide, which caused birth defects in thousands of children between 1957 and 1961 before health agencies recognized the problem and immediately banned the drug for use by pregnant women.

SCARES THAT FAIL TO SCARE

As we said, the 2009 H1N1 pandemic was an example of a short-lived health scare, but there have been even less successful ones. From an astronomer's viewpoint, the 1973 arrival of Comet Kohoutek was anything but a fizzle. As comets go, it was a fine one, yet the general public came to regard it as the celestial equivalent of the Edsel. The news media had predicted that it would be the most spectacular comet in all of human history, a mind-blowing New Age avatar, at least 25 times brighter than the best sightings of Halley's Comet. Fringe commentators in 1973 went even further, predicting worldwide catastrophes, political upheaval, and disease epidemics in Kohoutek's wake. It met all the criteria for a health scare, except for the fact that hardly anyone believed it.

Why disease epidemics? The prevailing pseudoscience in 1973 held that a comet's tail is full of drifting alien microorganisms, as evidenced by the fact that the Bible and other sacred texts reported major plagues following the appearance of comets in the heavens. Comets, among other things, were reported in the Middle Ages at the time of the bubonic plague epidemic now known as the Black Death. Yet Comet Kohoutek came and went, unattended by any unusual disasters, biological or otherwise. The comet itself was barely visible with the naked eye, on a clear night, for those who knew just where to look. Yes, there was a stock market crash in 1973–1974, and several places had floods, and let us not forget Watergate. But something happens every year.

SCARES OTHER THAN HEALTH SCARES

Y2K was a scare, and it certainly fizzled, but it seems inappropriate to call it a health scare. With self-designated experts predicting that technology and crops would fail, that airplanes would fall from the sky, and that civilization as we know it would cease to exist, it would have been superfluous to claim that Y2K might also make people sick. But scaremongers abhor a vacuum, and by 2010, the Large Hadron Collider (LHC), the impending 2012 Apocalypse, and the Apophis asteroid had long since replaced Y2K as popular sources of quasi-millennial terror. These are not health scares either, nor (on the basis of available facts) are they worth worrying about. The LHC is unlikely to create black holes that will swallow our planet, and if it does, no one will be left to assess the health impact anyway. Nor is there reason to believe that the ancient Mayans knew more about astronomy than we do; nor does Apophis appear likely to hit the Earth.

MORE TERMS

This book has a large glossary, but a few common terms may require advance warning. A *threat* is something that can harm human beings or their goods or environment. A *hazard* is similar to a threat, only less. Threats and hazards may be further designated as biological, chemical, radiological, sociological, or whatever, depending on their source (not their target). *Risk* is a measure of the expected loss resulting from a given threat or hazard, based on how severe the loss might be and how likely it is to occur.

Almost any imaginable action or object has some degree of associated risk, and the science of *risk management* seeks to identify, analyze, and minimize risk exposure. *Risk compression* refers to the frequent human tendency to overestimate rare risks and to underestimate common ones. For example, surveys of military personnel stationed in the Middle East during the first Gulf War showed that many of them feared venomous snakes and scorpions more than they feared the enemy's weapons, although the latter accounted for many more casualties.

The western world of the twenty-first century has often been called *a risk society*—that is, a society preoccupied with its own future safety, or more specifically with the analysis of risks that result from modernization. Governments that take this policy too far may become overly restrictive "nanny states," whereas those who fail to take it far enough may be accused of neglecting public health.

Another term that appears frequently in the risk literature is the *precautionary principle*. According to this guideline, it is often necessary for a regulatory agency to take immediate action without waiting for absolute proof. For example, if preliminary evidence suggests that a given chemical is harmful, the precautionary principle holds that the chemical should be banned as a temporary precaution while the parties slug it out in court. Depending on the outcome, the ban may become permanent. Even if further study exonerates the chemical, however, history shows that public opinion may outweigh the facts. Inevitably, the precautionary principle has led to some expensive and controversial mistakes, and some opponents interpret it to mean that the smallest risk outweighs even the greatest benefit.

The book presents 50 examples of recent and not-so-recent health scares, divided for convenience into seven categories:

- Medical interventions, such as vaccines and drugs.
- Infectious diseases or specific disease outbreaks.
- Food scares and recalls.
- Chemical additives in foods and beverages.
- Other potential biological hazards, such as spiders.
- Other chemical and radiological exposures, such as pesticides.
- Actions and reactions, such as lifestyle choices.

NOTES

1. J. R. Callahan, *Biological Hazards* (Oryx Press, 2002).
2. J. R. Callahan, *Emerging Biological Threats* (ABC-CLIO, 2009).

REFERENCES AND RECOMMENDED READING

Atkinson, H. G. "Internet Hosts Rumors and Hoaxes Galore." *Health News*, Vol. 7, 2001, p. 5.
Baum, A. "Stress, Intrusive Imagery, and Chronic Distress." *Health Psychology*, Vol. 9, 1990, pp. 653–675.
Brierley, S. "We're All Losing Faith in the Appliance of Science." *Marketing Week*, 18 July 2002.

Calman, K. "Beyond the 'Nanny State': Stewardship and Public Health." *Public Health*, Vol. 123, 2009, pp. e6–e10.

Collier, N., et al. "BioCaster: Detecting Public Health Rumors with a Web-Based Text Mining System." *Bioinformatics*, Vol. 24, 2008, pp. 2940–2941.

Colman, E. "Dinitrophenol and Obesity: An Early Twentieth-Century Regulatory Dilemma." *Regulatory Toxicology and Pharmacology*, Vol. 48, 2007, pp. 115–117.

Daley, J. "Overhyped Health Headlines Revealed." *Popular Science*, August 2009.

Ferriman, A. "An End to Health Scares?" *British Medical Journal*, Vol. 319, 1999, p. 716.

Filipkowski, K. B., et al. "Do Healthy People Worry? Modern Health Worries, Subjective Health Complaints, Perceived Health, and Health Care Utilization." *International Journal of Behavioral Medicine*, 9 September 2009.

Grace, K. M. "The Myth-Buster." *Alberta Report*, 18 December 2000.

Grant, T. 2007. *Health Matters*. Hoboken: John Wiley.

Hansen, S. F., et al. "Categorizing Mistaken False Positives in Regulation of Human and Environmental Health." *Risk Analysis*, Vol. 27, 2007, pp. 255–269.

Harteveldt, R. "Nurses Pay the Price for Media Health Scares." *Nursing Times*, Vol. 102, 2006, p. 14.

Haynes, S. "Health Scares: Unfair on the Public and on Health Professionals." *Professional Care of Mother and Child*, Vol. 10, 2000, pp. 30–31.

Hoffer, Eric. 1951. *The True Believer: Thoughts on the Nature of Mass Movements*. New York: Harper & Row.

Jochelson, K. "Nanny or Steward? The Role of Government in Public Health." *Public Health*, Vol. 120, 2006, pp. 1149–1155.

Johansson-Stenman, O. "Mad Cows, Terrorism and Junk Food: Should Public Policy Reflect Perceived or Objective Risks?" *Journal of Health Economics*, Vol. 27, 2008, pp. 234–248.

Kennedy, D. "Bathers Injured by Plague of Razor-Sharp Molluscs." *The Times*, 10 August 1998.

Killick, S. "Don't Be Scared." *Audit Unit News*, Vol. 1, 1996, p. 1.

Krimsky, S. "Risk Communication in the Internet Age: The Rise of Disorganized Skepticism." *Environmental Hazards*, Vol. 7, 2007, pp. 157–164.

Lieberman, A. J., and S. C. Kwon. "Facts Versus Fears: A Review of the Greatest Unfounded Health Scares of Recent Times." *American Council on Science and Health*, September 2004.

Martin, D. "Wash Your Hands Immediately After Reading This Story." *New York Times*, 17 August 1997.

Mayo, D. G., and R. D. Hollander. 1994. *Acceptable Evidence: Science and Values in Risk Management*. New York: Oxford University Press.

Miller, M. L. "Is Drycleaning the Next Big Health Scare?" *American Drycleaner*, June 1999.

Neth, M. "Danger in the Daily Diet." *Stars and Stripes*, 23 April 1982.

"The Price of Prudence." *The Economist*, 24 January 2004.

Ross, J. F. "Risk: Where do the Real Dangers Lie?" *Smithsonian*, November 1995.

Schmidt, C. W. "Communication Gap: The Disconnect between What Scientists Say and What the Public Hears." *Environmental Health Perspectives*, 1 December 2009.

Skenazy, L. "Mothering as a Spectator Sport." *Newsweek*, 7 May 2009.

Smith, D. F. "Food Panics in History: Corned Beef, Typhoid, and 'Risk Society.'" *Journal of Epidemiology and Community Health*, Vol. 61, 2007, pp. 566–570.

Spake, A. "Confusion in Spades: The Anthrax Scares Reveal a Public Health System in Disarray." *U.S. News and World Report*, Vol. 131, 2001, pp. 42–48.

Spinks, J. "Positive Practice: Another Scare Story? Don't Panic." *GP*, 14 January 2002.

Stocking, S. H. and L. W. Holstein. "Manufacturing Doubt: Journalists' Roles and the Construction of Ignorance in a Scientific Controversy." *Public Understanding of Science,* Vol. 9(1), 2009, pp. 23–42.

Ticktin, M. "Pills, Panics, Precautions." *Nursing Times,* Vol. 95, 1999, pp. 55–56.

Weinhouse, B. "The Truth Behind Health-Scare Stories." *Glamour,* August 1992.

Whelan, E. M. "Stop Banning Products at the Drop of a Rat." *Insight on the News,* 12 December 1994.

Whelan, E. M. "The Top Ten Unfounded Health Scares of the Year." *Medscape Journal of Medicine,* Vol. 10, 2008, p. 51.

Part One

Medical Interventions

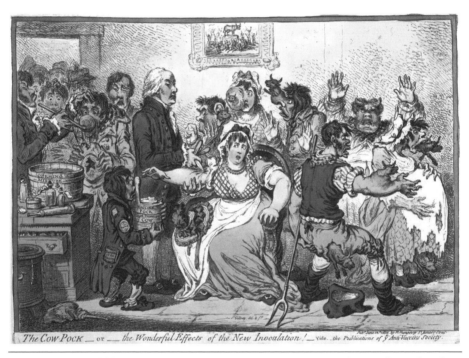

Figure 1   An 1802 cartoon that illustrates contemporary fears of vaccination.
(*Source*: United States Library of Congress.)

1

Measles Vaccine and Autism

We think of the key, each in his prison
Thinking of the key, each confirms a prison.

—T. S. Eliot, *The Waste Land* (1922)

SUMMARY

Many people believe that childhood vaccines are dangerous or ineffective. This chapter focuses on the widespread belief that the measles component of the MMR (measles-mumps-rubella) vaccine—or a mercury compound called thimerosal, which was formerly used in some other vaccines—can cause autism and related developmental disorders in children. The main source of this health scare is a single discredited 1998 study. Several other studies have demonstrated that no such link exists, but fear of autism has discouraged many parents from having their children vaccinated. This health scare has fizzled from a public health perspective, and in the minds of the majority of parents, but many continue to avoid the MMR vaccine. As a result, measles has made a comeback in some parts of the world, while rates of autism continue to increase for unknown reasons.

SOURCE

Unlike some health scares, this one has a source that is easy to pinpoint. As early as the mid-1970s, some doctors suspected that exposure to measles, rubella, mumps, or chickenpox—the diseases themselves, not the vaccines—might play a causal role in autism. In 1976, a German doctor speculated that smallpox vaccination might have a "starter function" for the onset of autism, but he concluded that any causal relationship was unlikely. In other words, vaccination might trigger the condition in a child who was already predisposed to it for some unknown reason. The important distinctions among association, causation, and the idea of a trigger function were all but forgotten in the debate that followed.

A 1979 study examined a sample of autistic children and found no clear association with any viral disease; but autism is a greatly feared disorder, and the search for risk factors continued. The bombshell came in 1998, when a medical research team in England, headed by Dr. Andrew Wakefield, reported evidence of a link between childhood autism and the measles component of the widely used MMR (measles-mumps-rubella) vaccine. This finding was published in the prestigious medical journal *Lancet*, and readers had no reason to doubt its validity. The article set off a storm of media controversy and litigation that has continued to the present day.

In 2004, several of the original authors of the 1998 study published a partial retraction of their findings. In 2010, the *Lancet* editorial staff published a full retraction of the article, twelve years after the fact. Yet in the minds of many parents, the vaccine would be forever linked with evil. Days after the 2010 retraction, CNN interviewed parents of autistic children who now felt doubly betrayed—first by doctors who had offered them closure, in the form of an explanation for their children's condition, and then by other doctors who claimed it was a mistake all along.

Contrary to rumor, the MMR vaccine never contained the preservative thimerosal. This aspect of the MMR health scare had a separate origin (see Chapter 2).

SCIENCE

Measles (rubeola) is a highly contagious airborne respiratory infection that was once a major scourge of childhood. It can lead to life-threatening pneumonia, meningitis, or other complications. The infectious agent is a virus that infects only humans, but it is closely related to the agents of several animal diseases. Measles should not be confused with German measles (rubella), an unrelated viral disease that causes a similar rash.

Although measles vaccines are widely available, and about 95 percent effective when given at the right age, nearly 200,000 children died of measles in 2008, most of them in the Third World. Crowding, malnutrition, and HIV infection are major risk factors for serious complications of measles. Obstacles to the use of this and other vaccines include poverty, distrust of medical science, complacence (in developed nations), fear of autism or other alleged side effects, and concerns about thimerosal—a mercury compound that was formerly added to some vaccines as a preservative. In about 2000, manufacturers in the United States stopped putting thimerosal in most pediatric vaccines, because some doctors and consumers suspected a link to a number of disorders, including autism. Despite this precaution, the autism epidemic in this country has continued, while the incidence of autism remains lower in some countries that still use thimerosal. Ironically, the MMR vaccine never contained thimerosal in the first place, but some activists apparently thought it did.

Autism is generally defined as a developmental disorder with impaired social interaction and communication. Its complexity far exceeds the scope of this book, and its cause remains a mystery, despite decades of research. Competing belief systems have further confused the issue; for example, in March 2008, an autism advocacy group falsely claimed that the Centers for Disease Control and Prevention (CDC) had confirmed the hypothesis that vaccines cause autism. In fact, a CDC spokesperson had simply told an interviewer that some children have an underlying mitochondrial disease that may produce some of the symptoms associated with autism when the children are stressed, by a fever or vaccination or any of a number of events. In other words, what we now call autism may turn out to have multiple causes, but there is no evidence that the MMR vaccine or thimerosal is among them. In March 2010, the U.S. Court of Federal Claims upheld that conclusion.

The present consensus is that neither the MMR vaccine nor thimerosal in other vaccines can cause autism. At most, vaccination might be one of several stressors that can trigger symptoms of autism in a child who (for unknown reasons) is already in the early stages of the disorder. Yet the controversy has continued, with some parents now blaming the MMR vaccine not only for autism, but also for epilepsy, arthritis, fatigue, attention deficit disorder, and other common health problems.

HISTORY

Fear of vaccination is nothing new. The 1802 cartoon at the beginning of this chapter (Figure 1) shows how people in that era felt about the cowpox vaccine that was used to protect against smallpox (Chapter 10). The cartoon shows small cows emerging from people's bodies, while a wall painting in the background depicts a Biblical story in which the followers of Moses abandoned God to worship the Golden Calf. Cartoonists were subtle in those days.

Measles is not nearly as deadly as smallpox, but neither is it a harmless childhood rash, contrary to the claims of some vaccination opponents. Before the measles vaccine was invented, thousands of children died of this disease every year. In 1941, for example, at least 2,279 American children died of measles, and thousands more developed measles-related encephalitis or other complications that damaged the brain, heart, or eyes. That is still a low percentage of the 894,134 cases of measles reported in the United States in 1941; the true number of cases was probably closer to 2 million, because virtually all children contracted measles before the vaccine was invented, and many cases were not reported. But however low the fatality rate might appear, even one preventable death is too many. Thanks to the vaccine, measles is now infrequent in this country. There were only 71 reported cases in the United States in 2009, but the disease could return at any time, and it remains far more dangerous than many Americans realize.

The first measles vaccine became available in 1963, and it greatly reduced the incidence of measles in developed nations. In the rest of the world, the vaccine was not widely available, and measles remained a serious public health problem in Africa and India until the 2001 Measles Initiative began its worldwide vaccination and health education campaign. The efforts of the Initiative—a partnership of the American Red Cross, CDC, UNICEF, the World Health Organization, and the United Nations—resulted in the rapid decline of measles deaths worldwide, from 757,000 deaths in 2000, to 410,000 in 2004, to 197,000 in 2007, to 164,000 in 2008. The goal of this program is to reduce measles deaths to 10 percent of the 2000 level by 2010. But even that 10 percent will keep the measles virus alive and able to reemerge wherever public health vigilance or public cooperation falters.

In light of these impressive numbers, what might interfere with the conquest of measles? Lots of things, including information overload and widespread distrust of medicine. As noted above, a single 1998 journal article that questioned the safety of the MMR vaccine was enough to partly reverse public health gains for several years, at least in developed nations where parents have enough leisure time to read tabloids and sign petitions. Then the pendulum swung the other way, and by 2009, the media were having a field day with Dr. Wakefield's alleged conflict of interest. Some journalists even accused him of fraud, while others insisted that his original conclusion was true, but that mysterious agencies forced his associates to retract it.

As noted earlier, suspicion regarding the MMR and other vaccines did not begin with the 1998 study. Vaccination rates were already on the decline in some countries. In 1989–1991, the United States had a measles epidemic, with about 55,000 cases and 135 deaths. Then Japan repealed its mandatory vaccination laws in 1994, and large measles epidemics soon returned to that country as well. In 2000, Japan had about 200,000 cases of measles and 88 deaths. In 2008, health officials reported that measles was once again endemic in Britain and showing "continuous spread," thanks to general apathy and scare campaigns about autism. In 2010, the Chinese government announced a new measles vaccination plan that many parents reportedly have opposed.

CONSEQUENCES

After publication of the 1998 Wakefield study, the fraction of children receiving the MMR vaccine in England reportedly fell from 92 percent to less than 80 percent. Although this might not sound too bad, 80 percent is far below the threshold needed for herd immunity—a phenomenon that occurs when a high enough percentage of a population is immune to a disease to prevent spread of that disease in the rest of the population. The baseline rate of vaccination, 92 percent, was already too low to achieve that result. This is why doctors have been unable to eradicate measles from the world, and why its incidence quickly rises whenever people stop vaccinating their children.

Since the combined MMR vaccine also protects children from mumps and rubella, these two diseases have shown a similar trend. For example, a recent study in Ireland and the UK showed an alarming increase in mumps-related testicle problems in young men. Moreover, some of the parents who allow their children to have the MMR vaccine apparently still believe it is harmful. A 2007 study of parents' attitudes showed that, in 2002, 24 percent of British mothers believed that the MMR vaccine was more dangerous than measles itself. By 2006, that fraction had dropped to 14 percent, but this is not exactly a vote of confidence. The percentage of mothers who absolutely rejected the MMR vaccine reportedly held steady at about 6 percent from 2002 to 2007. It is a highly vocal 6 percent.

This controversy took an ugly turn in March 2010, when a dubious press release claimed that one of the scientists who helped debunk the autism-vaccine connection had vanished with $2 million in grant money. Most news services ignored this story, while anti-vaccine bloggers plastered the Web with *ad hominem* attacks. At the time this book went to press, the facts were not yet in, but the story appeared to be a hoax, or at best irrelevant to the vaccine issue.

WHAT WENT WRONG?

Simply put, people cannot bear to do anything that might harm their children. For many parents, it seems preferable to avoid vaccination or any other medical treatment that sounds risky, thus leaving their children's health to God, fate, or random accident. In May 2010, a Harris poll showed that 48 percent of American parents were worried about serious adverse effects of vaccines. It is important to remember that many of today's parents and grandparents are measles survivors who remember the disease as a harmless rash, if they remember it at all. Those who died of measles, or suffered severe brain damage, are not in the debate.

Another problem is that the parents of autistic children are often under extreme financial and emotional stress that others fail to appreciate. A 2008 study showed that many of these parents must stop working to care for their children, while also facing high medical bills. In many cases, a large cash settlement from the National Vaccine Injury Compensation Program or a vaccine manufacturer could save their homes and greatly improve their lives. Thus, some of these parents become enraged when scientists dispute the connection between vaccines and autism.

Also, many people dislike the way scientists express their findings. We never seem to say "Drug X will absolutely cure Disease Z." Instead, we make statements such as: "The observed improvement in Disease Z patients in Group Q treated with Drug X is significant at the 0.05 level." In other words, if we had a big enough research grant to repeat the study many times, which we probably don't—and if all the experimental and control groups were comparable, which they probably aren't—then we are 95 percent confident that the observed improvement would turn out to be a nonrandom effect of Drug X. But people with sick children want reassurance and a cure, not a lesson in applied statistics. Doctors who administer a vaccine may consciously overhype its benefits to reassure patients, only to find themselves under fire. No, the MMR vaccine is not perfect. It prevents measles only 90 to 95 percent of the time. But it does not appear to harm children, and measles can.

A 2009 study offered subjects two hypothetical choices: a vaccine described as 100 percent effective against 70 percent of diseases, and a vaccine described as 70 percent effective against 100 percent of diseases. Not surprisingly, the first vaccine won by a landslide. Patients expect doctors to hit what they aim at, while the doctors themselves must often be content with just aiming at the right target. Many people want the kind of absolute binary perfection that religion can promise and medical science cannot. A faith healer who fails to cure a sick person can always find a graceful excuse, whereas a doctor with the same outcome must fall back on the numbers, which nobody liked in the first place.

The MMR scare and others like it have raised an important question. If researchers find what they truly believe is preliminary evidence of a threat to public health, how long should they keep it to themselves? In this case, the warning about the MMR vaccine turned out to be a false alarm. But suppose these scientists had instead chosen to sit on their findings for ten or twenty years, waiting for incontrovertible proof, and then it turned out that they were right all along? To coin a phrase, is it better to be safe or sorry?

REFERENCES AND RECOMMENDED READING

Baird, G., et al. "Measles Vaccination and Antibody Response in Autism Spectrum Disorders." *Archives of Disease in Childhood*, Vol. 93, 2008, pp. 832–837.

Begley, S. "Anatomy of a Scare." *Newsweek*, 2 March 2009.

Brownell, G., and D. Footes. "Is It Safe to Vaccinate?" *Newsweek*, 31 July 2000.

Burgess, D. C., et al. "The MMR Vaccination and Autism Controversy in United Kingdom 1998–2005; Inevitable Community Outrage or a Failure of Risk Communication?" *Vaccine*, Vol. 24, 2006, pp. 3921–3928.

Davis, N. F., et al. "The Increasing Incidence of Mumps Orchitis: A Comprehensive Review." *British Journal of Urology International*, Vol. 105, 2010, pp. 1060–1066.

Deer, B. "MMR Doctor Andrew Wakefield Fixed Data on Autism." *The Sunday Times*, 8 February 2009.

Deykin, E., and B. MacMahon. "Viral Exposure and Autism." *American Journal of Epidemiology*, Vol. 109, 1979, pp. 628–638.

Dobson, R. "Media Misled the Public over the MMR Vaccine, Study Says." *British Medical Journal*, Vol. 326, 2003, p. 1107.

Dyer, O. "GMC Clears GP Accused of Giving Court 'Junk Science' on MMR Vaccine." *British Medical Journal*, Vol. 335, 2007, pp. 416–417.

Geier, D. A., et al. "A Comprehensive Review of Mercury Provoked Autism." *Indian Journal of Medical Research*, Vol. 128, 2008, pp. 383–411.

Goodman, N. W. "MMR Scare Stories: Some Things are Just Too Attractive to the Media." *British Medical Journal*, Vol. 335, 2007, p. 222.

Guillaume, L., and P. A. Bath. "A Content Analysis of Mass Media Sources in Relation to the MMR Vaccine Scare." *Health Informatics Journal*, Vol. 14, 2008, pp. 323–334.

Halsey, N. A., et al. "Measles-Mumps-Rubella Vaccine and Autistic Spectrum Disorder: Report from the New Challenges in Childhood Immunizations Conference Convened in Oak Brook, Illinois, June 12–13, 2000." *Pediatrics*, Vol. 107, 2001, p. E84.

"Inquiry Planned into MMR Scare." United Press International, 23 February 2004.

Kalb, C., and D. Foote. "Necessary Shots?" *Newsweek*, 13 September 1999.

Kennedy, R. F., Jr. "Central Figure in CDC Vaccine Cover-Up Absconds with $2M." *Huffington Post*, 11 March 2010.

Kogan, M. D., et al. "A National Profile of the Health Care Experiences and Family Impact of Autism Spectrum Disorder among Children in the United States, 2005–2006." Pediatrics, Vol. 122, 2008, pp. e1149–e1158.

Li, M., and G. B. Chapman. "100% of Anything Looks Good: The Appeal of One Hundred Percent." *Psychonomic Bulletin and Review*, Vol. 16, 2009, pp. 156–162.

Murch, S. H., et al. "Retraction of an Interpretation." *Lancet*, Vol. 363, 2004, p. 750.

Offit, P. A., and S. E. Coffin. "Communicating Science to the Public: MMR Vaccine and Autism." *Vaccine*, Vol. 22, 2003, pp. 1–6.

Offit, P. A. 2008. *Autism's False Prophets: Bad Science, Risky Medicine and the Search for a Cure.* New York: Columbia University Press.

Patz, A. "Can You Spot Which Baby Hasn't Been Vaccinated?" *Baby Talk*, September 2009.

Salmon, D. A., and S. B. Omer. "Individual Freedoms Versus Collective Responsibility: Immunization Decision-Making in the Face of Occasionally Competing Values." *Emerging Themes in Epidemiology*, Vol. 3, 2006, p. 13.

Schmid, R. E. "Court Says Thimerosal Did Not Cause Autism." Associated Press, 12 March 2010.

"Scientists Retract Earlier MMR-Autism Tie." United Press International, 4 March 2004.

Smith, A., et al. "Tracking Mothers' Attitudes to MMR Immunisation 1996–2006." *Vaccine*, Vol. 25, 2007, pp. 3996–4002.

Speers, T., and J. Lewis. "Journalists and Jabs: Media Coverage of the MMR Vaccine." *Communication and Medicine*, Vol. 1, 2004, pp. 171–181.

Tuller, D. "An Ounce of Prevention: Sometimes the Public Health Field is a Victim of its Own Success." *California*, Summer 2010, pp. 27–29.

Wakefield, A. J., et al. "Ileal-Lymphoid-Nodule Hyperplasia, Non-Specific Colitis, and Pervasive Developmental Disorder in Children." *Lancet*, Vol. 351, 1998, pp. 637–641.

Wong, G. "China Mass Measles Vaccination Program Sparks Outcry." Associated Press, 12 September 2010.

2

Hepatitis B Vaccine and Multiple Sclerosis

A lie travels round the world whilst the truth is putting on its boots.

—Winston Churchill (1932)

SUMMARY

As discussed in the previous chapter, many people sincerely believe that vaccines are dangerous or ineffective or both. This chapter focuses on the widespread belief that the hepatitis B vaccine can cause multiple sclerosis or other chronic diseases. Hepatitis B itself is a serious disease that claims about 1 million human lives every year worldwide, yet it continues to spread, because many people are either unaware of the vaccine or refuse it on the basis of unsubstantiated rumors and fears. The hepatitis B virus (HBV) is about 100 times as infectious as HIV, and both children and adults are at risk, since HBV spreads by ordinary household contact as well as by fluid exchange. Hepatitis B has reached epidemic levels in some parts of the world and has contributed to the increasing rates of pancreatic and liver cancers. The fear of the HBV vaccine has fizzled in the sense that it no longer makes headlines, and the link to multiple sclerosis has been disproven, but vaccination rates remain low nevertheless.

SOURCE

Soon after the hepatitis B vaccine became available in 1982, doctors began to report isolated cases of neurological or other symptoms that developed within weeks or months after vaccination. This health scare went mainstream in the early 1990s, when the vaccine was suspected of causing several diseases. The hepatitis B vaccine was one of several that formerly contained the mercury compound thimerosal, and some doctors questioned the safety of that ingredient. The climax came in 2001, when a French court ordered a vaccine manufacturer to pay damages to two women who developed multiple sclerosis. A higher court overturned that judgment in 2004, and further studies of the vaccine have shown no connection to multiple sclerosis, but media coverage of the case increased public hostility toward vaccines in general. As in the case of the MMR vaccine (Chapter 1), many journalists and parents focused on the few studies that faulted the vaccine, while ignoring many others that reached the opposite conclusion.

It is possible that the hepatitis B vaccine may serve as a trigger for neurological problems in people who are already at high risk, but as of 2010 there is no conclusive proof of this effect. Almost any medical treatment has some associated risk, and doctors admit that about 1 in 600,000 persons who receive this vaccine may have an allergic reaction called anaphylaxis. The long-term consequences (if any) are unknown, but no one on record has died from this complication. Given a choice, a temporary, treatable allergic condition seems more acceptable than cancer, cirrhosis, liver failure, or other known consequences of hepatitis B.

SCIENCE

Like most human diseases, hepatitis B was probably a zoonosis (animal disease) at one time. Its agent, the hepatitis B virus, is similar to a virus that causes liver cancer in woodchucks. Another related virus causes hepatitis in ducks. HBV can survive on environmental surfaces for at least seven days, and there is even some evidence that mosquitoes may transmit this disease, at least in Africa. More common modes of transmission include sexual contact, needle sharing, wound infection, placental transfer from mother to fetus, and household contact involving contaminated objects.

As of 2009, about 400 million people worldwide have hepatitis B, one-third of them in China. An estimated 2 billion people either have the disease or have recovered from it, with or without liver damage. Recent estimates of annual hepatitis B deaths range from 500,000 to 1.2 million. Some of the health scares in later chapters of this book may sound like jokes, but hepatitis B is a deadly disease, and anything that discourages people from seeking vaccination is decidedly not funny. Besides being highly infectious, the hepatitis B virus is a known risk factor for liver cancer, pancreatic cancer, cirrhosis of the liver, and liver failure.

Reported new cases of hepatitis B in the United States declined sharply between 1995 and 2005, when the number reached the lowest level in the 40 years since the U.S. Centers for Disease Control and Prevention (CDC) started collecting data. The vaccine was probably responsible for the decline, since it was greatest in children and adolescents under age 15. The CDC estimates that there were about 43,000 new cases in the United States in 2007—many of them unreported—and that somewhere between 800,000 and 1.4 million Americans had chronic hepatitis B. The exact numbers are hard to determine, because many people with chronic HBV (about 20% of all cases) do not know they are infected until liver failure or other obvious symptoms appear. Meanwhile, they can infect other people, including their own unvaccinated children. Treatment for hepatitis B usually includes several weeks of antiviral drugs, which reportedly cause such severe side effects that many patients discontinue treatment.

As explained earlier, the main health scare involving the hepatitis B vaccine is the claim that it causes multiple sclerosis (MS), a chronic disease that affects the brain and spinal cord, progressively impairing the ability of nerve cells to communicate with one another. MS usually begins in early adulthood, and it affects an estimated 2.5 million people worldwide. Its cause is unknown at present, although various genetic, autoimmune, and environmental explanations have been proposed.

MS is not the only disease that some doctors have linked to the HBV vaccine. In 2009, a team of researchers examined reports of 32 patients who developed uveitis (a form of eye inflammation) days or weeks after hepatitis B vaccination between 1982 and 2009. But hundreds of millions of people received the vaccine during that 27-year period, and it is not clear how many of them would have developed uveitis anyway. Even if a direct causal relationship is eventually proven, uveitis is treatable and usually curable. Other doctors have proposed that the hepatitis B vaccine may be a risk factor for lupus erythematosus, myasthenia gravis, lichen planus, polyarthritis, pulmonary vasculitis, chronic fatigue syndrome, and several other conditions, but most of the published studies are based on small samples (often a single patient).

As noted earlier, the hepatitis B vaccine no longer contains the mercury compound thimerosal, which manufacturers formerly added to many vaccines to prevent contamination. There is no clear evidence that thimerosal was harmful in the first place, although some forms of mercury are known to be toxic (see Chapter 21). Countries that have stopped using thimerosal in vaccines have not reported a decrease in MS or autism.

HISTORY

When the hepatitis B vaccine became available to the public in 1982, it had already undergone several years of clinical trials. As with any new vaccine or drug, doctors were properly cautious, but the results were encouraging. The first reports of possible neurological problems associated with this vaccine appeared in the medical literature by 1983, and public concern was inevitable. Subsequent reports in the 1990s blamed the vaccine not only for multiple sclerosis, but also for arthritis, skin rashes, and even HIV transmission. None of these reports stood up to scrutiny, but alarming news is hard to retract or forget, and the cumulative weight of inconclusive reports made an impression. Finally, in the late 1990s, the French government yielded to public demand and stopped requiring adolescents to have this vaccine. Anti-vaccination groups in the United States followed suit, demanding an immediate moratorium on mandatory vaccination of children attending public schools.

In 1997, however, analysis of data from 60 million HBV vaccine recipients showed that the incidence of multiple sclerosis was actually slightly *lower* than in the general population. (Of course, this did not prove that the vaccine prevents MS; the difference was probably random.) The vaccination requirement was then reinstated in France. In the United States, the Medical Advisory Board of the National Multiple Sclerosis Society reached the same conclusion: there was no evidence of a statistical or causal link between the hepatitis B vaccine and MS. As of 2010, the American Medical Association recommends this vaccine for everyone under 18, and for adults at high risk. Other influential groups have issued similar statements, but in the minds of true believers, all vaccines are suspect. In a 2010 survey of U.S. parents, nearly 90 percent ranked vaccine safety as the most important topic in children's health research.

Some activists have actually suggested that the hepatitis B vaccine should be reserved for children in specific families or neighborhoods where allegedly high-risk behaviors and unsanitary practices are rampant. Most of the activists themselves, of course, feel that their own families cannot possibly be at risk. But who should have the task of going door to door, interviewing people and inspecting their homes to make this determination? The whole point of requiring everyone to be vaccinated, irrespective of socioeconomic status or lifestyle choice, is to avoid the connotation of blame and simply stop the disease. Anyone can get sick.

CONSEQUENCES

Although the hepatitis B vaccine has been available for nearly thirty years, many people avoid it because of these unproven health scares. By some estimates, about one-third of the global population—more than 2 billion people—are hepatitis B carriers who can transmit the disease to others by fluid exchange or household contact. In 2008, an Australian baby made world headlines when his parents concealed his whereabouts to shield him from mandatory hepatitis B vaccination. The mother already had the disease, and the child's future health was in immediate danger, yet public opinion favored the parents' right to refuse medical treatment.

There is no way to tell how many people have died needlessly from liver disease, or infected their own children, as a result of what now appears to be irresponsible scaremongering. The day after this book goes to press, someone may conclusively prove that the vaccine is dangerous. For the moment, however, we have no such proof, only an epidemic to fight.

WHAT WENT WRONG?

The 2001 French court case discussed earlier seemed to legitimize the hepatitis B vaccine health scare, when in fact judges are not doctors, and the evidence was extremely weak even before the judgment was reversed on appeal. Another factor that helps keep this scare alive is the catastrophic nature of multiple sclerosis, which (like autism) affects young people and is incurable at present.

The main problem, however, seems to be the usual gang of ambulance chasers and tabloid journalists who identify salable health scares and construct data to keep them going. Studies have shown that even healthcare workers in some countries now avoid hepatitis B vaccination because of perceived risk.

In 2004, for example, one vocal group that opposes hepatitis B vaccination claimed that the vaccine is more dangerous than the disease, citing "Merck's package insert showing the frequency of vaccine damage at a rate of 10.4%."[1] This statement would be alarming, if true—but if the vaccine predictably "damaged" 10 percent of recipients, it would not be on the market. In fact, the Merck package insert stated:

> Injection site reactions and systemic complaints were reported following 0.2% and 10.4% of the injections, respectively. The most frequently reported systemic adverse reactions (>1% injections), in decreasing order of frequency, were irritability, fever (>101°F oral equivalent), diarrhea, fatigue/weakness, diminished appetite, and rhinitis.[2]

These are minor side effects that last for a few hours or days, not for the rest of the person's life, and they are not necessarily related to the vaccine. In clinical trials, a comparable percentage of subjects who take a placebo report similar symptoms.

But if so many consumers reject the hepatitis B vaccine, what will happen if researchers someday develop an equally safe and effective vaccine to prevent HIV? The rejoicing will be premature, and decades of research effort will be in vain, if unfounded health scares block public acceptance of that vaccine too.

NOTES

1. Association of American Physicians and Surgeons, letter to Cook County Board of Commissioners, 10 March 2004.

2. Merck & Co., Inc., product information, Recombivax HB Hepatitis B Vaccine, December 2007.

REFERENCES AND RECOMMENDED READING

"Continue to Vaccinate against Hepatitis B." *Prescrire International*, Vol. 18, 2009, p. 131.

DeStefano, F., et al. "Hepatitis B Vaccine and Risk of Multiple Sclerosis." *Expert Review of Vaccines*, Vol. 1, 2002, pp. 461–466.

Duclos, P. "Adverse Events after Hepatitis B Vaccination." *Canadian Medical Association Journal*, Vol. 147, 1992, pp. 1023–1026.

François, G., et al. "Vaccine Safety Controversies and the Future of Vaccination Programs." *Pediatric Infectious Disease Journal*, Vol. 24, 2005, pp. 953–961.

Fraunfelder, F. W., et al. "Hepatitis B Vaccine and Uveitis: An Emerging Hypothesis Suggested by Review of 32 Case Reports." *Cutaneous and Ocular Toxicology*, 30 November 2009.

Gout, O. "Vaccinations and Multiple Sclerosis." *Neurological Sciences*, Vol. 22, 2001, pp. 151–154.

"Hepatitis B Vaccine Not Linked to MS." United Press International, 30 September 2008.

Herroelen, L., et al. "Central-Nervous-System Demyelination after Immunisation with Recombinant Hepatitis B Vaccine." *Lancet*, Vol. 338, 1991, pp. 1174–1175.

Kalb, C., and D. Foote. "Necessary Shots?" *Newsweek*, 13 September 1999.

Löbermann, M., et al. "Vaccination and Multiple Sclerosis." *Nervenarzt*, 17 October 2009. [In German]

MacIntyre, C. R., and J. Leask. "Immunization Myths and Realities: Responding to Arguments Against Immunization." *Journal of Paediatrics and Child Health*, Vol. 39, 2003, pp. 487–491.

Mikaeloff, Y., et al. "Hepatitis B Vaccination and the Risk of Childhood-Onset Multiple Sclerosis." *Archives of Pediatric and Adolescent Medicine*, Vol. 161, 2007, pp. 1176–1182.

Mikaeloff, Y., et al. "Hepatitis B Vaccine and the Risk of CNS Inflammatory Demyelination in Childhood." *Neurology*, Vol. 72, 2009, pp. 873–880.

Nadler, J. P. "Multiple Sclerosis and Hepatitis B Vaccination." *Clinical Infectious Diseases*, Vol. 17, 1993, pp. 928–929.

Offit, P. A. "Thimerosal and Vaccines—A Cautionary Tale." *New England Journal of Medicine*, Vol. 357, 2007, pp. 1278–1279.

Pless, R. P. "Recent Differing Expert Opinions Regarding the Safety Profile of Hepatitis B Vaccines: Is There Really a Controversy?" *Expert Opinion on Drug Safety*, Vol. 2, 2003, pp. 451–455.

Ramagopalan, S. V., et al. "Association of Infectious Mononucleosis with Multiple Sclerosis: A Population-Based Study." *Neuroepidemiology*, Vol. 32, 2009, pp. 257–262.

Rougé-Maillart, C. I., et al. "Recognition by French Courts of Compensation for Post-Vaccination Multiple Sclerosis: The Consequences with Regard to Expert Practice." *Medicine, Science and Law*, Vol. 47, 2007, pp. 185–190.

Tardieu, M., and Y. Mikaeloff. "Multiple Sclerosis in Children: Environmental Risk Factors." *Bulletin de l'Académie Nationale de Médecine*, Vol. 192, 2008, pp. 507–509. [In French]

Terney, D., et al. "Multiple Sclerosis after Hepatitis B Vaccination in a 16-Year-Old Patient." *Chinese Medical Journal*, Vol. 119, 2006, pp. 77–79.

Topuridze, M., et al. "Barriers to Hepatitis B Coverage among Healthcare Workers in the Republic of Georgia: An International Perspective." *Infection Control and Hospital Epidemiology*, Vol. 31, 2010, pp. 158–164.

3

Fear of Menopause and HRT

I died for Beauty—but was scarce
Adjusted in the tomb
When One who died for Truth, was lain
In an adjoining room.

—Emily Dickinson, "I Died for Beauty" (1862)

SUMMARY

This chapter describes what we in the trenches call a double fizzle with reverse. First, doctors promoted hormone replacement therapy (HRT) as a universal cure for the allegedly devastating cosmetic and health effects of menopause. Then studies showed that HRT itself was dangerous, because it increased the risk of cancer and heart disease. Then the alleged perils of menopause fizzled, as more doctors and patients accepted it as a natural process; then the alleged perils of HRT partly fizzled too. Finally, a new round of studies showed that HRT was largely ineffective anyway, and hardly worth the risk of catastrophic illness, except for those who find the threat of cancer and heart disease more acceptable than facial hair and hot flashes. There are hopeful signs that the oscillations of this health scare have begun to subside.

SOURCE

Fear of menopause, like fear of erectile dysfunction, has inspired a series of particularly nasty health scares that exploit the basic human reluctance to accept the ravages of time and the attendant loss of sexual appeal. Perhaps the most influential source of the HRT fad was a book published in the 1960s by an American physician, as discussed later, but it would be unfair to blame this health scare on a single publication. Ever since that landmark work, a series of journal papers, magazine articles, and books have slalomed back and forth between urging women to have HRT and warning them of the dire consequences. Does HRT cause cancer or prevent it? Ditto stroke, heart disease, and osteoporosis? Does it increase the sex drive? Does it prevent minor things like wrinkles and hot flashes? Can it postpone menopause indefinitely? We will briefly explore some of these claims. There are hopeful signs, however, that women (and men) have begun to view menopause not as a disease to be cured, but as an inevitable consequence of surviving past mid-life.

SCIENCE

Menopause, also called the climacteric, is the time in a woman's life when she stops having menstrual periods and ceases to be fertile without medical intervention. Usually this happens sometime between the ages of 40 and 60. Younger women go through the equivalent of menopause if their ovaries are removed surgically, but this discussion will focus on the natural event. Some women regard menopause as a frightening catastrophe and the end of their existence as a female being, whereas others can't wait for it to start. Still others are too busy with their families and careers to pay much attention to minor discomfort or a couple of chin hairs.

During most of a woman's life, the ovaries release two hormones called estrogen and progesterone. When the ovaries stop working at menopause, there is a sharp drop in the level of both these hormones. After decades spent becoming accustomed to fluctuating levels of these powerful chemicals, it is not surprising that women should undergo a kind of withdrawal syndrome when the supply is cut. The resulting level of discomfort is subjective and hard to estimate from survey data, because women have listened to horror stories about menopause for so many years that the power of suggestion undoubtedly plays a role. It would be insensitive to dismiss menopause as "natural," because negative events such as death and sickness are natural too. But for many women, particularly those in good health, menopause is barely noticeable. Survey data suggest that only about 5 to 10 percent of menopausal women have symptoms that are severe enough to require treatment.

Neither estrogen nor progesterone disappears entirely at menopause, because the adrenal cortex also makes these hormones (in both men and women). Milk, yams, and other foods contain chemicals similar to progesterone, and soy contains phytoestrogens (plant estrogens), but there is no clear evidence that these products can relieve menopausal symptoms. Some recent studies claim that soy is beneficial; others disagree. Many industrial products, including some pesticides and plastics, are related to estrogen, and some researchers suspect that the proliferation of such chemicals in the environment may even be harmful to human reproductive health. Contrary to popular belief, an herbal remedy called black cohosh (*Actaea racemosa*) sold in health-food stores apparently does not bind to estrogen receptors, and has no effect on menopausal symptoms.

HISTORY

Like many other drugs and procedures that later became health scares, HRT started small and grew by stages. In the 1930s, doctors gave women estrogen to relieve hot flashes and other minor, temporary symptoms that some women experience at menopause. Nobody pretended that this treatment would restore youth, erase wrinkles, or prolong life; it was more like taking aspirin for a headache. This practice continued for the next few decades.

In a 1960 syndicated health column, Dr. Herman Niels Bundesen (1882–1960), past president of the American Public Health Association and Chicago's Commissioner of Health for over 30 years, listed several rules to ease the process of menopause: accept the inevitable, eat a good diet, get enough sleep—and, *if necessary*, take an estrogen supplement to "make the transition more gradual, thereby eliminating the symptoms." His column emphasized that only a few menopausal women had symptoms severe enough to need estrogen, and then only for a short time.

This Dr. Bundesen was a major player in public health, who wrote several books and was an advocate for such modern concepts as indoor plumbing, pasteurization of milk, treatment of pertussis with antibiotics, and distribution of condoms to help prevent syphilis and other sexually transmitted diseases. Many of his ideas found favor with the medical establishment, and his advice on most subjects reflected the standard of care. But a new era was dawning, and doctors and pharmaceutical companies knew a good thing when they saw it. Estrogen treatment was a potential gold mine, but the part about "accepting the inevitable" had to go. If a few months or years of estrogen treatment could help relieve severe discomfort in a few women, why not give it to every woman, for the rest of her life?

In 1966, an American physician published a sensational book that urged all premenopausal women to seek hormone treatment, to avoid what he called "the horror of this living decay."[1] For that was the main point of this therapy—to postpone the outward appearance of aging and to preserve a woman's sex appeal, not to improve her health. Several celebrity doctors jumped on the bandwagon, and other books appeared, claiming that HRT would cure depression and obesity and discourage husbands from chasing their secretaries and bring about an Earthly paradise. A typical 1967 syndicated medical column stated that "the estrogen hormone may hold the secret for prolonged youthful appearance in women past the age of 40"[2] and held no risks whatsoever.

A good example of the popularity of HRT in that era is a 1972 episode of the TV sitcom *All in the Family*, in which Edith Bunker entered menopause, conducted herself like a raving dingbat, and finally went to her doctor for hormone pills. There was no need for the scriptwriter to tell the audience what the pills were for; everybody knew. When a woman reached menopause, that was what she did. Otherwise, her husband might get mad and leave.

Researchers now estimate that hormone replacement therapy caused more than 15,000 cases of endometrial (uterine) cancer in the United States between 1971 and 1975 alone. But the connection went unrecognized at the time, and HRT remained popular until about 2002, when long-awaited clinical trials showed that this treatment greatly increased a woman's risk of cancer, heart attack, stroke, and pulmonary embolism. Far from preserving a woman's beauty and femininity, it was more likely to make her terminally ill.

CONSEQUENCES

It would scarcely be original or constructive to belabor the point that thousands of women died, and that hundreds of thousands more were injured, by an inadequately tested therapy that served little purpose other than vanity. Consumers are ultimately responsible for their own health—if adequately informed of risk—and no drug or procedure can be absolutely proven safe before it is approved for general use. Vaccines, antibiotics, and other drugs all come with associated risks, and so does hormone replacement therapy. The main difference is that vaccines and antibiotics can prevent or cure life-threatening diseases, whereas HRT was intended mainly to prevent hot flashes, mood swings, and wrinkles. Was the anticipated benefit worth the risk? Looking back at the results, it's easy to say no.

Despite all the hype, medical consumers often made good choices. In reviewing two decades of survey data, we were impressed by the fact that so many women refused hormone replacement therapy even after the media bombarded them with messages about its benefits. In a 1993 Gallup poll of women aged 45 to 60, only 34 percent took estrogen at the time of the survey, and only 42 percent had ever taken it. In 1995, a new book by a physician expressed puzzlement about the fact that so few women took advantage of HRT and speculated that poor compliance with doctors' orders or unfounded "myths or fears" might be responsible. But in a 2002 Gallup poll—not long before release of the data that consigned the HRT experiment to the dung heap of medical history—its users still represented only 37 percent of the sample.

We will hasten to add that hormone replacement therapy has many legitimate uses, such as relieving the discomfort of a young woman who has lost her ovaries, or helping people in the process of gender reassignment. Modern pharmaceuticals used for such purposes are far safer than the older ones. But giving powerful, largely untested drugs to millions of healthy women was never a good idea, and in retrospect it's hard to believe that the medical community ever condoned the experiment.

Medical disasters such as the HRT scare do not improve the image of modern healthcare. Just how far do most people trust their doctors? In a 2002 Gallup poll, 66 percent of respondents said most physicians could be trusted, quite a high rating—but only 20 percent felt that most HMO (health maintenance organization) managers could be trusted. Only car dealers came in lower, at 15 percent. Since there is a general perception (whether true or false) that HMO managers, not doctors, decide the course of medical treatment, these numbers reflect a low level of public confidence. By 2009, things were worse; 65 percent still rated medical doctors' honesty and ethical standards as high or very high, but only 8 percent gave HMO managers that rating, as compared with 6 percent for car dealers.

WHAT WENT WRONG?

It's no news that women prefer to look young and beautiful, or that hot flashes are reputed to be uncomfortable.[3] But how could a generation of (mostly male) physicians take such a chance with women's lives? All we can say is that, at various times in history, men have done equally foolish things to themselves. Long before the HRT controversy, long before athletes began abusing anabolic steroids to gain muscle mass, thousands of perfectly rational-seeming men paid doctors to implant *goat testicles* in their bodies in the hope of improving their virility. This was, in fact, a primitive form of hormone replacement therapy for men during the early twentieth century. The results ranged from gangrene and lockjaw to bankruptcy and social ostracism, to say nothing of the emotional strain on the goats. Yet the question remains: Why didn't people learn from their mistakes? Although more sanitary and modern-sounding than the goat fad, the recent experiment with women's lives was nearly as dangerous, and far larger.

NOTES

1. R. A. Wilson, *Feminine Forever* (NY: M. Evans, 1966).
2. L. Coleman, M.D., "Hormones for the Menopause" (King Features Syndicate, 28 April 1967).
3. The author has never had one.

REFERENCES AND RECOMMENDED READING

Batt, S. "Health Protection Lessons from the Women's Health Initiative." *Women's Health Journal*, January–March 2003.

Beck, M. "Menopause." *Newsweek*, 25 May 1992.

Bluming, A. Z., and C. Tavris. "Hormone Replacement Therapy: Real Concerns and False Alarms." *Cancer Journal*, Vol. 15, 2009, pp. 93–104.

Briffa, J. "HRT Does More Harm than Good." *Epoch Times*, 14 June 2009.

Chen, F. P. "Postmenopausal Hormone Therapy and Risk of Breast Cancer." *Chang Gung Medical Journal*, Vol. 32, 2009, pp. 140–147.

Davis, M. E. "Estrogenic Therapy in Gynecology." *Journal of Clinical Endocrinology and Metabolism*, Vol. 13, 1953, pp. 1428–1431.

Davis, M. E. "Estrogens and the Aging Process." *Journal of the American Medical Association*, Vol. 196, 1966, pp. 219–224.

Dyer, O. "Another HRT Trial is Stopped Early." *British Medical Journal*, Vol. 328, 2004, p. 305.

Eagen, A. B. "Reconsidering Hormone Replacement Therapy." *Network News*, May–June 1989.

Gallagher, W. "Midlife Myths." *Atlantic Monthly*, May 1993.

Haimov-Kochman, R., and Hochner-Celnikier, D. "Hot Flashes Revisited." *Acta Obstetricia et Gynecologica Scandinavica*, Vol. 84, 2005, pp. 972–979.

Heinemann, K., et al. "Prevalence and Opinions of Hormone Therapy Prior to the Women's Health Initiative: A Multinational Survey on Four Continents." *Journal of Women's Health*, Vol. 17, 2008, pp. 1151–1166.

Henderson, V. W. "Estrogens, Episodic Memory, and Alzheimer's Disease: A Critical Update." *Seminars in Reproductive Medicine*, Vol. 27, 2009, pp. 283–293.

Huston, S. A. "Women's Trust in and Use of Information Sources in the Treatment of Menopausal Symptoms." *Women's Health Issues*, Vol. 19, 2009, pp. 144–153.

Kantrowitz, B., and P. Wingert. "HRT Hype: Why You Should Ignore Most Stories About Hormone Replacement Therapy." *Newsweek*, 2 January 2009.

Palacios, S. "Advances in Hormone Replacement Therapy: Making the Menopause Manageable." *BMC Women's Health*, Vol. 8, 2008, p. 22.

Saad, L. "Women Mostly Uncertain About Hormone Replacement Therapy." Gallup News Service, 26 August 2002.

Seaman, B. 2003. *The Greatest Experiment Ever Performed on Women: Exploding the Estrogen Myth*. New York: Hyperion Books.

Singer, N. "Medical Papers by Ghostwriters Pushed Therapy." *New York Times*, 4 August 2009.

Singer, N., and D. Wilson. "Menopause, as Brought to You by Big Pharma." *New York Times*, 12 December 2009.

Stramba-Badiale, M. "Postmenopausal Hormone Therapy and the Risk of Cardiovascular Disease." *Journal of Cardiovascular Medicine*, Vol. 10, 2009, pp. 303–309.

Sturmberg, J. P., and D. C. Pond. "Impacts on Clinical Decision Making—Changing Hormone Therapy Management After the WHI." *Australian Family Physician*, Vol. 38, 2009, pp. 249–251, 253–255.

Thomas, E. "Many Regard Menopause as Avoidable Disease." *Winnipeg Free Press*, 25 August 1967.

Wallis, C., et al. "The Estrogen Dilemma." *Time*, 26 June 1995.

Wren, B. G. "The Benefits of Oestrogen Following Menopause: Why Hormone Replacement Therapy Should be Offered to Postmenopausal Women." *Medical Journal of Australia*, Vol. 190, 2009, pp. 321–325.

4

The DES Generation

For the sins of your fathers you, though guiltless, must suffer.

—Horace, *Odes* (23 B.C.)

SUMMARY

If estrogen treatment can't make a woman young again, or prevent heart disease or stroke or cancer (Chapter 3), can it safely prevent miscarriage, or at least safely enhance the growth of beef cattle? No, apparently not. In the mid-twentieth century, doctors treated millions of pregnant women with a synthetic estrogen called diethylstilbestrol (DES) to alleviate the fear of premature delivery. As so often happens, one fear replaced another; many of the daughters of these women later developed a rare form of cancer. As a result, DES is no longer given to pregnant women or fed to livestock. This health scare was on the verge of fizzling until researchers found new evidence of health risks to DES sons as well as daughters, and possibly even to the grandchildren of the DES generation.

SOURCE

In 1970, the journal *Cancer* reported a cluster of seven cases of a rare vaginal cancer among adolescent girls in the northeastern United States. A review of their mothers' medical records revealed that most (probably all) had taken DES during pregnancy. Reports of other cases followed in 1971, together with concerns about the common practice of adding DES to livestock feed to enhance growth. By the mid-1970s, the media had focused public attention on these issues, and a full-fledged health scare was in progress. The U.S. Food and Drug Administration (FDA) banned DES as a drug for pregnant women in 1971, and as a livestock feed additive in 1979.

In theory, those actions should have ended the problem. As it turned out, however, the DES scare refused to die. Some sources now claim that the risk (if any) was low, and that scaremongering journalists and environmental activists exaggerated the facts. But many others, citing equally convincing numbers, claim that the use of DES was one of the worst medical blunders in recorded history and that generations of DES descendants will pay the price. As health scares go, this one is a dilly. The following sections will examine some of these claims.

SCIENCE

Estrogen is one of several hormones that a woman's body needs to conceive a child and carry it to term. Doctors have long suspected that low estrogen levels may contribute to premenstrual tension, premature birth, and other reproductive problems. The word estrogen is derived from two Greek words meaning "producer of frenzy."

Diethylstilbestrol (DES) is a synthetic estrogen compound that doctors routinely prescribed for pregnant women between 1940 and 1970, believing it would increase the likelihood of a full-term pregnancy. A woman's circulating estrogen level often fell before events such as premature delivery or fetal death, so doctors reasoned that keeping the estrogen level high would prevent these problems. Thus, they prescribed the new synthetic estrogen not only for women with a past history of miscarriage, but also for many healthy women who had never been pregnant before.

As early as 1952, some doctors questioned the value of DES during pregnancy, but for the majority it remained the standard of care. As it later turned out, the skeptics were right; DES did not work as expected, but apparently it took three decades for that fact to become apparent. An estimated 5 to 10 million Americans either received DES during pregnancy or were exposed to DES in the womb, but doctors also prescribed the same drug for many other purposes. Besides being one of the drugs used for hormone replacement therapy at menopause (Chapter 3), it was prescribed for relief of breast engorgement after childbirth, for treatment of prostate and breast cancers, as a contraceptive for use after unplanned sex, and even to prevent adolescent girls from growing too tall.

The widespread use of DES between 1940 and 1970 might seem to imply that researchers tested it extensively on animals before giving it to human beings. It is unclear, however, if adequate testing ever took place. Animal rights activists claim that animal experiments showed that DES was safe for humans when in fact it was not, and cite this example as proof that animal testing is unreliable and should be banned. Other sources, however, claim the opposite—that DES was not properly tested on *pregnant* animals before its approval for use on humans, and that such testing might have saved many human lives.

Studies have established (not to everyone's satisfaction) that the daughters of women who took DES during pregnancy are at risk for an otherwise rare form of vaginal cancer called clear cell adenocarcinoma. By one estimate, about one in every 1,000 to 1,500 DES daughters will eventually develop this cancer. Ironically, these DES daughters also appear to be at increased risk for premature delivery—the same problem that their mothers took DES to avoid. Both the DES daughters and their mothers also have higher-than-expected rates of breast cancer. Even DES sons have an increased incidence of certain reproductive tract anomalies, such as hypospadias (a defect in the lower surface of the penis), undescended testicles, and testicular cancer. At least one study concluded that DES sons show no reduction in actual fertility, but these birth defects are a matter of great concern nonetheless.

An even more disturbing discovery is that the grandchildren of women who took DES during pregnancy may also be at risk for certain cancers and other health problems. If confirmed, this finding implies that the drug not only damaged the developing fetus, but actually caused genetic damage (mutations) that could be passed on to the children of the DES daughter or son. In theory, unless such genetic changes caused a reduction in fertility, they would persist in the human population forever. Other sources attribute this third-generation effect to epigenetic inheritance—changes in gene function without changes in the DNA.

At the time this book was written, DES's effects on grandchildren had not been proven, but some laboratory findings were suggestive. For example, a 1999 study showed that 11 percent of mice whose grandmothers were exposed to DES developed cancers of the reproductive tract. A 2008 study found no such trend in a sample of human DES grandchildren, but research is continuing.

HISTORY

DES was not the first form of estrogen that doctors gave to pregnant women in the hope of preventing premature delivery. In the nineteenth century, doctors sometimes treated menopausal women with an oral drug prepared from the ground-up ovaries of a cow. This was, of course, a crude form of estrogen, but it is not clear if it had any effect when administered in this form. Later, pharmaceutical companies prepared estrogen drugs by extracting and purifying the hormone from the urine of pregnant female horses. Such drugs, known as conjugated equine estrogens, were far more expensive to manufacture than synthetic estrogens like DES, which was invented in 1938 by a team of English doctors and widely used by the early 1940s.

In 1954, the FDA approved DES for another use—as an additive in livestock feed to increase the growth rate of cattle. This practice continued even after DES was recognized as a carcinogen, despite the 1959 Delaney Clause, which normally prohibited FDA approval of any food additive that caused cancer in laboratory animals. In this case, however, the residual amount of DES found in meat by the time it reached the consumer was so low that the FDA did not consider it dangerous. DES was popular in the cattle industry, because it accelerated growth and saved an estimated 500 pounds of feed per animal. Even after 1979, when the FDA formally banned the use of DES in animal feed, some illegal use reportedly continued. Other, safer growth stimulation products have since been developed, such as zeranol, an estrogenic hormone derived from a fungus.

So is it a good idea to use estrogens to make cattle and other livestock gain weight faster, when exposure to these chemicals may interfere with human reproduction and cause cancer? It all comes back to the question of risk versus benefit. People want inexpensive meat, and as long as the demand continues, cattle producers must take reasonable shortcuts to stay in business. It is unclear if the consumption of hormone-treated beef adds significantly to our exposure to estrogens, which are also present in eggs and other foods.

CONSEQUENCES

No health scare is complete without one or more lawsuits. By 1982, the U.S. manufacturers E. R. Squibb and Sons Inc. (later Bristol-Meyers Squibb), Eli Lilly and Co., and Upjohn were under fire from hundreds of DES daughters. In the late 1990s, a new wave of claims followed reports that DES sons and grandchildren were also affected. At latest word, Squibb was still receiving an average of 100 new DES-related claims per year. To our knowledge, no class action suit was filed.

Many lessons can be drawn from the DES scare, depending on who spins the story. Is it an argument for or against laboratory animal testing of new drugs? Did it teach doctors to think twice before giving inadequately tested drugs to millions of unwitting volunteers? Did it teach people to be responsible consumers first and obedient patients second? Did it confirm what everyone already knew—that couples would risk almost anything to have babies, and that pharmaceutical companies and cattle ranchers cannot stay in business without turning a profit? Or did it simply drive malpractice insurance premiums through the roof, reduce the popularity of veal, and scare the hell out of millions of women (and men) for no valid reason?

WHAT WENT WRONG?

The initial mistake, as also discussed in Chapter 3, was the willingness of doctors to hand out estrogen like candy to female patients who complained of almost anything, from headaches to flat feet. The inability of a woman to carry a fetus to term is not in that category; it is a serious problem that can drive would-be parents (and their doctors) to acts of desperation. Another problem is that doctors, like patients, must often rely on the FDA approval process, and it is not clear why DES received approval for human use without stronger evidence that it was either safe or effective.

Finally, the news media must accept a share of the responsibility for exaggerating some research findings, thus setting the stage for new health scares in the form of urban legends. One such legend states that certain foods contain high levels of estrogen that can cause people to become homosexual. Buffalo wings are a favorite target, for some reason. This legend apparently started with media accounts of hormones in meat and their possible effect on sexual behavior. To our knowledge, no food or drug is likely to change a person's innate sexual orientation.

REFERENCES AND RECOMMENDED READING

Barber, H. R. "An Update on DES in the Field of Reproduction." *International Journal of Fertility*, Vol. 31, 1986, pp. 130–144.

Batt, S. "Health Protection Lessons from the Women's Health Initiative." *Women's Health Journal*, January–March 2003.

Bren, L. "Animal Health and Consumer Protection." *FDA Consumer*, January–February 2006.

Brown, H. "Beware of People." *Forbes*, 26 July 2004.

"Cattle Drug: 'No Evidence of Cancer Hazard.'" *Science News*, Vol. 111, 1977, pp. 102–103.

"DES Daughters." *Time*, 24 March 1980.

Dieckmann, W. J., et al. "Does the Administration of Diethylstilbestrol during Pregnancy have Therapeutic Value?" *American Journal of Obstetrics and Gynecology*, Vol. 66, 1953, p. 1062.

Giusti, R. M., et al. "Diethylstilbestrol Revisited: A Review of the Long-Term Health Effects." *Annals of Internal Medicine*, Vol. 122, 1995, pp. 778–788.

Herbst, A. L. "Stilbestrol and Vaginal Cancer in Young Women." *CA: A Cancer Journal for Clinicians*, Vol. 22, 1972, pp. 292–295.

Herbst, A. L. "Exogenous Hormones in Pregnancy." *Clinical Obstetrics and Gynecology*, Vol. 16, 1973, pp. 37–50.

Herbst, A. L. "Diethylstilbestrol and Other Sex Hormones During Pregnancy." *Obstetrics and Gynecology*, Vol. 58 (5 Suppl.), 1981, pp. 35S–40S.

Jensen, T. K., et al. "Do Environmental Estrogens Contribute to the Decline in Male Reproductive Health?" *Clinical Chemistry*, Vol. 41, 1994, pp. 1896–1901.

Kurman, R. J. "Abnormalities of the Genital Tract Following Stilbestrol Exposure in Utero." *Recent Results in Cancer Research*, Vol. 66, 1979, pp. 161–174.

Mascaro, M. L. "Preconception Tort Liability: Recognizing a Strict Liability Cause of Action for DES Grandchildren." *American Journal of Law and Medicine*, Vol. 17, 1991, pp. 435–455.

Mayo, D. G., and R. D. Hollander. 1994. *Acceptable Evidence: Science and Values in Risk Management*. New York: Oxford University Press.

National Women's Health Network. 1980. *DES (Diethylstilbestrol)*. Resource Guide 6.

Newbold, R. R. "Prenatal Exposure to Diethylstilbestrol (DES)." *Fertility and Sterility*, Vol. 89 (2 Suppl.), 2008, pp. 55–56.

Newbold, R. R., et al. "Environmental Estrogens and Obesity." *Molecular and Cellular Endocrinology*, Vol. 304, 2009, pp. 84–89.

Raun, A. P., and R. L. Preston. "History of Diethylstilbestrol Use in Cattle." *Journal of Animal Science* (online), 2002.

Rubin, M. M. "Antenatal Exposure to DES: Lessons Learned . . . Future Concerns." *Obstetrical and Gynecological Survey*, Vol. 62, 2007, pp. 548–555.

Schrager, S., and B. E. Potter. "Diethylstilbestrol Exposure." *American Family Physician*, Vol. 69, 2004, pp. 2395–2400.

"Stilboestrol and Cancer." *British Medical Journal*, 11 September 1971.

Titus-Ernstoff, L., et al. "Offspring of Women Exposed in Utero to Diethylstilbestrol (DES): A Preliminary Report of Benign and Malignant Pathology in the Third Generation." *Epidemiology*, Vol. 19, 2008, pp. 251–257.

Travis, J. "Modus Operandi of an Infamous Drug." *Science News*, 20 February 1999.

U.S. Department of Health and Human Services, Public Health Service, National Toxicology Program. Report on Carcinogens, Eleventh Edition, 2005.

5

Aspirin and Reye's Syndrome

The remedy is worse than the disease.

—Francis Bacon, *Essays* (1597)

SUMMARY

Reye's syndrome is a rare but potentially fatal disorder that sometimes follows a relatively minor childhood viral infection, such as chickenpox (varicella) or influenza. Giving a child aspirin to reduce fever and relieve pain appears to be associated with increased risk of Reye's syndrome, although there is no proven causal link. In the early 1980s, a generation that once relied on chewable orange-flavored aspirin as a harmless childhood comfort suddenly came to regard the familiar drug as poison. This health scare has fizzled only in the sense that the issue remains unresolved. Acetaminophen has replaced aspirin as the analgesic of choice for children, the aspirin industry has found new markets, and the topic is no longer in the news. Until the role of aspirin in Reye's syndrome is clarified, parents should not give their children aspirin (or any other drug) except on a doctor's instructions.

SOURCE

The source of this health scare is short and simple. In 1963, Australian physician Ralph Douglas Kenneth Reye (1912–1977) and his colleagues published the first generally recognized description of what is now called Reye's syndrome. The statistical link to aspirin did not receive wide publicity until about 1980, after publication of several studies. Then the news media and consumer groups properly called attention to these findings, in an effort to protect children. Most pediatricians switched their patients to acetaminophen (often sold under the brand name Tylenol), while a few continued to recommend aspirin for even the youngest children, citing the extreme rarity of Reye's syndrome and the weakness of the statistical link to aspirin. Some mistakes and exaggerations are inevitable at the start of any legitimate health scare, but this one did not exceed its quota.

SCIENCE

Reye's syndrome is a potentially fatal childhood disease that damages the brain, liver, and other organs, apparently by causing changes in liver mitochondria—symbiotic structures that resemble bacteria and serve the important function of producing chemical energy in cells. (Mitochondria are similar to the better-known "midiclorians" of the *Star Wars* universe, with two exceptions: mitochondria are real, and they cannot speak.)

Although Reye's syndrome causes multiple effects, the worst damage results from swelling of the brain and fatty degeneration of the liver. The first phase of this syndrome is usually an acute viral infection that does not appear to be serious, such as chickenpox, influenza, or even the common cold. In the second phase, several days later, the brain and liver become involved and mitochondrial failure is rapid. This progression appears to occur more often if the child takes aspirin (acetylsalicylic acid) to relieve fever and pain. Early symptoms may include vomiting, lethargy, confusion, and nightmares, often progressing to disorientation, liver failure, seizures, coma, and respiratory arrest. Low blood sugar (hypoglycemia) and very high levels of blood ammonia are also typical. Even with treatment, the death rate is as high as 20 to 30 percent. Some Reye's survivors may have permanent disabilities.

Inevitably, not all cases of Reye's syndrome fit the above description, nor is every victim a child. In 2009, Japanese researchers reported an apparent case in a 26-year-old woman who took aspirin while recovering from pertussis (whooping cough), a bacterial infection. In another reported case, a 33-year-old woman who had recently given birth took aspirin for a tonsil infection, and soon died of Reye's syndrome.

At the time this book was written, the role of aspirin in Reye's syndrome was not fully understood. Some pediatricians remained unconvinced of the connection, whereas others drew a distinction between Reye's syndrome and Reye's-*like* syndrome, which may result from an inborn error of metabolism. In other words, genetic abnormalities may predispose to Reye's syndrome, and aspirin may serve as a trigger. Nor is it clear why this syndrome often follows a viral infection, but the pattern underlines the importance of vaccinating children against chickenpox and influenza. (There are no confirmed cases of Reye's syndrome resulting from vaccination.)

A 2005 publication suggests that salicylate (a metabolite of aspirin) may damage the mitochondria of liver cells, causing them to swell and malfunction. This finding is consistent with early reports that the liver cells of Reye's patients contain fewer, larger mitochondria than normal liver cells. Nonsteroidal anti-inflammatory drugs (NSAIDs) other than aspirin, such as acetaminophen (Tylenol) and ibuprofen (Advil or Motrin), do not appear to be associated with Reye's syndrome.

Some authors have pointed out that the incidence of Reye's syndrome began to decline even before the FDA put warning labels on aspirin bottles, and that it declined even in countries where children continued to take aspirin. If confirmed, this finding suggests that additional risk factors remain undiscovered. Other studies have suggested a possible connection between Reye's syndrome and various environmental hazards, such as methylmercury compounds (Chapter 21) or the organophosphate pesticide malathion.

HISTORY

As anyone knows who has read *The Clan of the Cave Bear*, people have used extracts of willow bark to treat fever and pain for thousands of years. The Latin name for willow is *Salix*, the source of the chemical name salicylic acid, of which aspirin (acetylsalicylic acid) is a derivative. Although the original source was willow, chemists have prepared salicylic acid by synthetic means since the mid-nineteenth century.

Given this history, it is hard to tell which came first, Reye's syndrome or aspirin. It is entirely possible that both predate civilization. A 1929 article in the medical journal *Lancet*—written by a doctor with the appropriate surname Brain—described six cases of a childhood disease that was probably Reye's, but the syndrome was not formally described in the medical literature until 1963, with Dr. Ralph D. Reye's landmark publication. Starting in 1974, several groups of concerned citizens joined the effort to protect children by discouraging the use of aspirin. Dr. Reye died in 1977, the same year that the FDA recognized this new syndrome as one of the 10 leading causes of death among American children aged 1 to 10.

At first, many cases of Reye's syndrome were probably diagnosed as viral encephalitis or meningitis, until more reports appeared in the literature and pediatricians learned what to look for. The Reye's epidemic peaked in 1980, when doctors reported 555 cases in the United States. Since millions of children had viral diseases that year, the incidence of Reye's syndrome was quite low, with or without aspirin. But this was a case in which the precautionary principle clearly applied, and by the time the FDA required warning labels on aspirin bottles in 1986, the majority of American parents and their pediatricians had already heard of Reye's syndrome.

In 1982, just as families across America were adjusting to acetaminophen as a substitute for aspirin, the nation woke to a new problem. Seven people in Chicago had died after taking Tylenol (acetaminophen) capsules that contained potassium cyanide. The culprit who tampered with the pills was never identified, although a man was arrested for extortion. This incident did little to improve consumer confidence in Tylenol, but it had no bearing on the Reye's scare in progress, and aspirin sales continued to plummet. In 1983, aspirin accounted for 62 percent of the U.S. pain reliever market, but by 1988 it had fallen to about 40 percent.

Then, in 1988, the news media announced the results of a large and well-timed study that established aspirin as a near-panacea for middle-aged and older adults. For the next two decades, aspirin was marketed as a magic bullet that could prevent heart attacks and strokes, besides relieving the pain and inflammation of arthritis. Every right-thinking baby boomer started carrying a bottle of nostalgic baby-sized chewable aspirin.

CONSEQUENCES

The legal profession sometimes benefits from health scares, and Reye's syndrome was no exception. In 1984, the consumer advocacy group Public Citizen's Health Research Group (HRG) and the American Public Health Association reportedly sued the FDA in an effort to compel it to require warning labels on aspirin. That case was dismissed, but the FDA started requiring such labels in 1986 anyway. As recently as 2002, attorneys representing a 22-year-old English woman sued the British government for negligence that allegedly contributed to her permanent disability 16 years earlier. In March 1986, the Committee on Safety of Medicines had determined that parents must be warned not to give their children aspirin, but bureaucratic hang-ups delayed the warning until June 1986. Meanwhile, the plaintiff contracted chickenpox, and her mother gave her aspirin. The High Court rejected the claim on the grounds that the government's 11-week delay was not excessive.

Another consequence of the Reye's health scare is that most people stopped using aspirin routinely to treat headaches or fever. This trend has persisted, although Reye's syndrome is seldom in the news. Yet authorities have also expressed concern about the increased use of acetaminophen, which carries some risks of its own. At least one team of pediatricians has speculated that the rapid increase in asthma and other allergic diseases since the 1980s might be related to avoidance of aspirin. Acetaminophen, which has largely replaced aspirin as a pain reliever, does not have its anti-inflammatory effect.

Inevitably, some sources have even asked if increased acetaminophen use by children might be responsible for the autism epidemic. Many health scares focus on autism at some point, because it is one of the worst medical catastrophes of our time, and an explanation and cure must be found. If enough hypotheses are explored, perhaps one will turn out to be right.

WHAT WENT WRONG?

The healthcare industry and the media both handled this health scare fairly well, and in that sense nothing went wrong. Yet this health scare fizzled in the worst way, with the most important questions still unanswered. The causal link, if any, between Reye's syndrome and aspirin remains unknown. Are all children susceptible, or only those with an underlying genetic defect?

Lesser issues also continue to nag. For example, the chemical salicylic acid (a metabolite of aspirin) is also a component of some popular acne medications. Can these topical creams also serve as a trigger for Reye's syndrome? If so, should younger teenagers avoid treating their pimples while they have the flu?

REFERENCES AND RECOMMENDED READING

Battaglia, V., et al. "Oxidative Stress is Responsible for Mitochondrial Permeability Transition Induction by Salicylate in Liver Mitochondria." *Journal of Biological Chemistry*, Vol. 40, 2005, pp. 33864–33872.

Belay, E. D., et al. "Reye's Syndrome in the United States from 1981 through 1997." *New England Journal of Medicine*, Vol. 340, 1999, pp. 1377–1382.

Brain, W. R., et al. "Acute Meningo-Encephalomyelitis of Childhood: Report of 6 Cases." *Lancet*, Vol. 1, 1929, pp. 221–227.

Clauson, K. A., et al. "Evaluation of Presence of Aspirin-Related Warnings with Willow Bark." *Annals of Pharmacotherapy*, Vol. 39, 2005, pp. 1234–1237.

Daugherty, C. C., et al. "A Morphometric Study of Reye's Syndrome: Correlation of Reduced Mitochondrial Numbers and Increased Mitochondrial Size with Clinical Manifestations." *American Journal of Pathology*, Vol. 129, 1987, pp. 313–326.

Davis, D. L., and P. Buffler. "Reduction of Deaths after Drug Labeling for Risk of Reye's Syndrome." *Lancet*, Vol. 340, 1992, p. 1042.

Dyer, C. "Government Sued for 11 Week Delay in Warning About Aspirin." *British Medical Journal*, Vol. 324, 2002, p. 134.

Feder, B. J. "The Stock Impact of Aspirin Report." *New York Times*, 28 January 1988.

Glasgow, J. F. "Reye's Syndrome: The Case for a Causal Link with Aspirin." *Drug Safety*, Vol. 29, 2006, pp. 1111–1121.

MacDonald, S. "Aspirin Use to be Banned in Under 16 Year Olds." *British Medical Journal*, Vol. 325, 2002, p. 988.

McGovern, M. C., et al. "Reye's Syndrome and Aspirin: Lest We Forget." *British Medical Journal*, Vol. 322, 2001, pp. 1591–1592.

Monto, A. S. "The Disappearance of Reye's Syndrome—A Public Health Triumph." *New England Journal of Medicine*, Vol. 340, 1999, pp. 1423–1424.

Morris, L. A., and R. Klimberg. "A Survey of Aspirin Use and Reye's Syndrome Awareness among Parents." *American Journal of Public Health*, Vol. 76, 1986, pp. 1422–1424.

Orlowski, J. P., et al. "Is Aspirin a Cause of Reye's Syndrome? A Case Against." *Drug Safety*, Vol. 25, 2002, pp. 225–231.

Partin, J. S., et al. "Serum Salicylate Concentrations in Reye's Disease." *Lancet*, 23 January 1982, pp. 191–194.

Porter, J. D., et al. "Trends in the Incidence of Reye's Syndrome and the Use of Aspirin." *Archives of Disease in Childhood*, Vol. 65, 1990, pp. 826–829.

Pugliese, A., et al. "Reye's and Reye's-Like Syndromes." *Cell Biochemistry and Function*, Vol. 26, 2008, pp. 741–746.

Reye, R. D., et al. "Encephalopathy and Fatty Degeneration of the Viscera: A Disease Entity in Childhood." *Lancet*, 12 October 1963, pp. 749–752.

Schrör, K. "Aspirin and Reye Syndrome: A Review of the Evidence." *Paediatric Drugs*, Vol. 9, 2007, pp. 195–204.

Springen, K. "Is Daily Aspirin a Good Idea?" *Newsweek*, 18 January 2008.

van Bever, H. P., et al. "Aspirin, Reye Syndrome, Kawasaki Disease, and Allergies: A Reconsideration of the Links." *Archives of Disease in Childhood*, Vol. 89, 2004, p. 1178.

Varner, A. E., et al. "Hypothesis: Decreased Use of Pediatric Aspirin Has Contributed to the Increasing Prevalence of Childhood Asthma." *Annals of Allergy, Asthma and Immunology*, Vol. 81, 1998, pp. 347–351.

Viscusi, W. K. "Efficacy of Labeling of Foods and Pharmaceuticals." *Annual Reviews of Public Health*, Vol. 15, 1994, pp. 325–343.

Warwick, C. "Paracetamol and Fever Management." *Journal of the Royal Society for the Promotion of Health*, Vol. 128, 2008, pp. 320–323.

Part Two

Infectious Diseases

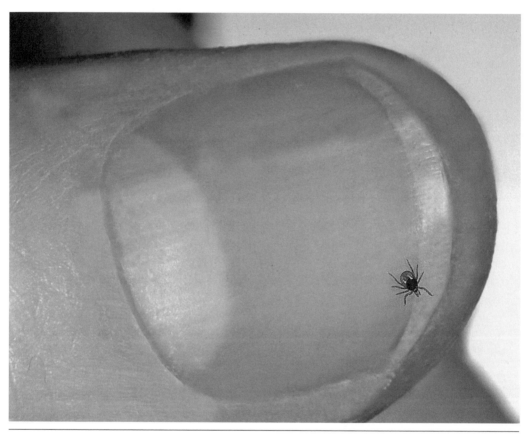

Figure 2   Immature *Ixodes* tick, the vector of Lyme disease.
(*Source:* U.S. Centers for Disease Control and Prevention, Public Health Information Library.)

6

Fear of Lyme Disease

This is one of those cases in which the imagination is baffled by the facts.
—Winston Churchill, *Remark in the House of Commons* (1941)

SUMMARY

Many people believe that chronic Lyme disease has reached epidemic proportions in the United States; that it is often incurable and ultimately fatal without years of antibiotic treatment and alternative medical practices; and that it can cause a bewildering range of disabling symptoms affecting virtually every organ in the body. Many other people, including most (not all) qualified researchers and physicians, regard Lyme as a treatable acute disease with specific symptoms and a good prognosis. In national opinion surveys, Lyme has emerged as one of the most feared of all infectious diseases, although its fatality rate is close to zero. Yet Lyme activists have opposed some of the most promising measures to combat the disease, including a vaccine (withdrawn from the market after consumer complaints) and proposals to control ticks by reducing deer populations. Although Lyme disease is real, and the controversy remains alive and well, the associated health scare appears to show a net fizzling trend.

SOURCE

Doctors first recognized Lyme disease while investigating an outbreak of what appeared to be juvenile rheumatoid arthritis in Connecticut in 1975. The news media picked up the story and ran with it. Lyme became a nationally notifiable disease in 1991, and some states have required reporting since the 1980s. The number of cases reported each year has risen steadily, for reasons that appear to include better diagnostic tests, more publicity, and a real increase associated with faulty wildlife management practices (see Science). Although Lyme is usually curable with antibiotics, and seldom (if ever) fatal, it has become a bandwagon, thanks to exaggerated urban legends and an aggressive publicity campaign. The Infectious Diseases Society of America insists that there is no such thing as chronic (long-term or lifelong) Lyme disease, but a number of highly vocal advocacy groups disagree. The health scare hinges largely on that point.

SCIENCE

The agent of Lyme disease is a spirochete (a type of bacterium) called *Borrelia burgdorferi*, but unlike some other spirochetes, it does not spread directly from one person to another. Instead, it enters the bloodstream with the help of an immature deer tick (Figure 2) that serves as a vector. These immature ticks live on mice, but they move to deer as adults, and deer are necessary for the ticks to complete their life cycle. Thus, the ticks have become more numerous as North American deer herds have grown larger, particularly in the northeastern states. Field studies have shown that reducing deer populations can also reduce the incidence of Lyme disease. Some sources indicate that mosquitoes and biting flies can also serve as vectors for this disease, at least in the laboratory. A pregnant woman infected with Lyme disease can transmit it to her fetus, and transfusions of infected donor blood may also spread the disease, although the risk is considered low.

In 2006, the Centers for Disease Control and Prevention (CDC) reported nearly 20,000 new cases of Lyme disease in the United States alone. This number does not include cases that are unrecognized, unreported, or self-diagnosed, so the true number may be higher. Many people become seropositive (develop antibodies) for Lyme disease without ever having symptoms, so they do not consult a doctor. Conversely, many people believe they have Lyme disease despite negative blood tests and the absence of any specific symptoms. Lyme disease is also common in several Canadian provinces and throughout Europe.

Like so many diseases, Lyme often starts like the flu, with low-grade fever, fatigue, headache, stiff neck, and muscle aches. Without treatment, these symptoms may last for several weeks, followed in some cases by persistent joint pain and swelling. The famous "bulls-eye" rash often appears at the location of the tick bite, but at least 10 percent of patients never develop this sign. Doctors have also reported some unusual presentations; in one case, epileptic seizures in an adolescent turned out to be the first sign of Lyme disease. The Web sites of Lyme advocacy groups present long lists of additional symptoms that members have reported. According to one such Web site, Lyme can cause weight gain, sexual dysfunction, "floaters" in the visual field, and a bad hangover after drinking alcohol.

It is unclear if Lyme can become a chronic infection or cause autoimmune disease, and we could fill another book (or several) with the arguments on both sides. The Infectious Diseases Society of America says no; the impassioned testimonials of advocacy groups say yes. A 2010 survey showed that only 2 percent of U.S. physicians regarded chronic Lyme disease as a legitimate diagnosis. As of 2009, the Social Security Administration does not list chronic Lyme disease as a recognized impairment, but many people have obtained disability benefits on the basis of more specific conditions that they believe result from Lyme. Suffice it to say that the potential long-term effects of this disease are not fully understood, and that accurate diagnosis and appropriate treatment are essential.

Two to four weeks of treatment with the right oral antibiotics can cure Lyme disease in about 95 percent of cases, if that is what the person really has. One problem is that many American doctors are unfamiliar with tickborne diseases other than Lyme, such as Rocky Mountain spotted fever, ehrlichiosis (anaplasmosis), babesiosis, and Colorado tick fever, which are more common than Lyme in some parts of the country and may require a different treatment regimen. Tick bites can also cause severe allergic reactions, including skin rashes and paralysis, which may be mistaken for an infection. In such cases, the solution is to find and remove the tick, which may be small and concealed by hair.

Some doctors have christened Lyme disease "The Great Imitator" or "The Easy Answer," names that reflect the confusion and frustration that has surrounded this disease since its discovery. Although Lyme is real and potentially devastating, its myriad symptoms and the difficulty of diagnosis have attracted a population of chronic patients who feel sick and believe they must have Lyme. When tested more carefully, many of these patients turn out to have some other disease, or none.

For example, a 1998 study showed that Lyme disease was vastly overdiagnosed in Oklahoma due to reliance on false-positive test results. Many cases turned out to be either ehrlichiosis or Rocky Mountain spotted fever; in that study, the investigators were unable to confirm even one case of true Lyme disease. Similarly, a 1998 study at Yale University reevaluated 209 patients who were diagnosed with Lyme disease elsewhere, and found that 60 percent showed no evidence of current or past infection.

When these 1998 studies were conducted, none of the widely available diagnostic tests actually detected the presence of *Borrelia burgdorferi*. Most blood tests simply detected antibodies to the bacterium, which prove nothing more than past exposure. False-positive tests for Lyme could result from antibodies to many other diseases, and false-negative tests soon after a tick bite might mean the immune system had not yet produced Lyme antibodies. Diagnostic testing has become far more accurate in the past ten years, but not everyone agrees with the results. As of 2010, CDC recommends a series of two tests for Lyme: the more sensitive ELISA (enzyme immunoassay) test, followed by the more specific Western blot test if the ELISA gives a positive result. For people who are not satisfied with this procedure, some laboratories reportedly offer alternative forms of Lyme testing that do not meet industry standards for accuracy.

HISTORY

Like many "emerging" diseases, Lyme has been with us for a long time, but has only recently attracted attention. European doctors described a similar disease before 1900 and associated it with tick bites in 1909, but the disease did not receive a name until 1975, after an outbreak of juvenile rheumatoid arthritis in the town of Lyme, Connecticut. In 1978, researchers proved that Lyme was a tickborne disease. In 1982, the spirochete was named *Borrelia burgdorferi* in honor of its discoverer, Dr. Willy Burgdorfer, an American scientist who was then director of the World Health Organization's Reference Center for Rickettsial Diseases at the Rocky Mountain Laboratory in Montana.

Lyme has become a greatly feared disease, particularly in the New England states. Thus, it is perhaps surprising that GlaxoSmithKline's 1998 discovery of a Lyme vaccine met with such resistance. The vaccine became available to the public in 1999, but the manufacturer pulled it off the market in 2002, citing low demand and poor sales. Reports indicate that it required a series of three shots and was about 80 percent effective. Certainly, this breakthrough did not inspire the same public enthusiasm as the Salk polio vaccine in the 1950s. On the contrary, media reports indicate that even the volunteers who tested the Lyme vaccine ended up suing the manufacturer for side effects, but the CDC investigated these claims and found them unsubstantiated. A 2006 *Nature* editorial cited the withdrawal of this vaccine as a prime example of "unfounded public fears" blocking vaccine development.

CONSEQUENCES

In a 2003 Gallup poll, 3 percent of a representative sample of Americans ranked Lyme as the disease they feared most. That might sound like a very small percentage, were it not for the fact that Lyme is curable and almost never fatal. Parkinson's disease, a devastating and incurable neurological disorder that afflicts millions, tied with Lyme disease in that same poll at 3 percent. No disease won a preponderance of votes; cancer was ranked highest, at 16 percent.

Some industries have benefited from this exaggerated perception of Lyme disease, such as those that manufacture tick repellants and control agents. Nobody really likes ticks, with or without Lyme disease; but the indiscriminate use of pesticides may also kill beneficial insects, and their overuse may ultimately result in resistant tick populations, just as unneeded long-term antibiotic treatment promotes the evolution of resistant bacteria.

Herbal remedies, poultices, and other alternative treatments for Lyme disease are widely marketed, although there is little evidence that they work. For example, there are claims that immediately cauterizing a tick bite by burning the skin with a hot object will prevent infection. This is unlikely to work, and can cause severe injury. We have also seen at least one book designed to help "patients who have been denied a Lyme diagnosis." But what is so great about a Lyme diagnosis? Perhaps a better goal would be an accurate diagnosis.

The emergence of Lyme disease has also added a few new terms and acronyms to the medical lexicon. As a possible solution to the controversy regarding the existence of chronic Lyme, one source proposes substituting the less attributive term "tick-associated polyorganic syndrome" or TAPOS. Others refer to this phenomenon as "post–Lyme disease syndrome." A Lyme-like rash after a tick bite in the absence of Lyme disease is sometimes called southern tick-associated rash illness (STARI).

Although the connection might not appear obvious, the Lyme disease epidemic has also increased tensions between animal rights activists and wildlife management agencies. Wherever humans "manage" natural resources, diseases find new hosts. There is solid evidence that the recent Lyme disease epidemic has resulted partly from the deer population explosion in the northeastern United States, because the ticks that serve as vectors spend part of their life cycle on deer. But most people like to look at deer, and hunters also like to shoot them, so the idea of simply reducing the number of deer is unpopular.

WHAT WENT WRONG?

Many people who feel genuinely sick are unable to obtain a useful diagnosis or effective treatment. This does not mean the people are crazy; it means that medicine is an inexact science, that the most treatable patients and those in immediate danger have the highest priority, and that access to good healthcare (at least in the United States) is at an all-time low. If the quality and affordability of healthcare continue to decline, more and more people will inevitably turn to alternative medicine, whether it works or not.

The alleged symptoms of chronic Lyme disease often include (but are not limited to) fatigue, headache, joint and muscle pain, numbness, weakness, palpitations, shortness of breath, difficulty in concentrating, and memory loss. These symptoms are real, but they might also characterize half the health scares in this book. Earlier generations called these symptoms neurasthenia, effort syndrome, or "the vapors." Newer terms include chronic fatigue syndrome, fibromyalgia, toxic mold exposure, depression—or, if anybody saw a tick, chronic Lyme disease. Patients often find themselves filing multiple insurance appeals and migrating from one specialist to another, finally settling on whichever diagnosis seems least objectionable to all parties. Those who cling to the medical roulette wheel long enough to land on chronic Lyme may find some comfort in the anti-inflammatory effect of antibiotics. Someday, doctors may be able to determine exactly what ails each person, but that day has not yet come.

REFERENCES AND RECOMMENDED READING

Baker, P. J. "Perspectives on 'Chronic Lyme Disease.'" *American Journal of Medicine*, Vol. 121, 2008, pp. 562–564.

Bellick, P. "Tick-Borne Illnesses Have Nantucket Considering Some Deer-Based Solutions." *New York Times*, 5 September 2009.

"Bugging Ticks for Profits." *Time*, 21 August 1989.

Carmichael, M. "The Great Lyme Debate." *Newsweek*, 22 August 2008.

Cowley, G., and A. Underwood. "A Disease in Disguise." *Newsweek*, 23 August 2004.

Feder, H. M., et al. "A Critical Appraisal of 'Chronic Lyme Disease.'" *New England Journal of Medicine*, Vol. 357, 2007, pp. 1422–1430.

Halperin, J. J. "A Tale of Two Spirochetes: Lyme Disease and Syphilis." *Neurologic Clinics*, Vol. 28, 2010, pp. 277–291.

Hoppa, E., and R. Bachur. "Lyme Disease Update." *Current Opinion in Pediatrics*, Vol. 19, 2007, pp. 275–280.

Hu, L. T., and M. S. Klempner. "Update on the Prevention, Diagnosis, and Treatment of Lyme Disease." *Advances in Internal Medicine*, Vol. 46, 2001, pp. 247–275.

Johnson, L., and R. B. Stricker. "Attorney General Forces Infectious Diseases Society of America to Redo Lyme Guidelines due to Flawed Development Process." *Journal of Medical Ethics*, Vol. 353, 2009, pp. 283–288.

Kalb, C. "Lyme Time in D.C.: Unraveling How to Best Treat the Disease." *Newsweek*, 30 July 2009.

Klempner, M. S., et al. "Two Controlled Trials of Antibiotic Treatment in Patients with Persistent Symptoms and a History of Lyme Disease." *New England Journal of Medicine*, 12 July 2001, pp. 85–92.

Landers, S. J. "Panel Hears Conflicting Views on Lyme Disease Treatment." *American Medical News*, 17 August 2009.

Lautin, A. "Lyme Disease Controversy: Use and Misuse of Language." *Annals of Internal Medicine*, Vol. 137, 2002, pp. 775–777.

Nau, R., et al. "Lyme Disease—Current State of Knowledge." *Deutsches Ärzteblatt International*, Vol. 16, 2009, pp. 72–81.

"New Symptoms in Disease." Associated Press, 1 June 1977.

"Region Linked to Disease." Associated Press, 23 May 1979.

Reid, M. C., et al. "The Consequences of Overdiagnosis and Overtreatment of Lyme Disease: An Observational Study." *Annals of Internal Medicine*, Vol. 128, 1998, pp. 354–362.

Shapiro, E. D. 2008. "Lyme Disease." *Advances in Experimental Medicine and Biology*, Vol. 609, 2008, pp. 185–195.

Sigal, L. H. "The Lyme Disease Controversy: Social and Financial Costs of Misdiagnosis and Mismanagement." *Archives of Internal Medicine*, Vol. 156, 1996, pp. 1493–1500.

Sigal, L. H. "Misconceptions about Lyme Disease: Confusions Hiding Behind Ill-Chosen Terminology." *Annals of Internal Medicine*, Vol. 136, 2002, pp. 413–419.

Steere, A. C. "Lyme Disease: A Growing Threat to Urban Populations." *Proceedings of the National Academy of Sciences U.S.A.*, Vol. 91, 1994, pp. 2378–2383.

Stricker, R. B., and L. Johnson. "Chronic Lyme disease and the 'Axis of Evil.'" *Future Microbiology*, Vol. 3, 2008, pp. 621–624.

Warner, R. "Ticks and Deer Team Up to Cause Trouble for Man." *Smithsonian*, April 1986.

Wormser, G. P., et al. "The Clinical Assessment, Treatment, and Prevention of Lyme Disease, Human Granulocytic Anaplasmosis, and Babesiosis: Clinical Practice Guidelines by the Infectious Diseases Society of America." *Clinical Infectious Diseases*, Vol. 43 (Supplement), 2006, pp. S123–S168.

7

Swine Flu 1976

The boy cried "Wolf, wolf!" and the villagers came out to help him.
—Aesop, *The Shepherd Boy and the Wolf* (circa 550 B.C.)

SUMMARY

In 1976, public health officials identified an unusual influenza virus at a military base in New Jersey and decided to vaccinate all Americans, in the hope of preventing a deadly epidemic. The virus was identified as swine flu, and researchers thought it was similar to the strain that caused the 1918 influenza pandemic. In fact, the two strains were quite different; the deadly 1918 virus was a form of bird flu, and the 1976 virus never posed much of a threat. It did not spread beyond the base, and only a few cases were ever identified. Worse, the swine flu vaccine had unexpected side effects that made several hundred people seriously ill and claimed at least 32 lives. The scare that fizzled was the flu epidemic itself, not the vaccine. Concern about the safety of that vaccine was justified, but over the years it has contributed to unwarranted fears regarding vaccines in general. Although largely forgotten today, the 1976 incident adversely impacted the credibility of other public health programs.

SOURCE

The immediate source of this health scare was highly specific, although some details are not entirely clear. In February 1976, a soldier at Fort Dix, New Jersey, somehow contracted an unusual form of influenza that doctors thought was similar to the strain that killed tens of millions of people in the 1918–1919 influenza pandemic. That soldier died within 24 hours, and several other soldiers at the same base were hospitalized. Experts studied the problem, and somebody—probably not the voice of the majority—calculated that this new influenza virus was likely to kill one million Americans. That estimate was highly quotable, and it leaked out. Fearing a deadly epidemic, the Ford administration made the controversial decision to immunize all Americans. Within a few weeks, the Food and Drug Administration (FDA) authorized vaccine manufacturers to gird for battle, and the news media announced that 50 to 100 million vaccine doses would be available by the fall of 1976. The stage was set, and the world held its collective breath. (Well, sort of.)

SCIENCE

Influenza (flu) is an airborne viral disease that usually starts abruptly, with a high fever, headache, and muscle pain. After a few days, these symptoms often subside, and the person develops a persistent dry cough, sore throat, and runny nose. The cough and general fatigue may last for weeks, and serious complications may develop, such as pneumonia or encephalitis. In a typical year, 10 to 20 percent of U.S. residents contract influenza, and some 200,000 are hospitalized with complications. About 36,000 to 40,000 die, usually as the result of a secondary infection such as bacterial pneumonia. Worldwide, there are about 500,000 to 1 million flu-related deaths in a typical year. In a pandemic (worldwide epidemic) year, these numbers usually rise, depending on the strains involved. Flu vaccines have been available since the 1940s, and antiviral drugs since the 1980s, but both are only partially effective.

Influenza A, the most common type of flu, affects not only humans but also birds, pigs, and other animals. Strains associated with birds and pigs are often called avian (bird) flu and swine flu, respectively; some of these strains can also infect humans. Some influenza viruses contain a mixture of components that are typical of both avian and swine flu. In 1976, when the Fort Dix outbreak took place, scientists were still learning how to identify influenza strains and subtypes, and they apparently overestimated the virulence of the new strain.

The news media and medical journals often describe influenza A viruses with acronyms such as H1N1 and H5N1. These antigenic subtypes get their names from the antigens (proteins) found on the surface of the virus. The letter H followed by a number identifies a glycoprotein called a hemagglutinin, and the letter N followed by a number identifies another glycoprotein called a neuraminidase. For example, H1N1 swine flu refers to a subtype with hemagglutinin 1 and neuraminidase 1. But these letters and numbers do not tell the whole story, because each subtype includes several strains. The 1918–1919 pandemic, the 1976 nonevent (this chapter), and the 2009 swine flu pandemic (Chapter 8) all resulted from quite different strains of H1N1 viruses.

Once a flu virus enters a human or animal population, what happens next depends on a number of factors, not all of them known or predictable. One factor is dumb luck; another is the basic reproductive rate (R_0) of the virus, which varies from one strain to another. This rate represents the average number of cases that will result from contact with one infected person, in a population with no immunity or treatment. If the number is higher than 1.0, the virus will probably spread, and if it is lower than 1.0, it probably won't. Scientists now know that the 1976 swine flu virus had a basic reproductive rate between 1.1 and 1.2, which meant it never had the potential to start much of an epidemic. By contrast, R_0 for the 1918 and 2009 pandemic viruses are estimated at about 3.0 and 1.5, respectively. For a discussion of the 2009 pandemic, see Chapter 8.

HISTORY

The Greek physician Hippocrates (460–375 B.C.) described a disease that sounds similar to influenza, but many upper respiratory infections have similar symptoms, so it is hard

Table 7.1. Influenza Pandemics

Date	Name	Estimated Deaths	Subtype
1580	None (Europe)	Unknown	Unknown
1729	Russian Flu	Unknown	Unknown
1782	Blitz Catarrh	Unknown	Unknown
1830	China Flu	1 to 2 million?	Unknown
1847	None (Europe)	<1 million	H1N1?
1889	Russian Flu	1 million	H3N8 or H2N2
1918	Spanish Flu	50 million	H1N1
1957	Asian Flu	2 million	H2N2
1968	Hong Kong Flu	1 to 2 million	H3N2
2009	H1N1 Pandemic	18 thousand	H1N1

to be certain. The word influenza appeared in Italian literature by 1504 and entered the English language in about 1743. The disease itself probably spread to the New World with one of the first waves of European settlers.

Between the isolation of the influenza virus in 1933 and the advent of HIV in 1981, influenza was perhaps the focus of more intensive study than any other viral disease. There were two influenza pandemics during that interval, in 1957 and 1968. Sources do not agree on the exact number of past pandemics, but there have been at least 10 since written records became available (Table 7.1).

Nobody knows exactly how many people died in the great influenza pandemic of 1918–1919, but with every passing year, the estimates grow larger. It is not clear if this trend represents improved statistical methods, retrieval of lost records, or the journalistic tendency to make a good story better. From the 1920s through the 1970s, the prevailing estimate was about 20 million. Later this was raised to 30 million, 50 million, or even 100 million, according to some authors. Whatever the real number, it was far too high; so when a similar-looking influenza virus unexpectedly appeared at Fort Dix in 1976, some degree of panic was inevitable. Many people still alive in 1976 remembered the 1918 pandemic, or had heard about it from their parents.

In an often-quoted February 1976 memo to the Office of Management and Budget, the U.S. Secretary of Health, Education, and Welfare reportedly wrote that "the projections are that this virus will kill one million Americans in 1976." Seasonal flu kills fewer than 40,000 Americans in a typical year, so this was an alarming projection. The memo leaked out, as memos do; and on 24 March 1976, President Gerald Ford announced the government's intention to inoculate every American against the new swine influenza.

Inevitably, some things went wrong. Most flu vaccines had always been grown in chicken eggs, but manufacturers found that the Fort Dix swine flu did not grow well in this medium, and yields were lower than expected. Then the insurance industry did its part, by refusing to insure the manufacturers against any claims of damage from the vaccine. To keep the program going, the government had to assume most of the liability.

By October 1976, the swine flu vaccine was ready, and an estimated 45 million people received it before the vaccination program was suspended due to unexpected side effects. Many public figures and celebrities were vaccinated, but apparently they were not among the several hundred people who developed neurological problems within a few weeks afterward, including the dreaded Guillain-Barré syndrome. This disorder also occurs in the general population, but it was seven times more common among people who had the 1976 flu vaccine. Many of the victims remained paralyzed for over a year, some were left with permanent disabilities, and at least 32 died. Some experts attributed these side effects to bacterial contamination of the vaccine, but others have claimed that all influenza vaccines may carry a similar risk. Ironically, the 1976 swine flu epidemic never materialized. Few cases were ever found, and no one knows how the virus reached Fort Dix in the first place. The debate continues to the present day.

CONSEQUENCES

There were lawsuits, of course; the federal government reportedly reached settlements with hundreds of people who developed Guillain-Barré syndrome or other problems attributable to the vaccine.

Although the late President Gerald Ford now enjoys favorable public ratings for his refreshing honesty and dignity, during his administration (1974–1977) he was unfortunately seen as something of a buffoon, who tended to trip over his own feet, grant questionable pardons, and make misstatements about Eastern Europe. The 1976 swine flu disaster only added to this negative perception, although the President really had nothing to do with it. The Fort Dix outbreak simply happened on his watch, and he followed the lead of his scientific advisors. Some have suggested that these advisors acted precipitously, but they were reacting to a potentially lethal change in the influenza virus, not to the death of one soldier. Somebody had to make the call, and it happened to be the wrong one in this case.

If the events of 1976 contributed to a general erosion of confidence in public health agencies and medical science in general, it also served to focus attention on Guillain-Barré syndrome and other potential side effects of vaccines. Before 1976, annual flu shots were generally assumed to be safe, but this disaster proved otherwise. Thus, when other batches of bad vaccine turned up, doctors were alert to the possibility. In 2000, for example, seasonal flu shots caused 960 cases of oculorespiratory syndrome (severe respiratory distress and eye irritation with facial swelling) in British Columbia. The problem was quickly traced to a bad batch of vaccine—unfortunately, about one-third of the 12 million doses distributed in Canada that season—and it did not recur the following year after the manufacturer changed its procedures. Also in 2000, a nasal influenza flu vaccine in Switzerland caused several cases of facial paralysis called Bell's palsy. Now drug manufacturers assume that every flu vaccine carries some risk and that a compensation program is necessary.

Knowledge is good, but it can backfire. Thanks to the news media, people are bombarded with scary information on every disease outbreak and often find it hard to make choices. Had the risks of smallpox vaccination been fully disclosed a century ago, many people would probably have refused to participate, and smallpox might still exist today.

Ironically, the 1976 swine flu vaccination program yielded one unexpected benefit, although it took many years to materialize. People who had their swine flu shots in

1976 had had partial immunity to the related virus that caused the 2009 H1N1 pandemic (Chapter 8).

WHAT WENT WRONG?

This is an unanswerable question. Given the perceived risk, could the CDC afford to wait and see what happened? Nobody could have predicted the abrupt disappearance of the swine flu strain found at Fort Dix, or the unusual side effects of the 1976 vaccine. Some public health experts prefer to regard the 1976 episode as a dress rehearsal or fire drill. The government may have reacted too quickly to the threat of swine flu in 1976, and too slowly to the threat of HIV in 1981. The next major opportunity to get it right came in 2009, as discussed in the next chapter.

But the 1976 swine flu debacle was not the first such dress rehearsal, and it is unlikely to be the last. During the Asian flu pandemic of 1957, a panel of medical experts concluded that mass influenza immunization made no sense. Dr. Ellis Sox, then San Francisco Health Director, made the following comment:

> Probably only 20 percent of the population will be hit. This means 80 [out] of 100 will not get Asian flu . . . the vaccine is only 50% effective and if it is given to the entire 100, only 10 of the 20 destined to get the flu will be protected. Of the 10, it is highly likely that some will be hit harder by the vaccine than they would have been by the disease.[1]

NOTE

1. "Experts See More Peril in Vaccine than in Flu" (*Washington Star*, 6 October 1957).

REFERENCES AND RECOMMENDED READING

Boffey, P. M. "Editorial Observer; Ruminating on Smallpox Vaccine and the Notorious Swine Flu Fiasco." *New York Times*, 27 October 2002.

Brown, D. "A Shot in the Dark: Swine Flu's Vaccine Lessons." *Washington Post*, 27 May 2002.

Dowdle, W. R. "Influenza Pandemic Periodicity, Virus Recycling, and the Art of Risk Assessment." *Emerging Infectious Diseases*, Vol. 12, 2006, pp. 34–39.

Dowdle, W. R., and J. D. Millar. "Swine Influenza: Lessons Learned." *Medical Clinics of North America*, Vol. 62, 1978, pp. 1047–1057.

Evans, D., et al. "'Prepandemic' Immunization for Novel Influenza Viruses, 'Swine Flu' Vaccine, Guillain-Barré Syndrome, and the Detection of Rare Severe Adverse Events." *Journal of Infectious Diseases*, Vol. 200, 2009, pp. 321–328.

Fineberg, H. V. "Preparing for Avian Influenza: Lessons from the 'Swine Flu Affair.'" *Journal of Infectious Diseases*, Vol. 197 (Suppl. 1), 2008, pp. S14–S18.

Fineberg, H. V. "Swine Flu of 1976: Lessons from the Past." *Bulletin of the World Health Organization*, Vol. 87, 2009, pp. 414–415.

"Flu Fight Plans Prepared." United Press International, 21 February 1976.

Greenstreet, R. "Adjustment of Rates of Guillain-Barré Syndrome among Recipients of Swine Flu Vaccine, 1976–1977." *Journal of the Royal Society of Medicine*, Vol. 76, 1983, pp. 620–621.

Iskander, J., and K. Broder. "Monitoring the Safety of Annual and Pandemic Influenza Vaccines: Lessons from the US Experience." *Expert Review of Vaccines*, Vol. 7, 2008, pp. 75–82.

Krause, R. "The Swine Flu Episode and the Fog of Epidemics." *Emerging Infectious Diseases*, Vol. 12, 2006, pp. 40–43.

Lessler, J., et al. "Transmissibility of Swine Flu at Fort Dix, 1976." *Journal of the Royal Society Interface*, Vol. 4, 2007, pp. 755–762.

Levine, A. J., and R. B. Trent. "The Swine Flu Immunization Program: A Comparison of Inoculation Recipients and Nonrecipients." *Evaluation & the Health Professions*, Vol. 1, 1978, pp. 195–215.

Miike, L. H. "Swine Flu Revisited." *Legal Aspects of Medical Practice*, Vol. 6, 1978, p. 5.

Neustadt, R. E., and H. V. Fineberg. 1978. *The Swine Flu Affair: Decision-Making on a Slippery Disease*. Washington, DC: U.S. Department of Health, Education and Welfare.

Puretz, D. H. "Some Thoughts on the 1976 Swine Flu Immunization Program: What Went Wrong?" *Journal of School Health*, Vol. 49, 1979, pp. 410–412.

Reismann, J. L., and B. Singh. "Conversion Reactions Simulating Guillain-Barré Paralysis Following Suspension of the Swine Flu Vaccination Program in the U.S.A." *Australian and New Zealand Journal of Psychiatry*, Vol. 12, 1978, pp. 127–132.

Vellozzi, C., et al. "Safety of Trivalent Inactivated Influenza Vaccines in Adults: Background for Pandemic Influenza Vaccine Safety Monitoring." *Vaccine*, Vol. 27, 2009, pp. 2114–2120.

Wade, N. "Swine Flu Campaign Faulted Yet Principals Would Do It Again." *Science*, Vol. 202, 1978, pp. 851–852.

Wecht, C. H. "The Swine Flu Immunization Program: Scientific Venture or Political Folly?" *American Journal of Law & Medicine*, Vol. 3, 1977–1978, pp. 425–445.

8

Swine Flu 2009

It is better to be a fool than to be dead.

—Robert Louis Stevenson, *Crabbed Age and Youth* (1877)

SUMMARY

At the time this book went to press in 2010, the H1N1 swine flu pandemic of 2009–2010 was already fading from memory, although the possibility remained that it might return in a more virulent form the following winter (or that aliens would land on Earth). Public health agencies took appropriate measures in 2009 to contain the pandemic, but made some inflated projections based on faulty data; the news media picked up the story and treated it like the Apocalypse. Even after the outbreak achieved technical pandemic status, polls showed that few Americans or Europeans took it seriously. By the time a vaccine was widely available, the peak of the pandemic had passed, and public interest was low. We should all be grateful that this health scare fizzled, instead of complaining about the unimpressive numbers.

SOURCE

In April 2009, the U.S. Centers for Disease Control and Prevention (CDC), the World Health Organization (WHO), and other public health agencies reported a cluster of unusual influenza cases in Mexico City. The virus was soon identified as a previously unknown strain of H1N1 swine flu, the same subtype—but not the same strain—that caused both the 1918 pandemic and the 1976 fiasco (Chapter 7). Press releases regarding the 2009 pandemic were accurate for the most part, but some exaggeration or misunderstanding was inevitable. For the next eight months, the world was bombarded with updates. There was no lack of information on the subject, but it is unclear if the majority of the population ever saw the pandemic as a real health scare.

SCIENCE

Chapter 7 contains a general discussion of influenza, including the associated numbers and terminology. There is some difference of opinion regarding the basic reproductive rate (R_0) of the 2009 H1N1 virus, but the most frequently quoted estimate is 1.5, or slightly higher than that of the 1976 bug.

HISTORY

Chapter 7 describes the general history of influenza and provides a summary of known pandemics (Table 7.1). As noted above, the 2009–2010 swine flu outbreak started near Mexico City in April 2009 and spread rapidly to the United States and other countries, with the press of the world hot on its tail. Perhaps the biggest change between the 1976 and 2009 swine flu outbreaks was the Internet, which enables both true and false information to circle the globe faster than ever before. The low point in the 2009 pandemic came early, when a major wire service allegedly quoted the World Health Organization (WHO) to the effect that the new influenza virus might physically blend with HIV (the agent of AIDS) to produce a deadly airborne threat that could "devastate the human race."[1] All the agency really said was that AIDS patients were at increased risk of complications if they also caught the flu; the H1N1 and HIV viruses cannot merge, but survey data suggest that a jaded public largely ignored the hype anyway. In June 2009, only 8 percent of Americans told the Gallup Organization that they were worried about the swine flu. That same month, WHO declared a pandemic.

Between April and October 2009, an estimated 22 million Americans contracted the H1N1 swine flu, and somewhere between 63,000 and 153,000 were hospitalized. Sources vary, but about 3,900 confirmed H1N1 deaths were reported in the United States during that interval. Later estimates of mortality for that time period, based on different assumptions, put the U.S. death toll from H1N1 at about 11,690 (range, 8,330–17,160). If these numbers sound scary, keep in mind that tens of thousands of Americans die from ordinary seasonal influenza every year. Europeans did not panic, either; in October 2009, a poll showed that only 12 percent of Germans intended to be vaccinated. As of August 2010, WHO reported a total of 18,449 confirmed H1N1 deaths worldwide—fortunately, just a small fraction of the toll for previous influenza pandemics. The number of cases peaked in October 2009 and had sharply declined by January 2010. In August 2010, WHO announced that the H1N1 pandemic was officially over.

Unlike the 1976 nonpandemic (Chapter 7), the 2009–2010 event was not marred by a defective vaccine with potentially deadly side effects—only by a vaccine that was somewhat late in production. It became available for high-risk groups (including children) in October 2009, the same month that the pandemic peaked and the number of cases began to decline. Since children needed two doses, two to four weeks apart, and it might take another six weeks for full immunity to develop, it is unclear how many cases of flu the vaccine actually prevented. In December 2009, the CDC estimated the rate of adverse events from the H1N1 vaccine as 82 per 1 million doses. By contrast, the rate of adverse events for the seasonal influenza vaccine used in 2009 was only 47 per 1 million doses. In both cases, problems were clearly quite rare. Also, about 95 percent of these adverse events were categorized as nonserious (e.g., sore arms) and 99.7 percent of adverse events were nonfatal.

Of 110 million H1N1 vaccine doses distributed in the United States between October 2009 and January 2010, only about 12 cases of Guillain-Barré syndrome were reported, and some of those were not confirmed. According to available records, a total of 13 people died soon after vaccination, but 9 of them already had serious underlying illness, and 1 died in a car accident. As of February 2010, only about 23 percent of Americans had received the H1N1 vaccine, and there was a lot of vaccine left over. By July 2010, an estimated 40 million doses had expired and were scheduled for burning.

CONSEQUENCES

When this book was written in 2010, it was too soon to assess the long-term medical or sociological consequences of the H1N1 pandemic. Did it increase public confidence in the healthcare system, or further erode it? We predict the former, because public health authorities clearly handled this pandemic better than the 1976 outbreak. Will those who received the vaccine suffer any long-term consequences? This appears highly unlikely, based on available data, but we have no crystal ball.

It is probably safe to say that the pandemic was a learning experience for all involved. The first reports in April 2009 greatly overestimated the mortality rate for this virus. By summer, the CDC predicted up to 90,000 H1N1 deaths in the United States alone; six months later, the total came in at more like 11,000. Some government spokesmen also made statements that did not help matters. Vice President Joseph Biden said he would avoid air travel during the swine flu epidemic, and British healthcare authorities even advised women to postpone pregnancy until after the threat of H1N1 flu had passed. A year later, the pandemic was technically still going, and the airlines and baby boutiques would be out of business had anyone followed this advice. Perhaps public figures should agree on a set of guidelines for future pandemics.

Then there was the hurry-up-and-wait principle. Everyone at risk (based on a rolling definition) was urged to seek vaccination as soon as possible, yet production of the vaccine was delayed until after the pandemic had already begun to wane. A Gallup poll released 10 November 2009 indicated that only 5 percent of Americans had received the vaccine, although about 50 percent wanted it. By the time enough vaccine was available for everyone, the show was mostly over. These contradictory messages caused initial panic in some people, while the majority rolled their eyes and switched channels. Not another media health scare!

WHAT WENT WRONG?

In retrospect, it's easy to dismiss the H1N1 pandemic as a tempest in a teapot—a claim that WHO has vehemently denied. Some conspiracy theorists even speculated that the government might have staged the pandemic as a distraction from the economic recession or the global climate controversy. Certainly, the body count was far lower than that of any previously recognized influenza pandemic (Table 7.1). But the low death rate should be cause for rejoicing, not for complaint. The vaccine shortage was a problem, but it resulted from production delays that were largely beyond the government's control. Improved vaccine production methods are definitely something to think about.

Clinics that ran short of vaccine turned to the antiviral drug Tamiflu, which can shorten the course of the disease by a few days, sometimes at the cost of major side effects. Many clinics reportedly gave this drug to people who were not at risk for serious complications, or had never even been tested for flu. Then predictable astonishment set in when the first patients turned up with H1N1 viruses that were resistant to Tamiflu. An estimated 98 percent of seasonal influenza viruses were already resistant to this drug, thanks to years of overuse.

If anything went wrong, it was the media hailstorm of confusing messages and contradictory updates. It almost seemed that too much information was available. The first reports insisted that young people were at greatest risk and had the highest priority for vaccination. Then it turned out that most H1N1 deaths in some states were actually among older people. Eventually, it became difficult to find out who should have the vaccine, or even who was eligible for it. At that point, a few people reportedly tried to steal the vaccine, but most just wished the pandemic would go away.

NOTE

1. M. Sieff, "Swine Flu–HIV Could Devastate Human Race" (UPI, 4 May 2009).

REFERENCES AND RECOMMENDED READING

Adams, J. "WHO Head Chan: Swine Flu Combined with HIV Poses Serious Threat." *San Francisco Examiner*, 4 May 2009.
"Another Run on Masks?" *Home Care Magazine*, 26 August 2009.
"Avoiding Panic in a Pandemic." *Lancet*, Vol. 373, 2009, p. 2084.
Bast, A. "United Nations Loses Count." *Newsweek*, 3 August 2009.
Brainard, C. "Media Hype Swine Flu Report." *Columbia Journalism Review*, 26 August 2009.
Brownlee, S., and J. Lenzer. "Does the Vaccine Matter?" *The Atlantic*, November 2009.
Castledine, G. "Swine Flu Panic is Being Spread by Ignorance." *British Journal of Nursing*, Vol. 18, 2009, p. 651.
Check, E. "Heightened Security After Flu Scare Sparks Biosafety Debate." *Nature*, Vol. 434, 2005, p. 943.
Enserink, M. "Experts Dismiss Pig Flu Scare as Nonsense." *Science*, Vol. 307, 2005, p. 1392.
Epstein, J. M. "Modeling to Contain Pandemics." *Nature*, Vol. 460, 2009, p. 687.
Fidler, D. P. "H1N1 After Action Review: Learning from the Unexpected, the Success and the Fear." *Future Microbiology*, Vol. 4, 2009, pp. 767–769.
Fillion, K. "Actual Flu Cases, a New Strain, Seems to Validate Our Fears, Not Just of Illness or Foreigners, but of Social Disruption." *Maclean's*, 11 May 2009.
Garrett, L. "The Path of a Pandemic." *Newsweek*, 2 May 2009.
Gillentine, A. "Deathly Flu Season Predicted." *Colorado Springs Business Journal*, 25 August 2009.
Henig, J. "Inoculation Misinformation." *Newsweek*, 19 October 2009.
"Is the U.S. Swine Flu Epidemic Over?" Associated Press, 6 February 2010.
Kalb, C. "Fighting Flu and Falsehoods." *Newsweek*, 27 October 2009.
Larson, H. J., and D. L. Heymann. "Public Health Response to Influenza A (H1N1) as an Opportunity to Build Public Trust." *Journal of the American Medical Association*, Vol. 303, 2010, pp. 271–272.
MacInnis, L. "WHO Says HIV Patients at Higher Risk from Flu." Reuters, 2 May 2009.

McNeil, D. G. "Debating the Wisdom of 'Swine Flu Parties.'" *New York Times*, 7 May 2009.

Shigemura, J., et al. "Responses to the Outbreak of Novel Influenza A (H1N1) in Japan: Risk Communication and Shimaguni Konjo." *American Journal of Disaster Medicine*, Vol. 4, 2009, pp. 133–134.

Sieff, M. "Swine Flu–HIV Could Devastate Human Race." United Press International, 4 May 2009.

Stafford, N. "Only 12% of Germans Say they will have H1N1 Vaccine after Row Blows Up over Safety of Adjuvants." *British Medical Journal*, 21 October 2009.

Stein, R. "Vaccine System Remains Antiquated." *Washington Post*, 24 November 2009.

U.S. Government, Executive Office of the President. "Report to the President on U.S. Preparations for 2009-H1N1 Influenza." President's Council of Advisors on Science and Technology, 7 August 2009.

World Health Organization. "Considerations on Influenza A (H1N1) and HIV Infection." News Release, 6 May 2009.

World Health Organization. "Transcript of Virtual Press Conference with Dr. Keiji Fukuda." News Release, 14 January 2010.

World Health Organization. "Pandemic (H1N1) 2009—Update 91." *Disease Outbreak News*, 12 March 2010.

Wyatt, H. V. "Ambiguities and Scares in Educational Material about AIDS." *AIDS Education and Prevention*, Vol. 1, 1989, 119–125.

9

Ebola Reston 1989

What is a virus but a colonizing force that cannot be defeated?
—Well-Manicured Man in *The X-Files: Fight the Future* (1998)

SUMMARY

On several occasions, starting (we think) in 1989, imported monkeys destined for laboratory experimentation died of Ebola hemorrhagic fever soon after their arrival at quarantine facilities in the United States. The health scares that followed were not extreme, but it was appropriate to wonder if the animal handlers who also became infected (without symptoms) might have spread this greatly feared disease to other humans or their pets and wildlife in nearby communities. The 1989 scare fizzled, in the sense that no outbreak resulted, and the press did not become too excited about it. Further study showed that the Ebola Reston virus (ERV) in its present form, although it is a form of Ebola, does not cause human disease. Similar incidents in 1990 and 1996 passed largely unnoticed, but public concern about biomedical laboratory accidents in general remains high.

SOURCE

In December 1989, an animal quarantine facility at a research laboratory in Reston, Virginia found Ebolavirus infection in a shipment of about 100 crab-eating macaque monkeys (*Macaca fascicularis*) imported from the Philippines. At that time, Ebola hemorrhagic fever was a greatly feared and relatively little-known disease, and the event caused public concern for a short time. Several animal handlers who worked with the monkeys also tested positive for Ebola, although none developed symptoms. As it turned out, the Reston strain—named for that outbreak, and now recognized as a separate species of Ebolavirus—in its present form does not pose a threat to humans, or at least not to those with healthy immune systems. Press releases emphasized the swift, decisive actions that were taken to contain the outbreak, such as improving safety measures, euthanizing all the exposed monkeys, and carefully monitoring the health of their human caretakers. So effectively did these measures contain panic that similar Reston Ebolavirus outbreaks at quarantine facilities in 1990 and 1996 passed nearly unnoticed.

SCIENCE

The virus family Filoviridae takes its name from the filamentous shape of its members, which belong to the genera *Ebolavirus* and *Marburgvirus*. Photomicrographs of these strange-looking viruses are familiar to anyone who saw the 1995 motion picture *Outbreak*. Tropical fruit bats serve as hosts for some (possibly all) of these viruses.

The genus *Ebolavirus* contains at least five species that cause hemorrhagic fevers, but until recently most sources referred to these species as strains, a term that implies a closer relationship:

- Zaire Ebolavirus (formerly called Ebola Zaire), discovered in 1976 in Zaire, which is now called the Democratic Republic of the Congo.
- Sudan Ebolavirus (formerly called Ebola Sudan), discovered in 1976 in the Republic of the Sudan.
- Bundibugyo Ebolavirus, found in the Republic of Uganda in 2007 and identified in 2008.
- Cote d'Ivoire Ebolavirus (formerly called Ebola Tai), found in the Ivory Coast in 1994.
- Reston Ebolavirus (formerly called Ebola Reston) from the Philippines, first found in imported monkeys after the 1989 outbreak in Virginia.

The first three Ebola species have all caused epidemics in humans and other primates in Africa. The fourth species apparently infects chimpanzees in the Ivory Coast, and it has also caused nonfatal illness in at least one exposed veterinarian. The Reston Ebolavirus occurs in the Philippines, where it occurs in monkeys, pigs, and (without symptoms) in humans. Most Reston-infected monkeys die, but pigs, like humans, can serve as carriers and transmit the disease to other animals.

The Zaire Ebolavirus is the one usually associated with the name Ebola, thanks to several sensational books and the motion picture *Outbreak*, which featured a fictitious Ebola-like disease called Motaba. Unlike Ebola, Motaba was not only airborne but also killed 100 percent of its victims. The real Zaire Ebolavirus spreads by contact with body fluids, so it is somewhat easier to contain than the fictional Motaba, and not everyone dies.

Ebola symptoms include a high fever, headache, vomiting, and diarrhea, often followed by bleeding from every orifice, multiple organ failure, and death in 50 to 90 percent of cases. As of 2009, the largest Ebola outbreak to date was in Uganda in 2000–2001, with 425 reported cases and 224 deaths (53%). Experimental Ebola vaccines have been effective in laboratory animals, but as of 2009, treatment of infected human patients focuses on supportive care and isolation. The closely related Marburg virus causes a similar hemorrhagic fever known as "green monkey disease."

Thanks to an overzealous press, many people think they are at risk for Ebola and related hemorrhagic fevers. In fact, these diseases seem hard to catch, even in areas where they are endemic. Visitors to Africa should avoid obvious hazards such as handling dead animals. In 2009, an American visiting Uganda became infected with the Marburg virus after touring a cave occupied by fruit bats. (He recovered, and none of his contacts became ill.)

HISTORY

Ebola was officially discovered in Zaire (Democratic Republic of the Congo) in 1976, but medical historians have found descriptions of similar diseases in ancient records. For example, in 430 B.C. a mysterious plague killed an estimated one-third of the population of Athens, Greece. The Greek historian Thucydides (460–395 B.C.) survived that plague and left a vivid account:

> People in good health were all of a sudden attacked by violent heats in the head, and redness and inflammation in the eyes, the inward parts, such as the throat or tongue, becoming bloody and emitting an unnatural and fetid breath. These symptoms were followed by sneezing and hoarseness, after which the pain soon reached the chest, and produced a hard cough . . . In most cases also an ineffectual retching followed, producing violent spasms, which in some cases ceased soon after, in others much later. Externally the body was not very hot to the touch, nor pale in its appearance, but reddish, livid, and breaking out into small pustules and ulcers. But internally it burned so that the patient could not bear to have on him clothing or linen even of the very lightest description . . . when they succumbed, as in most cases, on the seventh or eighth day to the internal inflammation, they had still some strength in them. But if they passed this stage, and the disease descended further into the bowels, inducing a violent ulceration there accompanied by severe diarrhoea, this brought on a weakness which was generally fatal.[1]

Although the prevailing view is that Thucydides was describing a smallpox epidemic, the frequency of hemorrhaging, diarrhea, and hiccup-like retching, plus the observer's unfamiliarity with the disease, seem more consistent with Ebola. Also, Thucydides wrote that the disease originated in Africa and spread through Egypt and Libya before reaching Greece.

More recently, American author Edgar Allen Poe (1809–1849) described a fictitious but seemingly Ebola-like disease in his 1842 short story, "The Masque of the Red Death":

> The "Red Death" had long devastated the country. No pestilence had ever been so fatal, or so hideous. Blood was its Avatar and its seal—the redness and the horror of blood. There were sharp pains, and sudden dizziness, and then profuse bleeding at the pores, with dissolution. The scarlet stains upon the body and especially upon the face of the victim, were the pest ban which shut him out from the aid and from the sympathy of his fellow-men. And the whole seizure, progress and termination of the disease, were the incidents of half an hour.[2]

Given this history, it is not surprising that the real Ebola hemorrhagic fever shocked the world when doctors discovered (or rediscovered) it in 1976. To most Americans, however, this disease seemed far away until 1989, when the monkeys began to die in Reston, Virginia. Suddenly, it was no longer just a scary story.

The CDC responded to the 1989 incident with tighter quarantine procedures for imported monkeys, and some facilities reportedly were closed. When the same thing happened again in 1990 and 1996, this time in Texas, the media barely blinked. As before, the monkeys died and the people seroconverted, but the disease apparently did not spread to animals outside the facility.

CONSEQUENCES

Sometimes it appears that people worry about the wrong things. The real scare should not be the death of laboratory monkeys—who were not destined for long lives under the circumstances anyway—but the recent discovery of an Ebolavirus in Philippine pigs, as reported by the World Health Organization and the news media in early 2009. Now the disease has officially entered the human food chain. Few people eat gorillas or chimpanzees on a regular basis, but hundreds of millions of people all over the world eat pork. Even some vegetarians handle raw meat, or live and work in close contact with pigs. At present, the Reston Ebolavirus does not seem to make people sick, but it could mutate to a more deadly form in pigs, just as the influenza virus has done.

Such news stories—mad cow disease, bird flu, and now this—may have driven some people to avoid meat. The controversial practice of transplanting organs between species may also encounter new hurdles. Doctors have long recognized the danger of introducing primate viruses into human populations, but pigs are considered less risky (not to mention less intelligent) and have been used extensively for medical purposes. Heart valves, blood vessels, skin, and other tissues have been transplanted from pigs to humans, and genetic modification of pig cells could soon make these procedures routine, in the absence of strong arguments to the contrary.

WHAT WENT WRONG?

There is no disease so bad that a dedicated science journalist can't make it sound even worse. Some popular books on Ebola, smallpox, and other diseases are graphic enough (or exaggerated enough) to scare the daylights out of readers. Unfortunately, laboratory accidents are inevitable. It is hard for any occupational group to be careful all the time, or for any safety procedure to be foolproof. Laboratory personnel get tired, distracted, and overconfident, just like everyone else. There have been highly publicized incidents in which respected researchers got in legal trouble for safety lapses that seemed innocent to their colleagues.

People who find their work rewarding often accept an element of risk. The primates in a lab, by contrast, are bored and challenged by the prospect of something to do, such as finding a way out of their cages and biting the people who put them there. With or without Ebolavirus, laboratory accidents are a disaster waiting to happen. Once the latest health scare fizzles, and exotic disease outbreaks cease to be news, the stage is set for more accidents.

NOTES

1. Thucydides, *The Peloponnesian War*, Second Book, Chapter VII, translated by R. Crawley (New York: Modern Library, 1951).

2. E. A. Poe, *Short Stories* (NY: Editions for the Armed Services, 1945).

REFERENCES AND RECOMMENDED READING

Barrette, R. W., et al. "Discovery of Swine as a Host for the Reston Ebolavirus." *Science*, Vol. 325, 2009, pp. 204–206.

Becker, S., et al. "Evidence for Occurrence of Filovirus Antibodies in Humans and Imported Monkeys: Do Subclinical Filovirus Infections Occur Worldwide?" *Medical Microbiology and Immunology*, Vol. 181, 1992, pp. 43–55.

Dalgard, D., et al. "Ebola Virus Infection in Imported Primates—Virginia, 1989." *Morbidity and Mortality Weekly Report*, 8 December 1989, pp. 831–832, 837–838.

"Ebola Reston in Pigs and Humans, Philippines." *Weekly Epidemiological Record*, World Health Organization, 13 February 2009.

"Ebola Virus Infection in Imported Primates—United States." *Canada Diseases Weekly Report*, Vol. 16, 1990, pp. 17–18.

Eisenberg, D. "Ebola is Back in the U.S., but Experts Say Humans have Nothing to Fear—Yet." *Time*, 29 April 1996.

Hayes, C. G., et al. "Outbreak of Fatal Illness Among Captive Macaques in the Philippines Caused by an Ebola-Related Virus." *American Journal of Tropical Medicine and Hygiene*, Vol. 46, 1992, pp. 664–671.

Jahrling, P. B., et al. "Preliminary Report: Isolation of Ebola Virus from Monkeys Imported to U.S.A." *Lancet*, Vol. 335, 1990, pp. 502–505.

Kilpatrick, K. "Canada's Ebola Scare Over but Questions Just Beginning." *Canadian Medical Association Journal*, Vol. 164, 2001, pp. 1031–1032.

Leroy, E. M., et al. "Fruit Bats as Reservoirs of Ebola Virus." *Nature*, Vol. 438, 2005, pp. 575–576.

Margasak, L. "Mishandling of Germs on Rise at U.S. Labs." Associated Press, 2 October 2007.

McNeil, D. G. "Pig-to-Human Ebola Case Suspected in Philippines." *New York Times*, 24 January 2009.

Meslin, F. X., et al. "Public Health Implications of Emerging Zoonoses." *Revue Scientifique et Technique*, Vol. 19, 2000, pp. 310–317.

Olson, P. E., et al. "The Thucydides Syndrome: Ebola Déjà Vu?" *Emerging Infectious Diseases*, Vol. 2, 1996, pp. 155–156.

Pearson, S., et al. "Ebola-Reston Virus Infection among Quarantined Nonhuman Primates—Texas, 1996." *Morbidity and Mortality Weekly Report*, Vol. 45, 1996, pp. 314–316.

Peterson, A. T., et al. "Ecologic and Geographic Distribution of Filovirus Disease." *Emerging Infectious Diseases*, Vol. 10, 2004, pp. 40–47.

"Rare, Deadly Virus Found in Monkey at Virginia Lab." *Washington Post*, 1 December 1989.

Roberts, J. A., and K. Andrews. "Nonhuman Primate Quarantine: Its Evolution and Practice." *ILAR Journal*, Vol. 49, 2008, pp. 145–156.

Singh, B. "Taking Down Goliaths: New Vaccines May Spell the End for Ebola, Marburg and Lassa Virus Infections." *Healthcare Quarterly*, Vol. 8, 2005, pp. 20, 22.

Snelson, H. "PRRS and Ebola Virus Reported in Philippine Pigs." News Release, American Association of Swine Veterinarians, 15 December 2008.

Sullivan, B. "Smallest Terrorist of Them All Plays Havoc with Health." Associated Press, 21 April 1977.

Towner, J. S., et al. "Newly Discovered Ebola Virus Associated with Hemorrhagic Fever Outbreak in Uganda." *PLoS Pathogens*, 21 November 2008.

Ungar, S. "Hot Crises and Media Reassurance: A Comparison of Emerging Diseases and Ebola Zaire." *British Journal of Sociology*, Vol. 49, 1998, pp. 36–56.

10

The Second War on Smallpox

Those things yonder are no giants, but wind-mills, and the arms you fancy, are their sails, which being whirled about by the wind, make the mill go.

—Miguel de Cervantes, *Don Quixote de la Mancha* (1605)

SUMMARY

The first conquest of smallpox is a story of human genius and courage, but the second conquest is harder to describe—mainly because, to paraphrase an old joke, we gave a war and nobody came. In 2002, after the events of September 11, 2001, and the anthrax mailings, the Bush administration decided to protect the American public from the possible resurgence of smallpox. The only reason given was that terrorists might obtain this virus, which has not existed in the wild since 1978, and reintroduce it to the world as an act of sheer mindless evil. But apparently there was never any real evidence that terrorists had access to the smallpox virus, or that they intended to deploy any biological agent. Thus, smallpox had its 15 minutes of fame, and the chief beneficiary was the vaccine manufacturer. It is always a good idea to be prepared for emergencies, but there are many diseases that might serve as biological weapons.

SOURCE

One probable source of the 2001 smallpox scare was an excellent 2000 biohazard book written by a public health expert in collaboration with a science journalist. The book dramatized its major points with a series of fictitious scenarios involving such props as renegade scientists and crop dusters. It was a real nail-biter, but its authors may have failed to consider how some world leaders might overreact to a vivid work of fiction.

Then came the postal anthrax incident in October 2001, which led some people to suspect that foreign terrorists had attacked the United States with biological weapons. The incident occurred only a few weeks after the destruction of the World Trade Center, and national security was on everyone's mind. Whenever one unusual event closely follows another, it is human nature to infer a connection. Thus, within days after the anthrax mailings, the news media erupted with speculation about bioweapons in general and smallpox in particular. It was unclear at the time, and has remained unclear, why an outbreak of anthrax from a probable domestic source made people worry about smallpox from a foreign source; but in November 2001, the Bush Administration signed a contract to buy 150 million doses of smallpox vaccine from a British firm. A year later, on 13 December 2002, the President announced a plan to vaccinate all military personnel and first responders.

Did the same sources that believed Iraq was hiding weapons of mass destruction also believe that some terrorist group or sponsoring nation had access to the smallpox virus? No, apparently not, for President Bush stated, in 2002: "Our government has no information that a smallpox attack is imminent."[1] At least two U.S. laboratories already had large stocks of smallpox vaccine that was made in the 1950s and apparently still retained its potency, but that was not good enough—we needed a new batch. Soon, a massive and expensive plan went into effect, sensational tabloid articles and TV programs about smallpox began to appear, and people of the author's generation began proudly displaying our decades-old smallpox vaccination scars and listening to *Fox News*. It was a strange time.

SCIENCE

The U.S. Centers for Disease Control and Prevention (CDC) classifies smallpox (variola) as a Category A bioterrorism agent. This category consists of high-priority diseases with the following characteristics:

- They are easily disseminated (by either natural or artificial means).
- They have a high death rate.
- They are likely to cause panic and social disruption.
- They require planning and action by public health agencies.

In addition to smallpox, other Category A diseases include anthrax, botulism, plague, smallpox, tularemia, and viral hemorrhagic fevers (filoviruses and arenaviruses). Within this group, smallpox is unique in at least three respects: it spreads directly from person to person more readily than the others; it is not a zoonosis (animal disease); and it is the only Category A agent that no longer exists in the wild.

The last known victims of smallpox were a Somali man named Ali Maow Maalin, who contracted smallpox and recovered in 1977, and Janet Parker, a British medical photographer who died in 1978 when smallpox virus escaped from a laboratory. Two known samples of the virus now reside in high-security laboratories in the United States and Russia, but other nations may have samples of their own. The World Health Organization (WHO) declared smallpox eradicated from the world in 1979, and manufacturers stopped making the vaccine. Between 1979 and 1984, WHO received and investigated 179 reports of suspected smallpox, but found that all were chickenpox or another similar-looking disease.

But when smallpox still existed, what was it really like? There were two general forms, variola minor and variola major, both spread by airborne transmission or direct contact. Variola minor was somewhat worse than a bad case of chickenpox, with many bumps, some scarring, and a fatality rate below 1 percent. Variola major is what we usually mean by smallpox; and here the confusion starts. Depending on which sources one believes, variola major is either a severe pustular disease that kills about 20 percent of untreated patients and disfigures many more; or else it is a science-fiction nightmare that flays its living victims into screaming puddles of soon-dead glop.

We will skip the last part, but here is a description written by public health professionals before 1975, when smallpox still existed in the wild:

> The 2 to 4 day pre-eruptive illness frequently resembles influenza. The temperature falls and a deep-seated rash appears. This rash passes through successive stage of macules, papules, vesicles, pustules and finally scabs, which fall off at the end of the third to fourth week; fever frequently intensifies after the rash has evolved to the pustular stage.[2]

Pretty weak stuff, huh? No bestseller there. But much of the media frenzy has focused on the rare hemorrhagic form of variola major, which historically occurred in only about 2 percent of cases and sounds a bit like Ebola (Chapter 9). For a more typical description of the smallpox experience, we will turn not to doctors or journalists, but to a Texas man named Charles Barber. In 1949, his mother Lillian became the last known American to die of smallpox, when an outbreak infected at least eight people in the Rio Grande Valley. The other seven survived, including Charles's severely ill father and a younger brother who had a milder case. Charles and two other family members never showed signs of smallpox, although they were quarantined in the same house:

> I had to put socks on his hands so that he wouldn't scratch himself. And I would change his sheets, and each time I would burn a double handful of scabs that came off his body. . . . My brother was very sick, but he didn't break out, not in one solid scab like my daddy.[3]

If that was smallpox, what was the vaccine like? Most people have heard the story of cowpox, a mild relative of smallpox that once protected English dairy workers from the real item. In 1796, Dr. Edward Jenner (1749–1823) recognized the protective effect of cowpox and conducted a clinical trial: he infected a number of children (including his own son) with cowpox and then exposed them to smallpox. The experiment was crude and reckless by modern standards, but it worked. The vaccinia virus, a cowpox derivative, has served as a smallpox vaccine ever since, despite some initial public skepticism (Figure 1). Ring vaccination, in which doctors vaccinate all known contacts of a smallpox patient, was the strategy that ultimately rid the world of this disease.

Of course, vaccinia is a disease in its own right, and it is not entirely harmless either. In the old days, out of every 1 million people who received this vaccine, about 1,000 could expect serious side effects, about 30 had potentially life-threatening reactions, and 1 or 2 died. It is not clear if the odds have improved over the years, but people who have been recently vaccinated against smallpox can still infect others who come in contact with their vaccination site. In one particularly unpleasant 2006 case, a woman contracted vulvar vaccinia (exactly what it sounds like) after sleeping with a military vaccinee. In parts of Europe and South America, cowpox and vaccinia viruses left over from the smallpox era have jumped their fences (so to speak) and run amok like feral pigs, causing recent disease outbreaks in humans, cats, and livestock.

HISTORY

At about the time of the 2001 anthrax mailings, the news media quoted a public health authority to the effect that starting a smallpox epidemic would be as easy as levelling the World Trade Center using planes hijacked with box cutters. Actually, it might be a good deal easier, if somewhat pointless. Reintroducing smallpox to an immunologically naïve world would probably harm the countries that traditionally sponsor terrorism more than it would harm prosperous societies that can afford the vaccine. In any case, the comment was probably intended as a hypothetical example rather than a prediction. Fighting bioterrorism was high on the public's list of things to do that year, and a number of dramatic books on the subject had already appeared in print in the years leading up to the millennium.

In a January 2003 Gallup poll, 63 percent of American respondents said they were either somewhat worried or very worried about smallpox. That was a significant increase from the previous November, when only 53 percent were somewhat or very worried. In January 2003, 53 percent said they would agree to smallpox vaccination, but not if their doctors refused it. As it turned out, the vaccine was not available to the general public anyway, and few healthcare workers wanted it. Military personnel had no choice, and by the end of 2003, some 500,000 had received the vaccine

Some military personnel reportedly suffered fatal heart attacks after receiving the smallpox vaccine, but it is not clear if the vaccine caused those events. Many others suffered chest pain due to inflammation in or around the heart, but these reactions were temporary. This vaccine, in other words, is not to be taken lightly. But it is not impossible that smallpox may return someday, and the events of 2001–2003 may serve as a dress rehearsal. The vaccine may also prove useful if monkeypox (Chapter 12) begins to spread.

CONSEQUENCES

Acambis, the small British biotechnology firm that made the smallpox vaccine, reportedly had its first profit as a result of its contracts with the United States and with several European countries. A 2003 press release indicated that the company planned to reinvest the profit in research on West Nile and other vaccines. In 2004, however, Acambis reported lower profit forecasts due to production delays and safety issues.

A 2005 report by the Institute of Medicine concluded that the smallpox vaccination program had damaged the CDC's credibility. The original goal was to vaccinate a total of 10 million civilian healthcare workers and first responders within a year. Instead, the program petered out after only about 40,000 civilians were vaccinated. At no time did the CDC or any other agency adequately explain the scientific justification for the smallpox program.

WHAT WENT WRONG?

The purpose of the National Smallpox Vaccination Program was to vaccinate healthcare workers and first responders who could safely care for smallpox patients in the event of an attack. It was a fine plan, with just one missing element—evidence that a smallpox outbreak was at all likely. Some vaccines are harmless, and it makes sense to have them as a precaution. Smallpox vaccination, however, is potentially risky and requires some justification.

This dread disease is one of many that terrorists (or laboratory accidents, or natural selection, or melting glaciers, or space debris) might someday unleash on the world. But knowing that the United States is now prepared to combat smallpox, why wouldn't the terrorists simply release something else? There is no shortage of diseases and toxins to choose from. Fear alone is probably the best weapon, not to mention the cheapest.

NOTES

1. Office of the Press Secretary, 13 December 2002.
2. Benenson, A. S. (Editor), *Control of Communicable Diseases in Man*, 12th Edition (Washington, DC: American Public Health Association, 1975), p. 288.
3. Brezosky, L. "Family Recalls Last Smallpox Outbreak." *Associated Press*, 17 December 2001.

REFERENCES AND RECOMMENDED READING

Agwunobi, J. O. "Should the U.S. and Russia Destroy their Stocks of Smallpox Virus?" *British Medical Journal*, Vol. 334, 2007, p. 775.
Barquet, N., and P. Domingo. "Smallpox: The Triumph Over the Most Terrible of the Ministers of Death." *Annals of Internal Medicine*, 15 October 1997, pp. 635–642.
Blendon, R. J., et al. "The Public and the Smallpox Threat." *New England Journal of Medicine*, Vol. 348, 2003, pp. 426–432.
Bowman, S. "Weapons of Mass Destruction: The Terrorist Threat." Congressional Research Service, 7 March 2002.
Broad, W. J. "Guide for Mass Smallpox Vaccinations: Recipe with Missing Ingredients." *New York Times*, 24 September 2002.
Calabresi, M., and M. August. "Was Smallpox Overhyped?" *Time*, 26 July 2004.
Cohen, J., and M. Enserink. "Public Health: Rough-and-Tumble Behind Bush's Smallpox Policy." *Science*, Vol. 298, 2002, pp. 2312–2316.
DeBoer, K. "Study: Should America Vaccinate?" *Michigan Daily*, 20 May 2002.
Hamilton, R., and R. McCain. "Smallpox, Risks of Terrorist Attacks, and the Nash Equilibrium: An Introduction to Game Theory and an Examination of the Smallpox Vaccination Program." *Prehospital and Disaster Medicine*, Vol. 24, 2009, pp. 231–238.
Hammond, E. "Should the U.S. and Russia Destroy their Stocks of Smallpox Virus?" *British Medical Journal*, Vol. 334, 2007, p. 774.
Ježek, Z., et al. "Smallpox and its Post-Eradication Surveillance." *Bulletin of the World Health Organization*, Vol. 65, 1987, pp. 425–434.
May, T., and R. D. Silverman. "Should Smallpox Vaccine be Made Available to the General Public?" *Kennedy Institute of Ethics Journal*, Vol. 13, 2003, pp. 67–82.
Meckler, L. "Government Buys 150 Million Doses of Smallpox Vaccine." *Associated Press*, 29 November 2001.
Pappalardo, J. "Public Would Ignore Authorities in Terror Event." *National Defense*, November 2004.

Perisic, A., and C. T. Bausch. "Social Contact Networks and Disease Eradicability under Voluntary Vaccination." *PLoS Computational Biology*, 6 February 2009.

Rauch, J. "Countering the Smallpox Threat." *Atlantic*, December 2001.

Sinclair, R., et al. "Persistence of Category A Select Agents in the Environment." *Applied and Environmental Microbiology*, Vol. 74, 2008, pp. 555–563.

Spake, A. "It Was Unbelievable." *U.S. News and World Report*, 14 March 2005.

Strikas, R. A., et al. "US Civilian Smallpox Preparedness and Response Program, 2003." *Clinical Infectious Diseases*, Vol. 46 (Suppl. 3), 2008, pp. S157–S167.

Tian, J., et al. "Accurate Multiplex Gene Synthesis from Programmable DNA Microchips." *Nature*, Vol. 432, 2004, pp. 1050–1054.

Tucker, J. "The Smallpox Destruction Debate: Could a Grand Bargain Settle the Issue?" *Arms Control Today*, March 2009, pp. 6–15.

Wharton, M., et al. "Recommendations for Using Smallpox Vaccine in a Pre-Event Vaccination Program." *Morbidity and Mortality Weekly Report, Recommendations and Reports*, Vol. 52, 2003, pp. 1–16.

Wortley, P. M., et al. "Predictors of Smallpox Vaccination among Healthcare Workers and Other First Responders." *American Journal of Preventive Medicine*, Vol. 32, 2007, pp. 538–541.

Zoler, M. L. "Smallpox Vaccine Linked to Myocarditis: Unexpected Complications." *Family Practice News*, 1 February 2004.

11

Fear of Flesh-Eating Bacteria

Is it not enough that I am devoured, without my being expected to bless the power that devours me?
> —Fyodor Dostoevsky, *The Idiot* (1868, English translation by E. Martin, 1915)

SUMMARY

Several species of bacteria can enter the body through a break in the skin and—in a very small percentage of cases—cause unexpectedly severe, rapid damage to the deeper layers of connective tissue. The resulting infection, called necrotizing fasciitis (NF), is an ancient problem that can result in limb amputation or death, even after minor or unnoticed injuries. The risk declined, but did not disappear, in most developed nations after the discovery of antibiotics. Now that some pathogens have become resistant to those antibiotics, and the press needs grotesque stories, these so-called flesh-eating bacteria have returned in spades. Group A streptococci and many other bacteria can cause this type of infection. The associated health scare has recently fizzled in the sense that others have replaced it in the limelight, but the more general problem of antibiotic-resistant bacteria is alive and well.

SOURCE

People have known for thousands of years that dreadful infections with rapid destruction of tissue and loss of life can sometimes follow even minor wounds or surgical operations. Doctors first described this condition in the mid-eighteenth century, and they have called it necrotizing fasciitis since 1952. (Necrosis means tissue death, and fasciitis means inflammation of the sheet of connective tissue that underlies the skin.) As far as we can tell, however, the term "flesh-eating bacteria" did not exist until British tabloids coined it in the early 1990s, after a highly publicized outbreak of bacterial infections near London that involved Group A *Streptococcus* (plural, streptococci).

Such infections were nothing new to doctors, who investigated the outbreak as a possible new strain of an old enemy. Meanwhile, across the pond, a New York firefighter's widow sued a hospital for negligence in the 1991 death of her husband from necrotizing fasciitis. Suddenly, journalists noticed that there were many such cases—an estimated 500 to 1,500 per year in the U.S. alone, with a death rate of about 20 percent. Since necrotizing fasciitis was not on the list of diseases that doctors were required to report to public health agencies, the full extent of the problem had gone unnoticed by the general public. Then, as so often happens, hundreds of individual events ceased to be cold statistics and merged to form a raging beast. Streptomania was born.

SCIENCE

About 15 to 30 percent of all people in the United States carry Group A streptococci in their bodies, either without symptoms or with only minor illness. Necrotizing fasciitis normally results only if these bacteria are themselves infected with a virus that causes them to produce a toxin. NF is not the only possible outcome; another invasive streptococcal infection that became a health scare in the 1980s is toxic shock syndrome, sometimes associated with tampon use. Conversely, many other types of bacteria can also cause NF, and the term no longer refers to the specific agent, but rather to the effects. In 2000, for example, a marine bacterium called *Photobacterium damsela* infected a wound on a Florida man's leg and caused a severe case of necrotizing fasciitis. Table 11.1 lists some of the bacterial species that are known to cause similar infections.

Once the process is underway, the bacterial infection spreads rapidly along the fascia, often destroying tissue at a rate of more than one inch per hour. Unless doctors recognize the problem quickly and take appropriate action, the patient dies. Even with the

Table 11.1. Some Bacteria That Can Cause Necrotizing Fasciitis

Aeromonas hydrophila

Bacteroides fragilis

Clostridium perfringens

Clostridium septicum

Escherichia coli

Haemophilus aphrophilus

Klebsiella sp.

Photobacterium damsela

Proteus sp.

Pseudomonas sp.

Ruminococcus (Peptostreptococcus) productus

Staphylococcus aureus (including MRSA)

Streptococcus pneumoniae

Streptococcus pyogenes

Vibrio vulnificus

best treatment available, the death rate may be as high as 20 to 25 percent. Treatment includes antibiotic therapy, hyperbaric oxygen treatment, and intravenous immuno-globulin (antibodies extracted from donor blood). Surgical removal of infected tissue and amputation of limbs may often be necessary.

Until recently, most streptococcal infections responded quickly to antibiotic treat-ment, but drug-resistant strains have appeared. As with many other bacteria, the main cause appears to be the overuse of antibiotics. Scottish scientist Alexander Fleming (1881–1955) discovered penicillin in 1928, and German chemists created the first sulfa drugs in 1932. Other "miracle drugs" followed in rapid succession. When these drugs first appeared, doctors and the general public tended to use them indiscriminately. But whenever populations of living organisms are exposed to a poison, resistance is likely to evolve. Some bacteria, for example, have genes that enable them to produce enzymes that break down the antibiotic molecule. Bacteria with this capability are more likely than others to survive and reproduce in the presence of antibiotics. Some antibiotic-resistant bacteria can even transfer the resistance genes to other species of bacteria.

As a result, many bacterial infections that were once treatable are now resistant to most or all antibiotics. In the United States alone, about 100,000 people die from drug-resistant bacterial infections every year. Certain resistant bacterial strains have become a major problem in U.S. hospitals, where these bacteria infect an estimated 2 million patients every year. Community-acquired drug-resistant infections (those acquired out-side hospitals) are also becoming increasingly common.

The fact that necrotizing fasciitis is a rare infection makes it harder to identify spe-cific risk factors. In about half the known cases, the patient is young and apparently in good health. In the other half, risk factors may include immune suppression, recent chickenpox, intravenous drug use with dirty needles, advanced age, diabetes, or simply having surgery in a hospital where antibiotic-resistant bacteria are likely to occur. Some researchers have claimed that the use of NSAIDs may be associated with invasive strep infections.

HISTORY

Since necrotizing fasciitis can follow even the most minor injuries, prehistoric humans probably saw it from time to time. Dogs and other animals get it too. According to the historian Flavius Josephus (A.D. 37–101), King Herod the Great of Judea—the same Herod who tried to kill baby Jesus—suffered from a similar disease that destroyed his genitals. At least one medical historian has identified this disease as a form of NF.

French doctors described a condition similar to necrotizing fasciitis in the mid-eighteenth century, and the first detailed descriptions appeared about 100 years later. At various times in history, doctors have referred to this condition as malignant ulcer, putrid ulcer, or hospital gangrene. In 1881, Jean Alfred Fournier (1832–1914) described the form now known as Fournier's gangrene, which invades the scrotum and may be the same disease that Herod had. This infection is now known to take several different forms, but what they all have in common is that the infection spreads quickly along fascial planes, causing rapid destruction of tissue. The more general form of the infection acquired its present name, necrotizing fasciitis, from a journal article published in 1952.

Necrotizing fasciitis made headlines many times during the late twentieth century. In 1994, a cluster of 18 cases in England resulted in 11 deaths, but no common risk factor was ever identified, except that several of the people had recent surgery. Sporadic cases have included so many famous and accomplished people that we are bound to leave somebody off the list: Former Quebec premier Lucien Bouchard and South African journalist R. W. Johnson each lost a leg to this disease, in 1994 and 2009, respectively. Nobel laureate Eric A. Cornell lost an arm and shoulder in 2004, but survived. Physicist Alexandru Marin and economist David Walton both died from necrotizing fasciitis, in 2005 and 2006, respectively.

CONSEQUENCES

In the last few years, many journalists have commented on the long waiting times in hospital emergency rooms and the suboptimal quality of healthcare in general. Many diseases and injuries can wait—and wait—and wait—but necrotizing fasciitis is not one of them. Major problems have occurred when hospital admissions personnel failed to recognize the condition for what it was, or when the line was simply too long. In 2008, a 62-year-old Canadian woman reportedly died of necrotizing fasciitis at a hospital, after waiting 21 hours for a doctor to examine her. (Similar problems have also occurred at hospitals in the United States and Great Britain.) As hospitals become more crowded and understaffed, and more people try to doctor themselves at home, deaths related to necrotizing fasciitis may increase. Fortunately, as we said, this condition is rare.

Not even a health scare as gruesome as flesh-eating bacteria is immune to the forces of urban legend. In 1999, email recipients around the world were treated to the following warning:

> Several shipments of bananas from Costa Rica have been infected with necrotizing fasciitis, otherwise known as flesh-eating bacteria. Recently this disease has decimated the monkey population in Costa Rica.[1]

The rest of the message was not at all funny, because it instructed people to burn their skin if they developed symptoms of infection. In fact, the city of Cartago, Costa Rica had an outbreak of necrotizing fasciitis in the summer of 1999, but there was no known link to bananas or monkeys. At one time, this rumor got so far out of hand that the U.S. Centers for Disease Control and Prevention (CDC) set up a dedicated banana hotline.

WHAT WENT WRONG?

Media accounts generally focus on the swift, unpredictable, and ugly way in which this disease can kill or maim. But the real problem with antibiotic-resistant bacteria is the death and disability they cause by multiple routes, not how ugly and scary they look in the process, or how many tabloid newspapers they sell. All the publicity about "flesh-eating bacteria" may have missed the mark, because these deaths represent only a small fraction of the millions of deaths related to resistant bacteria in general. Thus, while the NF scare fizzled, the bugs were fruitful and continued to multiply.

It may never be possible to eliminate necrotizing fasciitis from the world, because it existed long before antibiotics were invented. A good start, however, might be to reduce antibiotic use and also improve hospital sanitation procedures. Studies in Norway, Finland, and elsewhere have shown that the first objective is achievable, if only physicians can resist their patients' demands for unneeded antibiotics. Some hospitals have also succeeded in reducing their populations of MRSA (methicillin-resistant *Staphylococcus aureus*) and other resistant bacteria, given sufficient funds and motivation.

The Group A *Streptococcus* bacteria that cause necrotizing fasciitis are among the worst in the world, from a human perspective. At various times in history, these same bacteria caused epidemics of scarlet fever and rheumatic fever that took the lives of many children. The strains that cause those two diseases appear to have subsided for the time being, but if they ever return, we would like to be waiting with effective weapons.

NOTE

1. Author's in-box (2000) and Snopes.com Web site.

REFERENCES AND RECOMMENDED READING

Bartlett, J. G. "Methicillin-Resistant *Staphylococcus aureus* Infections." *Topics in HIV Medicine*, Vol. 16, 2008, pp. 151–155.

Bassetti, M., et al. "Why Is Community-Associated MRSA Spreading Across the World?" *International Journal of Antimicrobial Agents*, Vol. 34 (Suppl. 1), 2009, pp. S15–S19.

Baurienne, H. "Sur une Plaie Contuse qui s'est Terminée par le Sphacèle de Tout le Scrotum." *Journal de Médecine, de Chirurgie et de la Pharmacie*, Vol. 20, 1764, pp. 251–256.

Bellapianta, J. M., et al. "Necrotizing Fasciitis." *Journal of the American Academy of Orthopaedic Surgeons*, Vol. 17, 2009, pp. 174–182.

Berger, J. "Yellow Journalism." *Family Practice News*, 1 May 2000.

Bross, M. H., et al. "*Vibrio vulnificus* Infection: Diagnosis and Treatment." *American Family Physician*, Vol. 76, 2007, pp. 539–544.

Caher, J. "Suit in 'Flesh Eating Bacteria' Case Settled for $2.5 million." *Albany Times Union*, 21 July 1994.

Cheung, J. P., et al. "A Review of Necrotizing Fasciitis in the Extremities." *Hong Kong Medical Journal*, Vol. 15, 2009, pp. 44–52.

Hewitt, B. "A Common Germ Turns Deadly." *People Weekly*, 13 June 1994.

Kotrappa, K. S., et al. "Necrotizing Fasciitis." *American Family Physician*, Vol. 53, 1996, pp. 1691–1697.

Lemonick, M. D. "Streptomania Hits Home." *Time*, 20 June 1994.

Livaoğlu, M., et al. "Necrotizing Fasciitis with *Ruminococcus*." *Journal of Medical Microbiology*, Vol. 57, 2008, pp. 246–248.

Medina Polo, J., et al. "Gangrena de Fournier: Estudio de los Factores Pronósticos en 90 Pacientes." *Actas Urológicas Españolas*, Vol. 32, 2008, pp. 1024–1030.

Mendoza, M., and M. Mason. "Killer Superbug Solution Discovered in Norway." Associated Press, 31 December 2009.

Monaghan, S. F., et al. "Necrotizing Fasciitis and Sepsis Caused by *Aeromonas hydrophila* after Crush Injury of the Lower Extremity." *Surgical Infections*, Vol. 9, 2008, pp. 459–467.

Rehm, S. J. "*Staphylococcus aureus*: The New Adventures of a Legendary Pathogen." *Cleveland Clinic Journal of Medicine*, Vol. 75, 2008, pp. 177–180, 183–186, 190–192.

Sarani, B., et al. "Necrotizing Fasciitis: Current Concepts and Review of the Literature." *Journal of the American College of Surgeons*, Vol. 208, 2009, pp. 279–288.

Stout, D. "The Strep Danger: A Need for Vigilance, Not Panic." *New York Times*, 5 April 1995.

Ungar, S. "Hot Crises and Media Reassurance: A Comparison of Emerging Diseases and Ebola Zaire." *British Journal of Sociology*, Vol. 49, 1998, pp. 36–56.

Wilson, B. "Necrotizing Fasciitis." *American Surgeon*, Vol. 18, 1952, pp. 416–431.

Yamashiro, E., et al. "Necrotizing Fasciitis Caused by *Streptococcus pneumoniae*." *Journal of Dermatology*, Vol. 36, 2009, pp. 298–305.

12

Monkeypox 2003

Nature is often hidden; sometimes overcome; seldom extinguished.

—Francis Bacon, *Essays* (1597)

SUMMARY

Monkeypox is an African viral disease that can infect rodents, rabbits, monkeys, and humans. The disease is closely related to smallpox, but it is less infectious and less often fatal. A 2003 monkeypox outbreak among humans in the United States caused short-lived public concern, but there were no known deaths, and the event never erupted into a full-fledged health scare. Appropriate public health measures contained the outbreak, and restrictions on the import of African rodents reduced the probability of future outbreaks. We include this example mainly as proof that the story arc of a health scare is hard to predict. An exotic, potentially deadly, smallpox-like disease infected somewhere between 71 and 94 people in America's heartland, yet the media barely blinked, and the scare fizzled quickly.

SOURCE

In June 2003, the U.S. Centers for Disease Control and Prevention (CDC) investigated an outbreak of an exotic disease called monkeypox in several U.S. states. Sources do not agree as to the exact number of cases. The most widely cited total, originally published on the Medscape Web site, stands at 93 cases: 44 in Wisconsin, 24 in Indiana, 19 in Illinois, 4 in Ohio, and 1 each in Kansas, Missouri, and New Jersey (but these numbers add up to 94). The CDC itself reported 71 human cases as of July 2003. Whichever total is correct, most of the patients reported contact with pet black-tailed prairie dogs (*Cynomys ludovicianus*), which had caught the disease at a pet shop from imported African rodents called Gambian pouched rats (*Cricetomys gambianus*). Fortunately, doctors in the affected states reported the disease to CDC as required by law, and CDC made a thorough investigation. To this day, the official CDC fact sheet on monkeypox states that "several" Americans caught the disease in 2003. Even the name of the virus—monkeypox—probably helped alleviate panic, because it sounds vaguely silly, although the disease itself is serious. As a result, both the outbreak and the potential for media frenzy were nonstarters.

SCIENCE

Although an intensive public health campaign successfully eradicated smallpox (variola) from the world in 1978, closely related poxviruses still exist in wild and domestic animal populations, causing diseases with names such as cowpox, buffalopox, raccoonpox, and camelpox. Some of these diseases, including monkeypox, may also pose a threat to humans. Smallpox itself, like other human diseases, was most likely an animal disease at one time. According to one study, smallpox probably evolved thousands of years ago from a viral disease of African rodents. Since viruses are known to change over time, monkeypox and its relatives bear watching.

Despite its common name, monkeypox is not primarily a disease of monkeys; wild squirrels and other rodents serve as the main reservoir. Most human outbreaks to date have occurred in central Africa. Human monkeypox causes a rash similar to that of chickenpox (varicella) or a relatively mild case of smallpox, with raised pus-filled bumps covering part or all of the body. Some authoritative sources state that it is impossible to distinguish among these three diseases without laboratory testing, whereas others state that they are easy to distinguish. In fact, nobody expects to see smallpox in the present era, and chickenpox is rare in adults, so the diagnosis may default to monkeypox. The doctor who identified the first 2003 monkeypox case at a Wisconsin clinic stated that the patient had fewer lesions than chickenpox typically causes, and that she was not as sick as a smallpox patient. Also, monkeypox is more likely than the other two diseases to cause swollen lymph nodes. Other symptoms of monkeypox usually include eye irritation, fever, headache, muscle pain, chills, sweats, and sometimes a dry cough. The incubation period is usually 10 to 12 days.

The death rate for monkeypox in Africa appears to be about 15 percent for children, but only 1 to 10 percent for adults. These numbers prove that monkeypox is a dangerous disease, but not as bad as smallpox, which was fatal in about 20 to 25 percent of untreated patients. The death rate for monkeypox in the United States might be lower than in Africa, should it ever become established here, because many people are better nourished and have access to better medical care. In the 2003 U.S. monkeypox outbreak, there were no reported deaths. Also, the smallpox vaccine—of which the United States now has a large supply (see Chapter 10)—is about 85 percent effective in preventing the closely related monkeypox. Some antiviral drugs are also helpful in severe cases.

Monkeypox spreads by contact with body fluids or by airborne droplet transmission. Some doctors have speculated that the virus might someday move rapidly from person to person, migrate out of Africa, and cause worldwide epidemics, as smallpox did in earlier centuries. Recent studies suggest that this outcome is unlikely, because the secondary attack rate for monkeypox—the odds of catching the disease from an infected person—appears to be only about 9 percent for monkeypox, as opposed to 25 to 40 percent for smallpox. Only one or two cases in the 2003 monkeypox outbreak were known to result from transmission between humans. In other words, monkeypox is much harder to catch than smallpox.

HISTORY

Informal descriptions of a pox-like disease of African monkeys appeared in the veterinary literature as early as 1861. Scientists first discovered the monkeypox virus in 1958, in laboratory monkeys called crab-eating macaques (*Macaca fascicularis*), the same species that caused the 1989 Ebola Reston outbreak (Chapter 9). Monkeypox was not known to infect humans until 1970, when an outbreak occurred in Zaire (now called the Democratic Republic of the Congo). Several hundred more cases of human monkeypox occurred during the 1970s and 1980s, but the Western press paid little attention at the time. There were no prolonged epidemics, only short-lived outbreaks and sporadic cases, mostly in children who caught the disease while skinning infected animals caught in the forest.

In 1996, however, civil unrest in the Congo forced more people to hunt wild animals for food. New outbreaks of monkeypox occurred, and health officials noted that most of these cases were transmitted directly from one person to another. This new characteristic of the disease raised some concern about future outbreaks, and in fact monkeypox has continued to spread in Africa. Ironically, the conquest of smallpox has contributed to this trend. As noted earlier, the smallpox vaccine also protects against monkeypox; as a result, after the Democratic Republic of the Congo discontinued its smallpox vaccination program in 1980, confirmed monkeypox cases in that country increased 20-fold.

At the time this book was written, there had been no official reports of human monkeypox outside Africa since 2003, but the global demand for exotic pets may favor the spread of this disease. Accurate diagnosis has sometimes been a problem; one suspected monkeypox outbreak in 2007 turned out to be chickenpox, and the reverse error might happen on occasion.

CONSEQUENCES

Medical researchers have studied monkeypox since the 1970s, but it is probably fair to say that this 2003 outbreak in a developed nation has focused global attention on the disease. Although most sources do not regard monkeypox as a potential biological weapon, it clearly qualifies as an emerging human disease, and thus worthy of study. The results have included new vaccines and other promising discoveries.

The 2003 outbreak has also contributed an interesting footnote to the smallpox vaccination controversy. Since the monkeypox and smallpox viruses are closely related, a person who survives one will most likely gain lifelong immunity to the other. So if monkeypox is not dangerous (at least to well-nourished adults), and if the return of smallpox is as likely as a recent administration believed, then why not simply import some more sick rats and expose the entire U.S. population to a mild strain of monkeypox? Such a program would not only create a market for African rodents and benefit the exotic pet industry, but would also avoid the enormous cost and perceived risks associated with smallpox vaccination. By contrast with that artificial process, being bitten by a Gambian pouched rat or dormouse is an entirely natural experience that should meet the requirements of anti-vaccination crusaders.

Of course, we are joking—but something quite similar happened centuries ago in England, when milkmaids realized they were immune to smallpox (Chapter 10) because their work on dairy farms exposed them to a related but milder disease called cowpox. A derivative of the cowpox virus, first used in 1796 to induce immunity in people other than milkmaids, was called vaccinia—the source of today's smallpox vaccine, and the more general term vaccination, a medical breakthrough that has transformed public health. Alas, obstacles to such a plan in today's world include the fact that rat bites (like cow udders and dirty needles) can also transmit other diseases. Also, wild viruses are not subject to quality control measures, and like all living things they can mutate into more or less lethal forms.

WHAT WENT WRONG?

It might seem strange that the monkeypox outbreak of 2003 caused no obvious panic, although it came at a time when the threat of bioterrorism was near the top of the list of public priorities, thanks to the highly publicized smallpox vaccine controversy and the apparently unrelated anthrax mailings of 2001. A 2003 Gallup poll showed that 15 percent of Americans ranked bioterror agents (as a group) as the disease they feared most; only cancer came in higher, at 16 percent.[1] Yet the media in 2003 barely mentioned the usual suspects—terrorists—as the potential source of this unexpected outbreak of monkeypox, an exotic smallpox-like disease in America's heartland. Instead, the culprits were identified as sick rodents, and that was the end of it.

Inevitably, the 2003 outbreak caused some confusion and controversy. For example, the results of a mathematical simulation showed that a human monkeypox outbreak is unlikely to last longer than 14 generations. Some readers found this prospect alarming, because 14 human generations (assuming an average generation time of 25 years) meant the outbreak would last 350 years! Of course, the study was not referring to human generations; it meant generations of viral transmission. In this context, when Person A transmits the virus to Person B, that is one generation.

We admit to some puzzlement regarding the disease outbreaks that cause the greatest media flap. If the monkeypox outbreak had resulted in some deaths, might the public reaction have been different? Or is death a sufficient criterion for panic? As also noted in the Introduction, three California women died in 1999–2000 from an acute viral hemorrhagic fever that was traced to a little-known arenavirus. Related viruses include the agent of Lassa fever and other Category A bioterror agents, and the incident was never adequately explained. Yet media coverage was limited to a couple of short press releases, and no health scare resulted on that occasion either. Go figure.

NOTE

1. Gallup Organization (survey GO 138154).

REFERENCES AND RECOMMENDED READING

Abrahams, B. C., and D. M. Kaufman. "Anticipating Smallpox and Monkeypox Outbreaks: Complications of the Smallpox Vaccine." *Neurologist*, Vol. 10, 2004, pp. 265–274.

Altman, L. K. "Smallpox Vaccinations are Urged and Prairie Dogs are Banned to Halt Monkeypox." *New York Times*, 12 June 2003.

Altman, L. K. "Patient May Have Transmitted Monkeypox." *New York Times*, 13 June 2003.

Bartlett, J. "Monkeypox Review." *Medscape Today*, 15 July 2003.

Breman, J. G., and D. A. Henderson. "Poxvirus Dilemmas—Monkeypox, Smallpox, and Biologic Terrorism." *New England Journal of Medicine*, Vol. 339, 1998, pp. 556–559.

Carmichael, M. "The Prairie Dog Problem." *Newsweek*, 23 June 2003.

Chastel, C. "Human Monkeypox." *Pathologie-Biologie*, Vol. 57, 2009, pp. 175–185. [French]

Croft, D. R., et al. "Occupational Risk During a Monkeypox Outbreak, Wisconsin, 2003." *Emerging Infectious Diseases*, Vol. 13, 2007, pp. 1150–1157.

Di Giulio, D. B., and P. B. Eckburg. "Human Monkeypox: An Emerging Zoonosis." *Lancet Infectious Diseases*, Vol. 4, 2004, pp. 15–25.

Dubois, M. E., and M. K. Slifka. "Retrospective Analysis of Monkeypox Infection." *Emerging Infectious Diseases*, Vol. 14, 2008, pp. 592–599.

Essbauer, S., et al. "Zoonotic Poxviruses." Veterinary Microbiology, 26 August 2009.

Foster, S. O., et al. "Human Monkeypox." *Bulletin of the World Health Organization*, Vol. 46, 1972, pp. 569–576.

Guarner, J., et al. "Monkeypox Transmission and Pathogenesis in Prairie Dogs." *Emerging Infectious Diseases*, March 2004.

Hutson, C. L. "Monkeypox Zoonotic Associations: Insights from Laboratory Evaluation of Animals Associated with the Multi-State US Outbreak." *American Journal of Tropical Medicine and Hygiene*, Vol. 76, 2007, pp. 757–767.

Jezek, Z., et al. "Human Monkeypox." *Journal of Hygiene, Epidemiology, Microbiology, and Immunology*, Vol. 27, 1983, pp. 13–28.

Li, Y., et al. "On the Origin of Smallpox: Correlating Variola Phylogenetics with Historical Smallpox Records." *Proceedings of the National Academy of Sciences*, Vol. 104, 2007, pp. 15787–15792.

Ligon, B. L. "Monkeypox: A Review of the History and Emergence in the Western Hemisphere." *Seminars in Pediatric Infectious Diseases*, Vol. 15, 2004, pp. 280–287.

Moussatché, N., et al. "When Good Vaccines Go Wild: Feral Orthopoxvirus in Developing Countries and Beyond." *Journal of Infection in Developing Countries*, Vol. 2, 2008, pp. 156–173.

Nalca, A., et al. "Reemergence of Monkeypox: Prevalence, Diagnostics, and Countermeasures." *Clinical Infectious Diseases*, Vol. 41, 2005, pp. 1765–1771.

Parker, S., et al. "Human Monkeypox: An Emerging Zoonotic Disease." *Future Microbiology*, Vol. 2, 2007, pp. 17–34.

"Rare Virus May Have Caused Three Deaths in California." Associated Press, 4 August 2000.

Reed, K. D. "Monkeypox, Marshfield Clinic and the Internet: Leveraging Information Technology for Public Health." *Clinical Medicine and Research*, Vol. 2, 2004, pp. 1–3.

Rimoin, A., et al. "Major Increase in Human Monkeypox Incidence 30 Years after Smallpox Vaccination Campaigns Cease in the Democratic Republic of Congo." *Proceedings of the National Academy of Sciences U.S.A.*, 14 September 2010.

Sale, T. A., et al. "Monkeypox: An Epidemiologic and Clinical Comparison of African and U.S. Disease." *Journal of the American Academy of Dermatology*, Vol. 55, 2006, pp. 478–481.

U.S. Centers for Disease Control and Prevention. "Update: Multistate Outbreak of Monkeypox—Illinois, Indiana, Kansas, Missouri, Ohio, and Wisconsin, 2003." *Morbidity and Mortality Weekly Report*, 11 July 2003.

Part Three

Food Scares

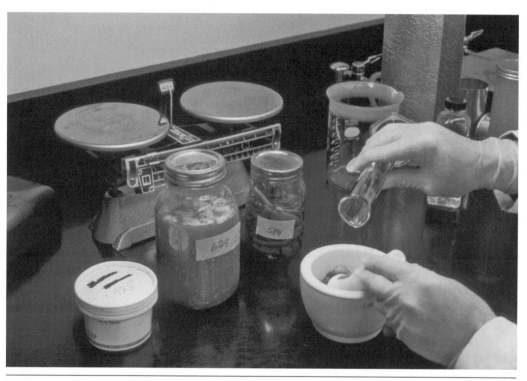

Figure 3   A technician prepares to extract botulin toxin from home-canned food. (*Source:* U.S. Centers for Disease Control and Prevention, Public Health Image Library.)

13

Fear of Canned Food

We may find in the long run that tinned food is a deadlier weapon than the machine-gun.
—George Orwell, *The Road to Wigan Pier* (1937)

SUMMARY

The invention of canned food in the nineteenth century solved some problems and created others. Many otherwise perishable foods could now be stored for long periods of time without refrigeration. Before commercial and home canning procedures were perfected, however, lead and tin poisoning and botulism were very real threats to public health, and many people were afraid of canned food. Improved methods have largely (though not entirely) solved these problems, and most consumers now take the safety of canned goods for granted, despite occasional product recalls and a few outbreaks involving home-canned food. This health scare has largely fizzled, only to be replaced by recent concerns about a plastic material used to line some cans.

SOURCE

The sources of this health scare are real disease outbreaks and product recalls, not rumors or urban legends. Of course, the rumor mill took a good story and made it better, but the underlying problem remained, and the news media made sure everyone heard about it. For example, an 1884 article in the *New York Times* displayed the eye-catching title "Are Canned Goods Poisonous?" The article itself was less inflammatory, claiming only that tainted meat should not be canned—sound advice—and also that manufacturers should be required to stamp cans with the date of sealing. (Nowadays most cans are stamped with the date of expiration, which is not quite the same thing, since the consumer still has no idea how old the contents might be.)

According to historian Gabriella Petrick, the shift to mass production of canned food after the American Civil War also contributed to anxiety about the food supply. In earlier centuries, most people grew their own food or bought it from local farms. Now people in cities had to deal with canned foods of unknown origin, and frequent outbreaks of botulism (Figure 3) and other foodborne diseases resulting from the new process only served to reinforce this anxiety. In fact, boiling food after removing it from the can is usually enough to prevent botulism, but people didn't know that. Also, it is not customary to boil certain foods, such as canned tuna fish.

SCIENCE

The *Free Dictionary* defines canning as "a preservation method in which prepared food is put in glass jars or metal cans that are hermetically sealed to keep out air and then heated to a specific temperature for a specified time to destroy disease-causing microorganisms and prevent spoilage." For some acidic foods, such as canned tomatoes or pineapple, the temperature of boiling water (212°F or 100°C) is usually high enough. For certain other foods with a lower pH, such as green beans or meat, higher temperatures are required to kill bacterial spores. People who can foods at home often use a pressure cooker to achieve the necessary heat.

The term botulism refers to poisoning by a toxin called botulin, which certain bacteria (*Clostridium botulinum*) release when they grow in the absence of oxygen. The interior of a can of food provides ideal growth conditions, if the contents do not become hot enough during preservation to kill all the bacterial spores. Symptoms of botulism, which may appear from six hours to two weeks after exposure, include blurred vision, difficulty swallowing, and muscle weakness, often progressing to paralysis of the muscles used in breathing. Without prompt medical care and respirator support, many patients die. A botulin antitoxin can help block the effects of the toxin if given soon enough.

As of the early twenty-first century, only about 100 cases of botulism are reported in the United States each year, many of them associated with home-canned food. Some infants also contract a form of botulism, usually from eating raw honey containing *Clostridium* spores that an adult's stomach acid would deactivate. Botulin toxin is so powerful that the U.S. government classifies it as a Category A bioterrorism agent. In theory, a small container of this toxin would be enough to kill everyone on Earth. (In practice, of course, delivery would pose logistic problems.)

Another chemical that sometimes contaminates canned food is lead, which was formerly used to seal some metal cans. American manufacturers voluntarily stopped using lead in the canning process in 1991, and the U.S. government banned the practice in 1995. This ban includes imported canned foods, but some foreign manufacturers have continued using lead. For example, a 1994 study of lead poisoning in Mexico City showed that at least one-third of food cans had unacceptably high lead levels, either because the cans had lead-soldered side seams or because the contents were contaminated by soil, air, or water before canning.

At one time in history, food cans were partly made of tin, and many people still refer to metal food containers as "tin cans" and the canning process itself as "tinning." Tin, like lead, is a potentially toxic metal if ingested in sufficiently large doses. Many cans still have a thin layer of tin on the exterior surface to prevent rust, but it does not come in contact with the food inside. In the 1960s, the advertising slogan "Tin cans are mostly made of steel" was intended to reassure consumers on that point.

Recent bad press about canned food has focused on the potential health effects of bisphenol A (BPA), a chemical used in the manufacturer of some plastic beverage containers and in the plastic linings of metal cans. At the time this book was written, this health scare had not yet fizzled and showed every sign of being legitimate. BPA belongs to a class of chemicals known as endocrine disruptors—chemicals that can bind to estrogen receptors and, in sufficiently high doses, may increase the risk of cancer and other health problems. When plastic containers are heated, BPA may leach into the contents. The U.S. Food and Drug Administration first approved BPA for use in food containers in 1963, so it was not subject to review under the Toxic Substances Control Act of 1976. The controversial issue is not whether BPA is an endocrine disruptor, but whether it leaches into foods and beverages at levels high enough to pose a health risk.

HISTORY

French confectioner Nicholas Appert (1749–1841) invented the first successful canning method in 1809. He and other early canners used glass containers, which were heavy and breakable, so manufacturers experimented with various procedures for making metal containers. Canned food was a great convenience for explorers and armies in the field, but sometimes the new invention backfired. For example, lead poisoning from canned food with lead-soldered seams probably killed some members of Sir John Franklin's 1845 Arctic expedition.

The 1847 invention of the stamped can marked a turning point in food preservation, but it also introduced new problems, as discussed above. Another turning point came in 1858 with the invention of the glass Mason jar that is often used for home canning. In 1876, a machine for shaping and soldering cans was exhibited at the Centennial Exposition at Philadelphia. An 1885 newspaper article describes the sealing process as follows:

> After being cooked a sufficient length of time a little puncture is made with an awl in the cover of the can, through which there will be a sudden gush of steam. A drop of solder is then placed over the hole. When withdrawn from the fire and allowed to cool, a partial vacuum is formed by the condensation taking place within, which will cause the end of the can to bend down or in.[1]

Despite major technical improvements to this crude-sounding process during the next century, inadequate heating or leaks still happen on occasion. In 2007, an outbreak of botulism associated with Castleberry brand chili sauce and canned meat products resulted in a massive recall that cost the company an estimated $78 million. The manufacturing plant had recently started using new equipment that apparently did not heat the product long enough or at high enough temperatures. This was the first U.S. botulism outbreak in over 30 years that was traced to commercially canned foods, but sporadic cases have occurred. In 1982, for example, one confirmed case of botulism traced to canned Alaskan salmon resulted in the recall of more than 50 million cans of this product. An investigation determined that the problem resulted from small holes punched in the cans by defective equipment. There was nothing wrong with the fish at the time it was canned, but the incident still dealt a major blow to the salmon industry.

CONSEQUENCES

The historic fear of canned food goes beyond a fear of contamination. When George Orwell wrote his famous statement on the subject (quoted at the beginning of the chapter), he was not talking about botulism, but rather about the less tangible danger inherent in allowing the human population to become dependent on mass-produced, spiritually bankrupt corporate food. How many science-fiction stories have featured millennial gangs of starving wretches who must dive into submerged radioactive cities to retrieve stale-dated canned food, simply because they have no idea how to grind their own grain or pluck a chicken? The efficiency of Big Food has become necessary because there are so many people in the world. But let the machinery falter or the delivery trucks run out of fuel, and the chain of being goes straight to hell.

In our disaster-minded society, it's common knowledge that every household should have enough canned food and bottled water to sustain the occupants for a few days (or weeks or months). But if canned food and plastic bottles of water may contain toxic chemicals, then what? Glass jars and bottles are clean but also heavy, and they break easily in many types of emergencies; that is why metal cans and plastic bottles were invented in the first place. A few manufacturers have profited from these fears by selling extremely expensive food and water in containers that they claim are safe. But how are consumers to verify these claims? Even beef jerky has been found to harbor *Salmonella*, *Listeria*, and other harmful bacteria. Freeze-dried foods are considered relatively safe if rehydrated in water hot enough to kill any surviving bacteria, but boiling water is often inconvenient in emergency situations.

WHAT WENT WRONG?

What went wrong was the human population explosion. Instead of a few million people living on farms and growing their own food or buying it locally, we have several billion people, more than half of them packed into cities and dependent on imported goods. The evolution of food preservation techniques, including canned food, has been a necessary learning process for everyone involved.

For example, until a few years ago, supermarkets sold marked-down food in badly dented cans with the promise that dented cans are just fine. Cheerful magazine articles advised senior citizens on fixed incomes to take advantage of these bargains. Then somebody figured out that denting sometimes caused the seams to open, and this policy was reversed. The same magazines and stores now advise consumers *not* to buy dented canned food.

Glass jars with vacuum-sealed lids have provided another learning experience. Who could have predicted that children playing in supermarkets would remove the lids just to hear them pop, or that their parents might do the same thing to inspect the contents? Safety seals on some products have reduced this problem, but nothing can be made 100 percent safe.

NOTE

1. "Canned Food" (*Newport Mercury*, 28 February 1885).

REFERENCES AND RECOMMENDED READING

"Are Canned Goods Poisonous?" *New York Times*, 20 November 1884.

Biello, D. "Plastic (Not) Fantastic." *Scientific American*, 19 February 2008.

"Canned Goods." *Newport Mercury*, 28 February 1885.

Cengiz, M., et al. "A Botulism Outbreak from Roasted Canned Mushrooms." *Human and Experimental Toxicology*, Vol. 25, 2006, pp. 273–278.

"Connors Bros. Rebuilds after Massive Recall." *Food Institute Report*, 14 April 2008.

Ginsberg, M. M., et al. "Botulism Associated with Commercially Canned Chili Sauce." *Morbidity and Mortality Weekly Report*, Vol. 56, 2007, pp. 767–769.

Hernberg, S. "Lead Poisoning in a Historical Perspective." *American Journal of Industrial Medicine*, Vol. 38, 2000, pp. 244–254.

Kurtzweil, P. "Sixth-Grader Opens Lid for FDA Investigation." *FDA Consumer*, September–October 1997.

Petrick, G. "Feeding the Masses: H. J. Heinz and the Creation of Industrial Food." *Endeavour*, Vol. 33, 2009, pp. 29–34.

Poole, A., et al. "Review of the Toxicology, Human Exposure and Safety Assessment for Bisphenol A Diglycidylether (BADGE)." *Food Additives and Contaminants*, Vol. 21, 2004, pp. 905–919.

Quitmeyer, A., and R. Roberts. "Babies, Bottles, and Bisphenol A: The Story of a Scientist Mother." *PLoS Biology*, 17 July 2007.

Romieu, I., et al. "Sources of Lead Exposure in Mexico City." *Environmental Health Perspectives*, Vol. 102, 1994, pp. 384–389.

"Salmon Scare." *Time*, 3 May 1982.

"Salmon Sales in the Pink Again." *Chain Store Age Supermarkets*, July 1983.

Schmit, J. "Management Problems Cited in Botulism Case." *USA Today*, 30 June 2008.

Scholliers, P. "Defining Food Risks and Food Anxieties Throughout History." *Appetite*, Vol. 51, 2008, pp. 3–6.

Segal, M. "Botulism in the Entire United States." *FDA Consumer*, January–February 1992.

Sekizawa, J. "Low-Dose Effects of Bisphenol A: A Serious Threat to Human Health?" *Journal of Toxicological Sciences*, Vol. 33, 2008, pp. 389–403.

Seltzer, J., et al. "Castleberry's 2007 Botulism Recall: A Case Study by the Food Industry Center." University of Minnesota, August 2008.

Sheehan, D. M. "Activity of Environmentally Relevant Low Doses of Endocrine Disruptors and the Bisphenol A Controversy: Initial Results Confirmed." *Proceedings of the Society for Experimental Biology and Medicine*, Vol. 224, 2000, pp. 57–60.

Smith, D. F. "Food Panics in History: Corned Beef, Typhoid, and 'Risk Society.'" *Journal of Epidemiology and Community Health*, Vol. 61, 2007, pp. 566–570.

Sobel, J., et al. "Foodborne Botulism in the United States, 1990–2000." *Emerging Infectious Diseases*, Vol. 10, 2004, pp. 1606–1611.

Summerfield, W., et al. "Survey of Bisphenol A Diglycidyl Ether (BADGE) in Canned Foods." *Food Additives and Contaminants*, Vol. 15, 1998, pp. 818–830.

vom Saal, F. S., and C. Hughes. "An Extensive New Literature Concerning Low-Dose Effects of Bisphenol A Shows the Need for a New Risk Assessment." *Environmental Health Perspectives*, Vol. 113, 2005, pp. 926–933.

Weber, H. A. "On the Occurrence of Tin in Canned Food." *Scientific American Supplement*, 21 November 1891.

14

Potatoes and Birth Defects

Beware lest you lose the substance by grasping at the shadow.

—Aesop, *The Dog and the Shadow* (circa 550 B.C.)

SUMMARY

During the second half of the twentieth century, there was a widespread belief that exposure of the human fetus to late blight, a common fungus-like organism that infests potato plants, could cause spina bifida and other major birth defects involving the brain and spinal cord. As a result, pregnant women were advised not to eat or handle any damaged-looking potatoes. As it turned out, certain dietary deficiencies may increase the risk of these birth defects, but potatoes and potato blight do not appear to be directly involved. Although the causal relationship was largely discredited by the mid-1970s, related fears persist in the form of urban legends, such as the notion that pregnant women should not boil potatoes. As recently as 2009, a popular nutrition Web site advised pregnant women that spina bifida could result from exposure to green potatoes—citing the outdated studies about late blight, which is not even the same thing. (But nothing can be absolutely disproven, and people are still responsible for their own decisions, so we are not advising anyone to eat potatoes or any other food.)

SOURCE

According to two sources, a researcher named Guzman was the first to point out a possible link between potato blight and birth defects, in a paper published in a Mexican journal in 1969. We have been unable to find that paper, but the idea next surfaced in 1972, in the first of a series of papers published by British geneticist James Harrison Renwick (1926–1994), who believed it was possible to prevent 95 percent of neural tube defects just by avoiding potatoes. His papers cited both epidemiologic studies and animal experiments, and made an impressive case for the hypothesis.

There was no reason for other doctors or consumers to doubt the veracity of these findings, and it is best to err on the side of caution whenever the safety of unborn children may be at stake. As recently as 2002, a reprint edition of a 1988 textbook contained the following warning:

> Pregnant women have been warned recently by American press and a well-known British geneticist against the use of blighted potatoes. Such potatoes might cause serious birth defects like incomplete development of the spinal cord of the foetus. They have also been advised (i) not to peel potatoes without wearing gloves; (ii) not to inhale the steam of boiling potatoes, (iii) and not to use decayed, discoloured or bruised potatoes.[1]

This was not crackpot advice by any means; Dr. Renwick was an eminent scientist who based his conclusions on the best data available in the early 1970s. Within the next few years, however, other researchers determined that the earlier studies suffered from experimental design problems, and that there was no clear evidence that either potatoes or late blight was associated with human birth defects. In 1975, the *British Medical Journal* published an editorial with the self-explanatory title "End of the Potato Avoidance Hypothesis." Essentially, it said that the evidence was inconclusive and that the cited studies were not repeatable. But it was not the end for everyone, and occasional worrisome studies have continued to appear in the medical literature.

SCIENCE

Late blight is a fungus-like organism (an oömycete) called *Phytophthora infestans*, which literally means "devastating plant destroyer." This plant disease lived up to its name in the 1840s by destroying most of the Irish potato crop, causing a famine that killed about one million people and forced another million to emigrate. By requiring farmers to use high levels of fungicides, late blight also makes potato farming expensive and drives up prices. The disease now costs the potato industry an estimated $3 billion per year ($300 million per year in the United States alone), plus $100 to $200 per acre for fungicide treatment. Late blight is arguably the worst crop disease in the world, infecting potato crops in cool, humid regions of every continent. It also attacks other crops, such as tomatoes and peppers.

Late blight was already quite bad enough, in other words, when it came under suspicion for another reason. Some doctors thought exposure to late blight, or to the potato crops it infected, might damage the human fetus, causing neural tube defects—malformations involving the brain or spinal cord, such as anencephaly (absence of all or part of the brain) or spina bifida. These conditions were more common in Ireland than elsewhere in the world, and it was perhaps natural to think of potatoes.

No one really knows what causes spina bifida, but dietary deficiencies as well as genetic factors appear to be involved. Most doctors now advise pregnant or soon-to-be pregnant women to take a folic acid supplement. As usual, there is a tradeoff: a 2004 study shows that high levels of folic acid may increase the mother's risk for breast cancer while protecting the fetus from spina bifida. Other studies have suggested that dietary zinc deficiency may play a role in some of these birth defects, and that blight may contribute indirectly by reducing the zinc content of potatoes.

HISTORY

Long after the Irish famine ended and potatoes ceased to represent the food of poverty, some people suspected that evil still lurked in the fields. The Scots reportedly never trusted potatoes because the Bible did not mention them, and the English disliked potatoes because of their association with the Irish. Potatoes were blamed for flatulence and poor work habits.

Next, blighted potatoes were said to be dangerous because of toxins released by the blight, or from the potatoes' efforts to defend themselves against blight by producing toxins of their own. Then suspicion fell on any potatoes, blighted or otherwise. That fear merged with the unrelated fear of green spots on potatoes—parts of the potato that contain solanine, which can make people sick if ingested in large quantities. Then it was suddenly dangerous for a pregnant woman even to peel potatoes, or inhale the steam from boiling potatoes, much less to eat them.

The proposed link between late blight and birth defects came as bad news to the potato industry, because late blight exists wherever potatoes grow. In 1971, the Idaho Potato Commission reportedly funded a related study by St. Luke's Presbyterian Hospital in Chicago, and also established a research laboratory in Idaho for the same purpose. In 2004, when several industries noted that low-carb diets could promote spina bifida by reducing dietary intake of folic acid, the Idaho Potato Commission again came to the rescue, this time with a plan to promote the nutritional value of potatoes.

In reviewing the history of this health scare, we noticed a familiar pattern—the gradual transformation of a specific evildoer to a more general evildoer, to a whole group of evildoers, and finally to a powerful friend. The same thing happened with tomatoes, for example, which were first considered poisonous, and now are said to cure everything (Chapter 16); and with alcohol, which was the demon rum for centuries, until somebody decided that it might prevent heart disease (Chapter 47). Nobody likes late blight, of course, but the popular image of potatoes has steadily risen, culminating in the United Nations International Year of the Potato in 2008. In 2009, this health scare appears to be fizzling at last. Some Web sites even promote the belief that inhaling the steam from boiling potatoes can relieve asthma.

CONSEQUENCES

Dr. Renwick's 1972 warning about potatoes did no harm, except to the extent that it might have compounded the guilt trip that already consumes many expectant mothers. If the child has a birth defect, might she have somehow caused it by eating, doing, or thinking the wrong thing? Suddenly, even McDonald's french fries were suspect.

In nineteenth-century Ireland, it was hard for pregnant women to avoid potatoes, for the simple reason that other foods were scarce. In most modern societies, however, a more diverse diet is available, and there is no urgent reason to overcome this health scare. If a woman wishes to be extra careful, she can stop buying potatoes for nine months (or for a lifetime) without major inconvenience.

But we should not dismiss the potato scare out of hand, because ongoing studies suggest that the answer is not quite so simple. For example, Chinese researchers in 1993 reported that solanine or other glycoalkaloid chemicals found in potato sprouts caused neural tube defects in mouse embryos. This finding, if confirmed, would implicate the potato itself rather than late blight, except in the sense that potatoes may produce toxins to combat the blight. A study of human birth defects in China, published in 2008, showed that eating sprouted potatoes was one of several factors associated with neural tube defects. Related studies are ongoing.

WHAT WENT WRONG?

In this case, we would say that nothing went wrong. Some fairly convincing data suggested that potatoes, or blighted potatoes, might be harming unborn children. It would have been irresponsible for doctors to keep this suspicion to themselves, or for pregnant women to ignore the warning.

To the extent that there was a problem, it was a common one known as statistical confounding. In other words, people who are exposed to blighted potatoes are also exposed to many other things, such as poverty and famine in some eras and pesticides and plastics in others, plus a host of cultural practices and genetic factors. It can be hard to sort out these factors, or to get people to report them accurately. Also, there is the basic CYA principle. Nobody, including authors and publishers, will come right out and say: "It's safe, go ahead and eat it." Nothing in life is entirely safe, and we will continue to watch the biomedical literature for the latest findings on potatoes.

NOTE

1. O. P. Sharma, *Textbook of Fungi* (McGraw-Hill, 1988, p. 95).

REFERENCES AND RECOMMENDED READING

Allen, J. R., et al. "Teratogenicity Studies on Late Blighted Potatoes in Nonhuman Primates (*Macaca mulatta* and *Saguinus labiatus*)." *Teratology*, Vol. 15, 1977, pp. 17–23.

"Blighted Potatoes and Birth Defects." Associated Press, 9 August 1972.

"Blighted Potatoes, Blighted Fetus?" *Canadian Medical Association Journal*, Vol. 107, 1972, p. 1160.

Borman, B., and C. Cryer. "Fallacies of International and National Comparisons of Disease Occurrence in the Epidemiology of Neural Tube Defects." *Teratology*, Vol. 42, 1990, pp. 405–412.

Elwood, J. M. "Anencephalus, Spina Bifida, and Potato Blight in Canada." *Canadian Journal of Public Health*, Vol. 67, 1976, pp. 122–126.

Emanuel, I., and L. E. Sever. "Questions Concerning the Possible Association of Potatoes and Neural-Tube Defects, and an Alternate Hypothesis Relating to Maternal Growth and Development." *Teratology*, Vol. 8, 1973, pp. 325–331.

"End of the Potato Avoidance Hypothesis." *British Medical Journal*, Vol. 4, 1975, pp. 308–309.

Kinlen, L., and A. Hewitt. "Potato Blight and Anencephalus in Scotland." *British Journal of Preventive and Social Medicine*, Vol. 27, 1973, pp. 208–213.

Korpan, Y., et al. "Potato Glycoalkaloids: True Safety or False Sense of Security?" *Trends in Biotechnology*, Vol. 22, 2004, pp. 147–151.

Masterson, J. G., et al. "Anencephaly and Potato Blight in the Republic of Ireland." *British Journal of Preventive and Social Medicine*, Vol. 28, 1974, pp. 81–84.

Nevin, N. C., and J. D. Merrett. "Potato Avoidance During Pregnancy in Women with a Previous Infant with Either Anencephaly and/or Spina Bifida." *British Journal of Preventive and Social Medicine*, Vol. 29, 1975, pp. 111–115.

Nordby, K. -C., et al. "Indicators of Mancozeb Exposure in Relation to Thyroid Cancer and Neural Tube Defects in Farmers' Families." *Scandinavian Journal of Work, Environment, and Health*, Vol. 31, 2005, pp. 89–96.

"Potato Disease, Birth Defects Related?" Associated Press, 30 September 1974.

Renwick, J. H. "Hypothesis: Anencephaly and Spina Bifida are Usually Preventable by Avoidance of a Specific but Unidentified Substance Present in Certain Potato Tubers." *British Journal of Preventive and Social Medicine*, Vol. 26, 1972, pp. 67–88.

Renwick, J. H. "Potato Babies." *Lancet*, 12 August 1972.

Renwick, J. H. "Prevention of Anencephaly and Spina Bifida in Man." *Teratology*, Vol. 8, 1973, pp. 321–323.

Renwick, J. H., et al. "Potatoes and Spina Bifida." *Proceedings of the Royal Society of Medicine*, Vol. 67, 1974, pp. 360–364.

Renwick, J. H., et al. "Neural-Tube Defects Produced in Syrian Hamsters by Potato Glycoalkaloids." *Teratology*, Vol. 30, 1984, pp. 371–381.

Ristaino, J. B. "Tracking Historic Migrations of the Irish Potato Famine Pathogen, *Phytophthora infestans*." *Microbes and Infection*, Vol. 4, 2002, pp. 1369–1377.

Scholliers, P. "Defining Food Risks and Food Anxieties Throughout History." *Appetite*, Vol. 51, 2008, pp. 3–6.

Sever, J. L. "Potatoes and Birth Defects: Summary." *Teratology*, Vol. 8, 1973, pp. 319–320.

Sharma, R. P., et al. "Teratogenic Potential of Blighted Potato Concentrate in Rabbits, Hamsters, and Miniature Swine." *Teratology*, Vol. 18, 1978, pp. 55–61.

Spiers, P. S. "Spina Bifida, Anencephaly, and Potato Blight." *Lancet*, 24 February 1973.

Ulman, C., et al. "Zinc-Deficient Sprouting Blight Potatoes and their Possible Relation with Neural Tube Defects." *Cell Biochemistry and Function*, Vol. 23, 2005, pp. 69–72.

Wang, X. G. "Teratogenic Effect of Potato Glycoalkaloids." *Zhonghua Fu Chan Ke Za Zhi*, Vol. 28, 1993, pp. 73–75, 121–122. [In Chinese]

15

Fear of Oleomargarine

Flavor so good I feel like a queen!

—Imperial Margarine Commercial (1957)

It's not nice to fool Mother Nature.

—Chiffon Margarine Commercial (1972)

You call it corn, we call it maize.

—Mazola Margarine Commercial (1976)

SUMMARY

Margarine has outsold genuine butter in most industrialized nations since the 1950s, and the great oleomargarine wars of the past are all but forgotten. Yet an older generation remembers the days when state and federal laws required margarine sold in stores to be white or pink, to avoid the illusion that it was butter, and consumers had to add a tablet or stir in a little packet of orange goop to make the margarine turn yellow. The dairy industry fought long and hard to retain its market share, and yellow journalism earned its name. For a time, popular opinion shifted in the direction of margarine, both because of its lower cost and because it is made from "natural" vegetable oil. More recently the scales have tipped in favor of butter, which is made from equally "natural" cow's milk. In the end, yellow fats are just yellow fats, humans are omnivores, and the longstanding fear of margarine has largely fizzled, except in the form of occasional anti-margarine blogs published by butter advocates.

SOURCE

As soon as manufacturers began to sell oleomargarine as a cheaper substitute for butter, the dairy industry knew it was in trouble and made sure consumers heard about it. An 1884 *New York Times* article described how the availability of yellow margarine drove down the price of butter—not because margarine served the same purpose at lower cost, but because margarine labeled as butter allegedly made people sick, thus reducing consumer confidence in any yellow fat product.[1] In 1911, the same newspaper brought audiences the inside story of "butter moonshining," a sinister practice in which "thousands of tubs, unstamped by the revenue collectors, have been filled with a substance colored to the golden tint of fresh butter."[2] Although more profound contemporary issues have replaced yellow fats as objects of global paranoia, editorials on the relative merits of butter and margarine have continued to the present day.

SCIENCE

Chemically, margarine is a mixture of vegetable oil or animal fat with skimmed milk or buttermilk and water, plus other ingredients such as food coloring, salt, emulsifiers (chemicals to disperse the oil droplets in water), and vitamins A and D.

Chemists classify fats or lipids in several ways. Those that are liquid at room temperature are usually called oils, and most of today's margarines contain vegetable oils rather than solid animal fats. The oils most commonly used in margarines are corn, safflower, sunflower, soybean, cottonseed, rapeseed, and olive oil. Margarine ingredients are further classified by the types of fat molecules that they contain. Beef fat and lard, for example, are high in saturated fat, whereas olive oil is high in monounsaturated fat, and soybean oil is an example of a product that is high in polyunsaturated fat. These terms refer to the number of double bonds in the molecule. Vegetable oils can also be partially hydrogenated in the laboratory so that their melting point is higher.

Until recently, most margarine commercials focused on the polyunsaturated fat content of their products, but studies in the past decade have shown that another fat characteristic might have a greater health impact. Nearly everyone has heard of trans fat, which is a type of saturated fat with a specific molecular structure called a transisomer fatty acid. Other saturated fats have cis-isomer fatty acids and are known as cis fats. It is unclear why trans fats tend to cause health problems, and there is even some evidence that they don't, as discussed below.

The first margarines were made partly from beef fat and other animal products, and they do not sound particularly appetizing. An 1880 *New York Times* article describes how margarine was produced in large tanks of caul fat—in other words, the fatty membrane that surrounds the internal organs—reassuringly described as "the cleanest and least fibrous part of the cow."[3] In these tanks, the oil and tallow separated, and the oil was combined with milk to make margarine, while the tallow became the world's worst-smelling candles.

Contrary to popular opinion, margarine was scarcely more heart-healthy than dairy butter until the late 1990s, when margarine manufacturers started removing trans fats and other objectionable compounds from their products. As a result, studies of the effects of margarine consumption can be hard to interpret. For example, a 2009 study showed that children born in the 1990s and later who ate margarine every day had lower IQs by three points than those who did not. Horrors! In fact, diets high in trans fats have been linked to memory problems in animal experiments, and until recently most margarines contained up to 17 percent trans fats. But intelligence testing is far from an exact science, and even the brightest people probably have a hard time remembering how much margarine they ate years ago. A difference as small as three IQ points means essentially nothing. Similarly, a study published in 2003 showed that women who ate margarine had a higher risk of heart disease than those who ate butter. Again, however, most people use both products in various proportions, and the formulation of margarine has changed over the years.

According to an even more surprising research paper published in 2010, dietary intake of high levels of saturated fat was *not* related to risk of coronary heart disease, stroke, or cardiovascular disease in a meta-analysis (literature review) of previously published studies. If verified, this finding turns several decades of conventional wisdom on its ear, and it renders the margarine-butter debate largely moot. The study was partly funded by the National Dairy Council and Unilever, historical opponents in the oleo war.

HISTORY

In 1813, French chemist Michel-Eugène Chevreul (1786–1889) isolated a new fatty acid that formed lustrous pearl-like drops. He named it margaric acid, from the Greek word *margaritēs*, meaning pearl. In the late 1860s, another French chemist named Hippolyte Mège-Mouriés (1817–1880) combined this chemical with beef fat, milk, and salt water to create margarine as a butter substitute in the late 1860s. According to one story, French President Napoleon III (1808–1873) had offered a prize for the best butter substitute, and this new product was the winner. A few years later, a corporate ancestor of today's Unilever started producing margarine in Europe, and several American companies followed suit.

By the mid-1880s, what might be called yellow backlash was in full swing, with several states prohibiting the manufacture or sale of yellow margarine and the federal government imposing stiff taxes to discourage competition with butter. During the first four decades of the twentieth century, things looked bad for margarine, until improved advertising and wartime butter shortages turned the tide. Many of today's familiar margarine brands existed by 1950. By 1951, stores could legally sell yellow margarine. In 1967, Wisconsin became the last state to repeal its laws restricting the sale of margarine.

Recent trends in margarine and butter consumption are complex enough to fill a much longer chapter. Many people now use both products. For example, in 2002, about 70 percent of United Kingdom residents ate butter, but by 2004 this statistic had declined to 55 percent. However, butter's actual share of the UK yellow fats market increased from 39 percent in 2002 to 43 percent in 2004. In the United States, the dollar value of butter and margarine sales was about equal in 2004; but since butter is more expensive, margarine sales accounted for 2 ½ times the volume of butter. This is great stuff, but our point is that consumers have clearly overcome the historic fear of margarine.

Health scares often generate urban legends, and the great oleo war was no exception. According to one such story, margarine—like several other politically incorrect, highly processed foods—is chemically very similar to plastic. Another story claims that margarine was originally invented as a feed supplement to fatten turkeys. Both stories appear to be false.

CONSEQUENCES

Margarine is dangerous under specific circumstances—for example, if you smear it on the soles of your shoes. Earlier forms of margarine were not as healthy as they might have been, before their reformulation to eliminate trans fats. Otherwise, margarine is just another yellow fat, seemingly unworthy of the century-long debate it has inspired.

Some people prefer the taste of butter, whereas others prefer margarine. Margarine in its modern form is probably better for your arteries; butter has a texture that probably makes better cookies. And then there are the philosophical arguments. On the one hand, margarine is more natural than butter, in the sense that it is a derivative of vegetable oil. Vegetables served as food for primordial humans, but bovine milk probably did not. On the other hand, butter is more natural (or at least more traditional) than margarine, in the sense that it appeared on the menu at an earlier stage in human history. But what possible difference does it make?

Rhetoric aside, margarine and butter are both highly unnatural, in the sense that they are both extracted from natural materials using sophisticated equipment and stringent quality control measures. They do not ooze from trees or scamper through the woods. Of course, it is possible to make butter in a wooden churn instead of a Space Age laboratory, but the end product is the same, possibly with a few splinters.

WHAT WENT WRONG?

The argument could be made that nothing went wrong. Sellers of competing products will always say bad things about each other, and the oleo wars served to showcase all that is best and worst about the free enterprise system. As in any war, the real victims were mostly innocent bystanders—in this case, consumers, who were left to sort out a host of contradictory claims about these products while government agencies and industry lobbyists traded salvos.

NOTES

1. "Butter and Milk Cheap" (*New York Times*, 6 August 1884).
2. "The Butter Moonshiners" (*New York Times*, 23 July 1911).
3. "Oleomargarine: Congressmen Shown How the Article is Manufactured" (*New York Times*, 22 March 1880).

REFERENCES AND RECOMMENDED READING

Barnard, H. E. "Effect of Food Control on the Food Supply." *American Journal of Public Health*, Vol. 9, 1919, pp. 203–206.

"Butter and Milk Cheap: Effect of the Oleomargarine Bill Signed by Gov. Cleveland." *New York Times*, 6 August 1884.

"The Butter Moonshiners." *New York Times*, 23 July 1911.

"Court Dismisses CSPI's Trans Fat Suit Against BK." *Nation's Restaurant News*, 5 January 2009.

Dupre, R. " 'If It's Yellow, It Must Be Butter': Margarine Regulation in North America Since 1886." *Journal of Economic History*, Vol. 59, 1999, pp. 353–371.

"Feeding Oleo to the Navy." *Cass City Chronicle*, 10 November 1905.

Gattereau, A., and H. F. Delisle. "The Unsettled Question: Butter or Margarine?" *Canadian Medical Association Journal*, Vol. 103, 1970, pp. 268–271.

Gifford, A. "Whiskey, Margarine, and Newspapers: A Tale of Three Taxes." *In* Shugart, W. F. (Ed.). *Taxing Choice: The Predatory Politics of Fiscal Discrimination.* New Brunswick, NJ: Transaction Publishers, 1997.

Hamm, Richard F. 1995. *Shaping the Eighteenth Amendment: Temperance Reform, Legal Culture, and the Polity.* University of North Carolina Press.

Lupton, J. R., et al. "Letter Report on Dietary Reference Intakes for Trans Fatty Acids." Washington, DC: National Academy of Sciences, Institute of Medicine, 2002.

Macrae, F. "You'd Butter Believe It: Margarine Consumption is Linked to Lower IQs in Children." *Daily Mail*, 29 September 2009.

O'Connor, A. "The Claim: Margarine is Healthier than Butter." *New York Times*, 16 October 2007.

"Oleomargarine: Congressmen Shown How the Article is Manufactured." *New York Times*, 22 March 1880.

"Position Paper on Trans Fatty Acids." *American Journal of Clinical Nutrition*, Vol. 63, 1996, pp. 663–670.

Riepma, S. F. 1970. *The Story of Margarine.* Washington, DC: Public Affairs Press.

Scholliers, P. "Defining Food Risks and Food Anxieties Throughout History." *Appetite*, Vol. 51, 2008, pp. 3–6.

Siri-Tarino, P. W., et al. "Meta-Analysis of Prospective Disease Cohorts Evaluating the Association of Saturated Fat with Cardiovascular Disease." *American Journal of Clinical Nutrition*, 13 January 2010.

Strey, G. "The 'Oleo Wars': Wisconsin's Fight over the Demon Spread." *Wisconsin Magazine of History*, Vol. 85, 2001, pp. 2–15.

Theodore, R. F. "Dietary Patterns and Intelligence in Early and Middle Childhood." *Intelligence*, Vol. 37, 2009, pp. 506–513.

van Stuijvenberg, J. H. (Ed.) 1969. *Margarine: An Economic, Social, and Scientific History, 1869–1969.* Toronto: University of Toronto Press.

"Yellow Margarine: I Can't Believe It's Not Legal." *USA Today*, 16 December 2008.

Zevenbergen, H., et al. "Foods with a High Fat Quality are Essential for Healthy Diets." *Annals of Nutrition and Metabolism*, Vol. 54 (Suppl. 1), 2009, pp. 15–24.

Zock, P. L., and M. B. Katan. "Butter, Margarine and Serum Lipoproteins." *Atherosclerosis*, Vol. 131, 1997, pp. 7–16.

16

Fear of Tomatoes

I know I'm gonna miss her
A tomato ate my sister.

—Attack of the Killer Tomatoes (1978)

SUMMARY

According to a well-known story, everybody in the world believed that tomatoes were poisonous until 1820, when a free-thinking American tomato lover ate a tomato on the steps of a county courthouse in the presence of a gasping crowd of onlookers. The real story of universal tomato acceptance is more complicated, as of course we will explain, and the 1820 incident appears to be the fabrication of a twentieth-century journalist. Tomatoes are closely related to poisonous plants called nightshades, and some parts of the tomato plant are not edible, but there is nothing wrong with the fruit itself, except that it tends to squirt and is confusingly known as a vegetable. The fear of tomatoes (other than non-fried green ones) fizzled long ago, only to be replaced by the more recent belief that tomatoes contain powerful health-giving substances.

SOURCE

Colonel Robert Gibbon Johnson (1771–1850), an entrepreneur and onetime president of the Salem, New Jersey Horticultural Society, was destined for rebirth as a culture bearer in the tradition of Johnny Appleseed. After graduating from Princeton University in 1790, Johnson became Army paymaster in New Jersey under General Joseph Bloomfield at the time of the Whiskey Rebellion. The young paymaster rose quickly through the ranks, becoming a Captain in 1796, Major of Cavalry in 1798, Lieutenant Colonel in 1809, and finally Colonel in 1819 after serving in the War of 1812. In 1821 he was elected to the New Jersey State Assembly, a post that he held until 1826. In 1833 he became a judge in Salem, New Jersey, and in 1839 he published a book on the history of that city. He served as vice president of the New Jersey Historical Society from 1845 until his death in 1850. Yet none of these achievements compares with the single act that immortalized him in American folklore, if in fact it ever took place: On 28 September 1820, Col. Johnson stood (or in some versions sat) on the steps of the county courthouse, and before an assembled crowd of hundreds (perhaps thousands) of jeering spectators, did eat a tomato, or according to some sources an entire basket of tomatoes. Thus, the world learned for the first time that tomatoes are not poisonous.

Clearly, there are several things wrong with this story. Why were tomatoes so widely cultivated if everybody thought they were poisonous? The species makes a nice ornamental shrub, for those who do not mind having inedible rotting tomatoes all over the yard; the foliage was also used as an insect repellent at one time. More to the point, why was the story of Robert Gibbon Johnson not published anywhere for more than 80 years after the alleged event? The earliest related publication we could find was a 1908 newspaper article, which simply stated that Robert Gibbon Johnson *brought* tomatoes to Salem, New Jersey, in 1820. Even Col. Johnson's own 1839 book fails to mention the "courthouse steps" incident.

The main source of the 1820 tomato story appears to be a 1937 book by Joseph S. Sickler, an amateur historian and onetime postmaster of Salem, New Jersey. Sickler took the story to the next level by claiming not only that Johnson ate a tomato in public, but that he spent years afterwards patiently educating the natives to enjoy the wondrous red fruit (or vegetable or whatever). Finally, in 1949, the incident was dramatized in a popular American television program called *You Are There*.

SCIENCE

Tomatoes belong to a plant family called Solanaceae, which includes many poisonous plants and also many edible ones, such as potatoes, pepper, and eggplant. The scientific name of the tomato plant, *Lycopersicon esculentum*, literally means "edible wolf peach." For reasons that are not entirely clear, "wolf peach" was once a common name for the tomato. An earlier synonym, *Solanum lycopersicum*, means "wolf peach nightshade."

The main toxin found in the tomato plant is not solanine (see Chapter 14), but a related glycoalkaloid compound called tomatine. Its most common form, called alpha-tomatine, is about 100 times less poisonous than the solanine found in green parts of potatoes. Most of the tomatine is in the tomato flowers and leaves; the fruit contains only a little to begin with, and even that declines by about 50 percent as the tomato ripens and the color changes from green to red. Contrary to rumor, frying a green tomato will not destroy the toxin it contains, but the level is too low to be harmful anyway. In nature, the color red is sometimes a warning of danger or toxicity, but red tomatoes owe their color to two important nutrients called lycopene and beta-carotene. These compounds are also available in tablet form as dietary supplements, for those who prefer expensive sources or are allergic to tomatoes.

HISTORY

If the story of Robert Gibbon Johnson is not the real history of the tomato, then what is? Despite their association with spaghetti sauce, tomatoes are not native to Italy, any more than potatoes are native to Ireland. Both are New World plants; the tomato originally grew on the western coast of South America and was probably first cultivated in Mexico. In the early sixteenth century, explorers introduced the tomato to Europe, where it was a near-instant hit. Recipes for tomato catsup appeared in cookbooks before 1812. In 1821, an ad in the *Edinburgh Advertiser* offered for sale "Conserve of TOMATOES, prepared by the celebrated Monsieur Appert."

According to some sources, Europeans regarded the tomato as an aphrodisiac and dubbed it *pomme d'amour* ("love apple"), but others dismiss this story as a deplorable bit of folk etymology. At least one source claims that residents of New Orleans started using tomatoes in the late eighteenth century because their red color somehow showed support for the French Revolution. Still another source claims that George Washington's cook tried to kill him by feeding him tomatoes, but this appears to be an intentional work of fiction. By the 1830s, patent medicine dealers took the next logical step and sold tomato pills by newspaper advertisement as a substitute for calomel, a dangerous mercury-based drug that was formerly used to treat syphilis. By 1835, at least one American doctor claimed that tomato extract would also prevent cholera.

In colonial North America, some people ate tomatoes and others did not, a tradition that has continued to the present day. President Thomas Jefferson (1743–1826) reportedly ate tomatoes and grew them in his garden long before Robert Gibbon Johnson was a gleam in his father's eye. Some people in that era might have avoided tomatoes because of their reputation as an aphrodisiac, rather than any fear of poison, but President Jefferson evidently had no such qualms. Today, the typical American consumes about 80 pounds of tomatoes per year (including catsup), and it is one of the most common plants grown in home gardens.

Tomatoes have, on occasion, been associated with legitimate health problems. A minor health scare resulted in 1981 when President Ronald Reagan supposedly decreed that tomato catsup should count as a vegetable for purposes of school lunch program reimbursement. Some parents took that ruling as an endorsement of bad nutrition in public schools, but it appears that a USDA panel made the decision, and the president himself was not in the loop. Also, some outbreaks of food poisoning have been traced to *Salmonella* bacteria and other pathogens on tomatoes and other fresh produce (Chapter 23). These bacteria sometimes contaminate water used for irrigation or washing, and are not unique to tomatoes.

CONSEQUENCES

The source of our chapter epigraph is the 1978 motion picture *Attack of the Killer Tomatoes*, in which a crack team of government experts investigates violent assaults by mutant tomatoes—clearly the result of scientists meddling with forces best left alone. Sequels to date include *Return of the Killer Tomatoes* (1988), *Killer Tomatoes Strike Back* (1990), and *Killer Tomatoes Eat France* (1991). These movies also spawned at least two video games (1986 and 1991) and an animated TV series (1990).

Like many foods that somebody once regarded as dangerous, tomatoes have metamorphosed into a magic cure—most recently, for disorders of the prostate gland, until a 2007 study apparently dashed that hope. Lycopene has also been investigated for its possible protective effect against some forms of radiation.

The very idea of any danger inherent in tomatoes now seems hilarious and outrageous. Comedians throw them; health-food advocates argue about them; home gardeners who grow tomatoes brag about the results and display them on Web sites, although tomatoes are considered easy to grow. Grainger County, Tennessee, has an annual Tomato Festival, complete with a "Tomato Wars" event. Spain also has an annual tomato-throwing event called La Tomatina. It is not clear what the Earth's starving millions think of cultures that can afford to waste hundreds of tons of tomatoes every year as projectiles.

When a biotechnology firm allegedly started growing square tomatoes in 1994, a degree of public outrage resulted. Consumers had a delayed reaction to the wider implications of genetic engineering (Chapter 33), but a square tomato was just plain *wrong*. (In fact, despite rumors, the genetically engineered Flavr Savr tomato had a prolonged shelf life but was not square. The "square tomato" was an earlier strain, developed in the 1950s by selective breeding for easier packing in square boxes.)

WHAT WENT WRONG?

Nothing really went wrong. New and unfamiliar foods are often suspect, and rightly so. How many American or European tourists visiting Thailand for the first time would immediately eat a fried tarantula or scorpion? These foods are said to be good, but *wow*. By the same token, people in the eighteenth century already knew enough about botany to be particularly cautious when dealing with plants in the family Solanaceae, which includes some of the world's most dangerous plants, such as nightshade, belladonna, Jimson weed—and tobacco.

REFERENCES AND RECOMMENDED READING

Alexander, R. F., et al. "A Fatal Case of Solanine Poisoning." *British Medical Journal*, Vol. 2, 1948, p. 518.

Allen, A. "A Passion for Tomatoes." *Smithsonian*, August 2008.

Asano, N., et al. "The Effects of Calystegines Isolated from Edible Fruits and Vegetables on Mammalian Liver Glycosidases." *Glycobiology*, Vol. 7, 1997, pp. 1085–1088.

Barceloux, D. G. "Potatoes, Tomatoes, and Solanine Toxicity." *Disease-a-Month*, Vol. 55, 2009, pp. 391–402.

Donnelly, L. "Killer Tomatoes." *East Hampton Star*, 12 August 2008.

Farmer's Wife (Anon.). "Recipe to Destroy or Drive Away Bed Bugs." *Republican Compiler* (Gettysburg, PA), 15 May 1822.

Ferrer, A., et al. "Antigenic and Allergenic Differences Between Green and Mature Tomatoes." *Journal of Investigational Allergology and Clinical Immunology*, Vol. 18, 2008, pp. 411–412.

Friedman, M. "Tomato Glycoalkaloids: Role in the Plant and in the Diet." *Journal of Agricultural and Food Chemistry*, Vol. 50, 2002, pp. 5751–5780.

Friedman, M., et al. "Tomatine-Containing Green Tomato Extracts Inhibit Growth of Human Breast, Colon, Liver, and Stomach Cancer Cells." *Journal of Agricultural and Food Chemistry*, Vol. 57, 2009, pp. 5727–5733.

Kavanaugh, C. J., et al. "The U.S. Food and Drug Administration's Evidence-Based Review for Qualified Health Claims: Tomatoes, Lycopene, and Cancer." *Journal of the National Cancer Institute*, Vol. 99, 2007, pp. 1074–1085.

Lee, M. R. "The Solanaceae: Foods and Poisons." *Journal of the Royal College of Physicians of Edinburgh*, Vol. 36, 2006, pp. 162–169.

McGee, H. "Accused, Yes, but Probably Not a Killer." *New York Times*, 28 July 2009.

Morrow, W. J., et al. "Immunobiology of the Tomatine Adjuvant." *Vaccine*, Vol. 22, 2004, pp. 2380–2384.

Osterballe, M., et al. "The Prevalence of Food Hypersensitivity in Young Adults." *Pediatric Allergy and Immunology*, Vol. 20, 2009, pp. 686–692.

Peralta, I., and D. Spooner. "History, Origin and Early Cultivation of Tomato (Solanaceae)." In Razdan, M. K., and A. K. Mattoo (Eds.). 2007. *Genetic Improvement of Solanaceous Crops*, Vol. 2. Enfield: Science Publishers, pp. 1–27.

Redenbaugh, K. 1992. *Safety Assessment of Genetically Engineered Fruits and Vegetables: A Case Study of the Flavr Savr Tomato*. Boca Raton, FL: CRC Press.

Scholliers, P. "Defining Food Risks and Food Anxieties Throughout History." *Appetite*, Vol. 51, 2008, pp. 3–6.

Sickler, J. S. 1937. *The History of Salem County, New Jersey*. Salem, NJ: Sunbeam Publishing, p. 198.

Sickler, J. S. 1949. *The Old Houses of Salem County*. Salem, NJ: Sunbeam Publishing, p. 40.

Smith, A. F. "The Making of the Legend of Robert Gibbon Johnson and the Tomato." *New Jersey History*, Vol. 108, 1990, pp. 59–74.

Smith, A. F. 1994. *The Tomato in America: Early History, Culture, and Cookery*. Columbia: University of South Carolina Press.

Smith, A. F. "False Memories: The Invention of Culinary Fakelore and Food Fallacies." In Walker, H. (Ed.). 2001. *Proceedings of the Oxford Symposium on Food and Cookery 2000*. Devon, UK: Prospect Books.

Taylor, J. M. "Toxic Tomato Leaves." *New York Times*, 4 August 2009.

Wolf, T. H. "How the Lowly 'Love Apple' Rose in the World." *Smithsonian*, August 1990.

17

Fear of Watercress

Watercress is of a warm nature. When it has been eaten, it is not of much use or much harm to a person.

—Attributed to Hildegard von Bingen (A.D. 1098–1179)

SUMMARY

During the first half of the twentieth century, many people avoided eating watercress because of highly publicized disease outbreaks associated with this leafy green vegetable. There is nothing wrong with watercress itself, but the plant has often been gathered from slow streams and roadside drainage ditches of doubtful purity. Typhoid fever, amebic dysentery, and several other greatly feared diseases came to be associated with consumption of raw watercress. Once sanitation standards and production methods improved, this scare fizzled into history. Of course, waterborne pathogens can still contaminate almost any food, but properly cultivated and washed (or cooked) watercress no longer stands out as an exceptional risk. The safety of wild watercress depends mainly on the water where it grows.

SOURCE

There is no single historic event that stands out as the principal source of this health scare. One incident that probably made a major contribution was a 1913 wedding breakfast in Philadelphia, at which 19 persons ate watercress sandwiches and 18 of them—including the bride and groom—later developed typhoid fever. After an account of the incident appeared in the *Journal of the American Medical Association*, the wire services picked it up and published the details in the *New York Times* and other newspapers. Similar stories appeared from time to time at least through the 1940s, as discussed in the History section. Thus, like most pre-Internet health scares, this one spread mainly through the medium of print and by word of mouth.

Minor disease outbreaks leading to recalls of various food products are almost a routine occurrence in today's society (Chapter 23). Every year, the news media spend a few weeks or months on the latest foodborne disease scare and then quickly move on to the next. If people worried about all these food scares to the same extent that they once worried about watercress, it would be impossible to eat anything. In the old days, fewer food-related outbreaks were reported, mainly because infectious diseases were so widespread that a specific source was often hard to pinpoint. Watercress may have served as a focus for these fears partly because it was easily eliminated from the menu—unlike staples such as dairy products, meat, or grain, which also served as vehicles for disease in the old days. Watercress, in a word, was expendable.

Before we hear from the watercress lobby, let us hasten to add that watercress is a delicious and healthful vegetable that is as safe as any other food when grown, harvested, and prepared under reasonably sanitary conditions.

SCIENCE

The fear of watercress apparently has no technical name, so we will give it one: rorippa-phobia. Watercress (*Rorippa nasturtium-aquaticum* or *Nasturtium officinale*) is a common aquatic plant with hollow, floating stems and compound leaves that have a distinctive peppery flavor. This plant belongs to the same family as wild mustard and several cultivated cruciferous vegetables, such as cabbage, broccoli, and radishes. Watercress is native to Europe, but like many European plants it has become established in North American streams and ponds, and is also grown in hydroponic culture. It is an excellent source of several vitamins and minerals.

Many foodborne pathogens may occur in the water where this plant grows, and many disease outbreaks have been associated with consumption of watercress. It is not clear if most of these outbreaks result from actually eating the plant or from gathering it from a stream by hand and then transferring polluted water from hand to mouth. Some of these diseases are rare in North America at present, but their range and incidence may increase as a result of global climate change:

- *Typhoid fever.* In the past, this was the disease most often associated with watercress, but typhoid from any source has become rare in developed countries as a result of improved sanitation and water treatment systems. The disease causes high fever, headache, and intestinal damage, and the death rate is as high as 10 percent. On average, there are about 20 million cases of typhoid every year worldwide, but only about 400 in the United States. The agent is a bacterium (*Salmonella typhi*) that usually spreads by contaminated water or food.

- *Leptospirosis.* Participants in triathlons and other cross-country races sometimes contract this disease by splashing through polluted streams, with or without watercress. Often called swine fever, leptospirosis infects many species, including man. The agents include a long list of spirochetes in the genus *Leptospira*, and symptoms range from a mild flu-like illness to possible liver and kidney damage. Contact with rat urine is a risk factor for leptospirosis; in 2008, health authorities warned the public not to eat watercress gathered from a rat-infested stream in England.

- *Campylobacteriosis.* The agent is a bacterium (*Campylobacter jejuni*) that causes an estimated 2 million cases of acute diarrhea every year in the United States alone. Only a few of these cases result from eating watercress, and it is usually a self-limiting disease.

- *Listeriosis.* The bacteria (*Listeria monocytogenes* and related species) that cause this dangerous foodborne disease have been found on the leaves of watercress, but we are not aware of any actual outbreaks that have been traced to this plant. About 2,500 Americans contract listeriosis every year, and about 20 percent of them die. Symptoms often include high fever, headache, and nausea. In a pregnant woman, listeriosis can also cause birth defects or stillbirth.
- *E. coli infection.* Toxin-forming strains of the intestinal bacterium *Escherichia coli* (E. coli for short) have caused many outbreaks of bloody diarrhea and kidney failure in recent years. The usual source is contaminated food or water, but only a few cases have been associated with watercress.
- *Fascioliasis.* To understand this disease, think of two-inch-long flatworms colonizing your liver. The big liver fluke (*Fasciola hepatica*) lays its eggs in water, and although its usual hosts are sheep and cattle that drink from streams, people may swallow fluke eggs that cling to the leaves of watercress. In 1993, the CDC's International Task Force for Disease Eradication specifically noted that uncooked watercress is a potential source of this parasite. It is common in the tropics worldwide, but it also occurs in North America and Europe, and its prevalence may be increasing as a result of global climate change.
- *Cyclosporidiosis or cyclosporiasis.* The agent is a protozoan parasite called *Cyclospora cayetanensis* that can occur in even the cleanest-looking streams or in tap water. It infests ducks and wild mammals as well as humans, causing diarrhea and nausea. About 16,000 Americans contract this waterborne or foodborne disease every year, and watercress has been implicated in some cases.
- *Cryptosporidiosis.* The agent, a protozoan parasite called *Cryptosporidium parvum*, turns up in about the same places as *Cyclospora* (above) and causes a similar illness. There are about 300,000 human cases per year in the United States alone, and the oocysts have been found on watercress leaves.
- *Giardiasis.* Another protozoan parasite (*Giardia lamblia* and related species) causes this disease. It commonly occurs in streams and lakes, and it causes severe diarrhea that may last for as long as six weeks. Investigators have found *Giardia* cysts on watercress leaves, but this source accounts for only a few of the 2 million cases that occur every year in the United States alone.
- *Amebic dysentery.* A protozoan called *Entamoeba histolytica* causes this unpleasant disease, which involves severe bloody diarrhea with possible damage to the colon and liver. The ameba has a dormant form, called a cyst, that can survive outside the body in contaminated water, soil, or food, until a new host comes along and swallows it. These cysts have been found on watercress and other aquatic plants.

Infectious diseases and parasitic infestations are not the only problems that can result from improperly gathered watercress. Lead poisoning is also possible, if the stream or ditch contains high levels of lead pollution. Watercress often grows near poisonous plants, such as water hemlock (*Cicuta maculata*), and people gathering watercress have sometimes eaten a poisonous plant by mistake.

Some sources claim that watercress itself can cause bladder irritation, kidney disorders, inflammation of the throat and stomach, or aggravation of an existing thyroid disorder. By contrast, at least one study found that watercress tended to protect against breast cancer. Other, less formal studies have shown that watercress has an aphrodisiac effect, or the opposite. Still other sources go clear around the bend and claim that it protects against evil. Watercress clearly is powerful stuff.

HISTORY

The Greek general and historian Xenophon (430–354 B.C.) wrote that children fed on watercress would grow taller and have active minds, as in fact most children do. The plant is a good source of vitamin C, so it probably helped those with scurvy, but the early Greeks used it to treat almost everything. The Roman scholar Pliny the Elder (A.D. 23–79) wrote that watercress "purges the head of ill-humour" and even cured baldness.

Watercress was a popular "yarb" with early American settlers, and it retained its loyal following through the food shortages of the two World Wars and the Great Depression, despite increasing public awareness of disease risk. A 1916 syndicated newspaper column advised readers to wash watercress and then soak it in a vinegar solution for an hour and a quarter to prevent typhoid fever. A 1933 study found E. coli on most samples of watercress purchased from vendors in Chicago, and cited a number of earlier studies with similar findings. In 1938, the *British Medical Journal* reported an outbreak of four cases of leptospirosis that were all traced to the same stream in England. Only one of the four patients in that case had handled watercress; unfortunately, he was the one who died, and newspapers picked up the story.

In 1947, U.S. wire services ran a piece entitled "Watercress Fever Kills Clyde Man." An Ohio man and his son contracted typhoid fever after gathering watercress from a stream, but the press gave the disease a new name that stuck. By the 1950s, however, typhoid from any source was becoming rare in the United States, and watercress was already evolving from a controversial garnish into an established health food.

CONSEQUENCES

Today, there are clubs and newsletters devoted to the practice of gathering wild watercress. There are entire restaurants that specialize in watercress dishes. The wonder weed is even a key component of an anti-cancer patent medicine called Essiac Herbal Tonic. (Unfortunately, a 2006 study at Lawrence Livermore showed that Essiac can actually stimulate the growth of human breast cancer cells.) It's an old story: a powerful enemy becomes a powerful friend. In fact, in the present case it would be more accurate to say that a plant that formerly grew in dangerous places is now a fine salad or soup ingredient, if properly washed.

WHAT WENT WRONG?

As far as we can tell, watercress has outlived its bad reputation. When people get sick, they look for a culprit, but watercress was more like an innocent bystander. It is always risky to splash around in warm ponds and slow-moving streams where animals urinate and defecate and drink. People who gather watercress simply need to wash it—and their hands. We will conclude with some good advice from a recent watercress newsletter: "Pond water can carry Weil's disease [leptospirosis] but this is not a problem if hands are kept away from mouths, eyes and noses until they have been washed when the event is finished."[1]

NOTE

1. *Watercress Wildlife Association Newsletter*, Summer 2008.

REFERENCES AND RECOMMENDED READING

Alwi, S., et al. "In Vivo Modulation of 4E Binding Protein 1 (4E-BP1) by Watercress: A Pilot Study." *British Journal of Nutrition*, Vol. 104, 2010, pp. 1288–1296.

Ayala-Gaytán, J. J., et al. "Cyclosporidiosis: Clinical and Diagnostic Characteristics of an Epidemic Outbreak." *Revista de Gastroenterología de México*, Vol. 69, 2004, pp. 226–229. [Spanish]

Bundesen, H. N. "The Control of Foods Eaten Raw." *Journal of the American Medical Association*, Vol. 85, 1925, pp. 1285–1289.

Cook, N., et al. "Development of a Method for Detection of *Giardia duodenalis* Cysts on Lettuce and for Simultaneous Analysis of Salad Products for the Presence of *Giardia* Cysts and *Cryptosporidium* Oocysts." *Applied and Environmental Microbiology*, Vol. 73, 2007, pp. 7388–7391.

de Oliveira, C. A., and P. M. Germano. "Presence of Intestinal Parasites in Vegetables Sold in the Metropolitan Area of São Paulo-SP, Brazil. II—Research on Intestinal Protozoans." *Revista de Saúde Pública*, Vol. 26, 1992, pp. 332–335. [Portuguese]

Edmonds, C., and R. Hawke. "Microbiological and Metal Contamination of Watercress in the Wellington Region, New Zealand—2000 Survey." *Australian and New Zealand Journal of Public Health*, Vol. 28, 2004, pp. 20–26.

Fröder, H., et al. "Minimally Processed Vegetable Salads: Microbial Quality Evaluation." *Journal of Food Protection*, Vol. 70, 2007, pp. 1277–1280.

Gill, C. I., et al. "Watercress Supplementation in Diet Reduces Lymphocyte DNA Damage and Alters Blood Antioxidant Status in Healthy Adults." *American Journal of Clinical Nutrition*, Vol. 85, 2007, pp. 504–510.

Hoffman, G. L. "Control Methods for Snail-Borne Zoonoses." *Journal of Wildlife Diseases*, Vol. 6, 1970, pp. 262–265.

Kulp, K. S., et al. "Essiac and Flor-Essence Herbal Tonics Stimulate the In Vitro Growth of Human Breast Cancer Cells." *Breast Cancer Research and Treatment*, Vol. 98, 2006, pp. 249–259.

Mailles, A., et al. "Commercial Watercress as an Emerging Source of Fascioliasis in Northern France in 2002: Results from an Outbreak Investigation." *Epidemiology and Infection*, Vol. 134, 2006, pp. 942–945.

Meerburg, B. G., et al. "Rodent-Borne Diseases and their Risks for Public Health." *Critical Reviews in Microbiology*, Vol. 35, 2009, pp. 221–270.

Minette, H. P. "Leptospirosis in Poikilothermic Vertebrates. A Review." *International Journal of Zoonoses*, Vol. 10, 1983, pp. 111–121.

Morgan, M. "Rat Illness Fear from Beck Watercress." *Evening Gazette*, 5 August 2008.

Plummer, H. C. "A Washington Daybook." Oakland Tribune, 19 February 1929.

Robertson, K. M. "Four Cases of Weil's Disease Infected from the Same Stream." *British Medical Journal*, Vol. 2, 1938, pp. 1300–1304.

Rondelaud, D., et al. "Changes in Human Fasciolosis in a Temperate Area: About Some Observations Over a 28-Year Period in Central France." *Parasitology Research*, Vol. 86, 2000, pp. 753–757.

Scholliers, P. "Defining Food Risks and Food Anxieties Throughout History." *Appetite*, Vol. 51, 2008, pp. 3–6.

Snyder, W. R. "Wild Watercress." *WSJ Magazine*, 20 May 2009.

Tanner, F. W. "Microbiological Examination of Fresh and Frozen Fruits and Vegetables." American Journal of Public Health, Vol. 24, 1933, pp. 485–492.

"Vinegar Prevents Typhoid." *Stevens Point Daily Journal*, 23 September 1913.

"Watercress Fever Kills Clyde Man." *Evening Independent*, 29 May 1947.

"Wedding Guests Stricken: Bride and Bridegroom also Attacked by Typhoid after Eating Watercress." *New York Times*, 30 July 1913.

18

Fear of Beef

If beef is your idea of "real food for real people," you'd better live real close to a real good hospital.

     —Neal D. Barnard, M.D. (quoted in *The Buffalo News*, 1 December 1995)

SUMMARY

Since long before Pleistocene artists painted the leaping aurochs on their cave walls for future generations to admire, cattle have played an important role in human cultures. Yet in the last few decades, beef has come under fire as a vehicle for several major infectious diseases, a contributing factor in cardiovascular disease and cancer, an unwelcome contributor to global warming, a source of potentially harmful hormones and antibiotics used to promote growth, and an inefficient use of the Earth's finite resources. Nutritionists and fast-food restaurants have long pushed chicken and turkey as more healthful alternatives to beef, while the pork industry offered "the other white meat." The beef industry has responded with an advertising campaign that makes steak and hamburger look delicious enough to die for. Whether the fear of beef has truly fizzled is largely a matter of perspective, but our guess is that the cow has a few rounds left.

SOURCE

No single event sounded the death knell for the sacred cow. Instead, a long series of unfortunate discoveries during the twentieth century gradually chipped away at the popular image of beef, despite continued demand for dairy products. The use of hormones and antibiotics to enhance cattle growth, the advent of bovine spongiform encephalopathy (BSE, or "mad cow" disease) in England and its apparent transmission to humans, the all-too-frequent outbreaks of severe food poisoning traced to ground beef used in fast-food hamburgers, the ongoing controversy regarding the role of saturated fat in cardiovascular disease, and even the potential contribution of flatulent cows to the greenhouse effect and global warming—all these issues have made headlines in recent decades.

Starting in about 1986, the beef industry countered with rhetoric of its own, such as the famous slogans "Real food for real people" and "Beef, it's what's for dinner." This advertising campaign faltered when two of its celebrity spokespersons revealed potential conflicts of interest, but (to coin a phrase) all publicity is good publicity. One beef spokesperson, actress Cybil Shepherd, confided to the media that she tried to avoid eating red meat for health reasons. Another, actor James Garner, reportedly took time out of the beef campaign for quintuple bypass surgery.

SCIENCE AND HISTORY

Back in the 1970s, when so-called hippies first began to publicize environmental issues such as global warming and stratospheric ozone depletion, cattle emerged as one potential source of concern. According to the U.S. Environmental Protection Agency (EPA), ruminant livestock (mainly cows) produce an astonishing 80 million metric tons of methane gas every year worldwide, or nearly one-third of the methane attributable to human activities. This is bad news at a time when governments are beginning to acknowledge that global climate change is real and that excess methane and other gases are partly responsible for it. Of course, the digestive processes of livestock are not entirely under human control, despite continuing efforts to develop genetically engineered low-methane cows. But without the beef and dairy industries, the few wild cattle on Earth would be far less numerous and less flatulent than the existing herds. Another negative aspect of livestock farming in general is that it makes inefficient use of land. For example, one acre of beef cattle can provide enough food to keep a man alive for four months, whereas one acre planted in soybeans can feed a man for six years.[1]

Also in the 1970s, the widespread practice of adding hormones and antibiotics to beef cattle feed began to draw criticism. The purpose of these chemicals was to enhance growth and hold down the price of meat, but many scientists pointed out that chemical residues in meat might be harmful to consumers (Chapter 4). The U.S. Food and Drug Administration (FDA) banned the use of synthetic estrogen as a livestock feed additive in 1979, but some scientists continued to worry, because it seemed that many strange things were ending up in cattle feed.

Some farms claim that their cows eat nothing but nature's own grass, and those farms tend to charge above-average prices for their meat to offset higher production costs. Until recently, many other farms saved money and made their cows bulk up quickly by feeding them such unusual supplements as chicken manure, beef bone meal, and ground-up dead sheep. According to a 2005 journal article, some British farmers in the 1950s even fed their cattle a mixture of human remains imported from India. Although it would be hard to explain exactly what is wrong with these practices, such publicity has no doubt inspired many vegetarians.

But the controversy over "unnatural" cattle feed is no longer an aesthetic debate, because many (not all) scientists attribute the 1986–1993 mad cow disease epidemic in England to infected animal products used as cattle feed supplements. Mad cow disease, also called bovine spongiform encephalopathy (BSE), is a poorly understood brain disease that appears to be associated with nonliving proteins called prions. About ten years after the British epidemic, a number of humans developed a similar prion disease called new variant Creutzfeldt-Jakob disease (vCJD). At present, these diseases are fatal and there is no known treatment. BSE is considered dangerous enough to be classified as a biosecurity threat under the U.S. Bioterrorism Protection Act of 2002.

The segue from mad cow disease to the "downer cow" controversy is a natural one, but the issues are different. A downer cow is simply a live cow that is unable to walk as a result of disease or injury. Many cattle diseases, and all injuries, are not communicable to humans; but just to be on the safe side, most stockyards do not allow downers to enter the food supply. It would simply be too expensive to hospitalize and diagnose each sick cow, so most are slaughtered and incinerated, while a few are probably coaxed to get up and become meat. The advent of BSE, however, makes it more urgent than ever to avoid selling downer animals as food.

Just as mad cow disease was fading from the headlines, a new problem was gaining momentum. Bacteria called *Escherichia coli* (E. coli for short) are normal inhabitants of human and cattle intestines, but some of these bacteria, such as the highly publicized O157:H7 strain, can produce deadly toxins. A cow can harbor these bacteria without becoming sick, but humans are not so resistant. After an animal is slaughtered, its meat may become contaminated with bacteria from its own or other animals' intestines. A solid cut, such as a steak or roast, is easily washed off; but the process of grinding beef can quickly spread these dangerous bacteria through a large volume of hamburger meat, destined for American's fast-food restaurants. Heat kills the bacteria, but if the meat is undercooked, people can die. Toxigenic (toxin-producing) E. coli were first reported in about 1982, and meat is not the only vehicle; some outbreaks have involved milk, well water, or even contaminated sawdust. The most widely publicized American cases, however, were those involving hamburgers, such as the 1993 outbreak that sickened hundreds of customers at Jack-in-the-Box restaurants in several western states. Four children died, and the problem was traced to contaminated beef. The famous 1984 Wendy's slogan "Where's the beef?" took on a whole new meaning.

People have known for thousands of years that rotten meat does not smell quite right, but that distinctive road-kill aroma often has nothing to do with actual food safety. Fresh meat may contain dangerous pathogens, and road kill can be reasonably safe to eat (although we do not recommend it). Fast-food hamburgers contaminated with toxigenic E. coli smell and taste exactly like hamburgers. Until recently, doctors believed that the toxicity of rotten meat resulted from something called "ptomaine poisoning." The theory was that bacteria decompose proteins in the meat, and that this process releases certain chemicals that cause illness. In fact, we now know that the symptoms of food poisoning—usually diarrhea and nausea—result from the bacteria themselves or from the toxins they produce.

As if these concerns were not enough to discourage consumption of beef, doctors have warned for decades that people whose diet is high in saturated fats—such as those found in marbled beef and whole milk—have an inside track for cardiovascular disease. In recent years, these warnings have shifted to a specific type of saturated fat called a trans fat (see also Chapter 15). Yet a 2010 study concludes that dietary intake of high levels of saturated fat may not be related to cardiovascular disease after all. If verified, this finding may help improve the tarnished reputation of beef.

CONSEQUENCES

Inevitably, the fear of beef has resulted in many lawsuits, many of them legitimate. Minor stomach upset is a fact of life, but eating hamburgers at a chain restaurant should not endanger children's lives. Ground beef recalls due to E. coli contamination remain frequent in the United States, with eight separate recalls totaling over 6 million pounds of beef in 2007 alone.

Although we have found no survey data on the subject, it seems likely that the various beef-related problems of the last half-century may have reduced the popularity of steak tartare—raw ground beef, sometimes mixed with raw egg white, often spread on little crackers and sprinkled with salt or simply served in a garnished heap on a plate. It seems hard to understand how anyone ever ate this stuff, but apparently it is still popular in some countries. A less accessible version of steak tartare consists of raw horse meat.

Another consequence of beef anxiety may be the meteoric rise of Gardenburger and similar products that offer low-fat substitutes for meat. The high cost of beef and fear of premature death may be other factors contributing to this trend. Yet the quest for the perfect hamburger continues. According to a 2001 study, mixing ground beef with finely ground prunes (dried plums) may kill most of the E. coli, but has the disadvantage of making the meat taste like prunes.

WHAT WENT WRONG?

Many food scares and other public health problems are a direct result of human population growth. To provide affordable food to billions of people, food growers and processors often cut corners or simply make mistakes. Beef that is produced without high-protein feed supplements of dubious origin, synthetic hormones, or other growth enhancers usually costs more than standard issue, for the simple reason that the animals grow more slowly and require more expensive food.

Restaurant safety is also a numbers game. An estimated 40 million Americans eat fast food hamburgers every day. In other words, these restaurants serve more than *14 billion* hamburgers every year. In a hamburger universe that large, it is inevitable that some of the patties will not stay on the griddle long enough to cook through and that some employees will forget to wash their hands.

NOTE

1. J. R. Callahan, *Emerging Biological Threats* (ABC-CLIO, 2009), p. 248.

REFERENCES AND RECOMMENDED READING

Begley, S. "The End of Antibiotics." *Newsweek*, 28 March 1994.

Belay, E. D., and L. B. Schonberger. "The Public Health Impact of Prion Diseases." *Annual Review of Public Health*, Vol. 26, 2005, pp. 191–212.

Callaway, T. R., et al. "Forage Feeding to Reduce Preharvest *Escherichia coli* Populations in Cattle, a Review." *Journal of Dairy Science*, Vol. 86, 2003, pp. 852–860.

Colchester, A. C., and N. T. Colchester. "The Origin of Bovine Spongiform Encephalopathy: The Human Prion Disease Hypothesis." *Lancet*, Vol. 366, 2005, pp. 856–861.

Epstein, S. S. "Unlabeled Milk from Cows Treated with Biosynthetic Growth Hormones: A Case of Regulatory Abdication." *International Journal of Health Services*, Vol. 26, 1996, pp. 173–185.

Etherton, T. D., et al. "Recombinant Bovine and Porcine Somatotropin: Safety and Benefits of These Biotechnologies." *Journal of the American Dietetic Association*, Vol. 93, 1993, pp. 177–180.

Garber, K. "Food Safety's Dirty Little Secret." *U.S. News and World Report*, 15 September 2008.

Grobe, D., et al. "A Model of Consumers' Risk Perceptions Toward Recombinant Bovine Growth Hormone (rBGH): The Impact of Risk Characteristics." *Risk Analysis*, Vol. 19, 1999, pp. 661–673.

Hanson, C. "Despite Warnings, Meat Inspection Reform is Elusive." *Seattle Post-Intelligencer*, 15 March 1993.

Hedges, S. J. "Recalls Lead Consumers to Question Meat Safety." *Chicago Tribune*, 24 June 2007.

Higgins, K. T. "Minimum Processes, Maximum Hurdles." *Food Engineering*, January 2009.

Hussein, H. S. "Prevalence and Pathogenicity of Shiga Toxin-Producing *Escherichia coli* in Beef Cattle and their Products." *Journal of Animal Science*, 23 October 2007.

Juskevich, J. C., and C. G. Guyer. "Bovine Growth Hormone: Human Food Safety Evaluation." *Science*, Vol. 249, 1990, pp. 875–884.

Lasmeras, C. J. "The Transmissible Spongiform Encephalopathies." *Revue Scientifique et Technique*, Vol. 22, 2003, pp. 23–36.

Leonard, C. "Beef Industry Woes Could Mean Lesser-Quality Meat." Associated Press, 20 October 2010.

Lockary, V. M., et al. "Shiga Toxin-Producing Escherichia coli, Idaho." *Emerging Infectious Diseases*, Vol. 13, 2007, pp. 1262–1264.

MacKenzie, D. "New Twist in Tale of BSE's Beginnings." *New Scientist*, 17 March 2007, p. 11.

Marks, S., and T. Roberts. "E. coli O157:H7 Ranks as the Fourth Most Costly Foodborne Disease." *Food Safety*, September-December 1993.

McLaughlin, J. J. "Mystery in the Meat." *Restaurant Business*, 20 March 1995.

Moser, P. W. "Maybe It Was Something You Ate." *Saturday Evening Post*, May-June 1987.

Muniesa, M., et al. "Occurrence of *Escherichia coli* O157:H7 and Other Enterohemorrhagic *Escherichia coli* in the Environment." *Environmental Science and Technology*, Vol. 40, 2006, pp. 7141–7149.

Paulson, T. "Investigators Track Killer Bacteria." *Seattle Post-Intelligencer*, 15 March 1993.

Pennington, H. "Origin of Bovine Spongiform Encephalopathy." *Lancet*, Vol. 367, 2006, pp. 297–298.

Schneider, J., et al. "*Escherichia coli* O157:H7 Infections in Children Associated with Raw Milk and Raw Colostrums from Cows—California, 2006." *Morbidity and Mortality Weekly Report*, Vol. 57, 2008, pp. 625–628.

Scholliers, P. "Defining Food Risks and Food Anxieties Throughout History." *Appetite*, Vol. 51, 2008, pp. 3–6.

Schuff, S. "Drug-Resistant Salmonella Found in Recalled Beef." *Foodstuffs*, 10 August 2009.

Smith, P. G. "The Epidemics of Bovine Spongiform Encephalopathy and Variant Creutzfeldt-Jakob Disease: Current Status and Future Prospects." *Bulletin of the World Health Organization*, Vol. 81, 2003, pp. 123–130.

Varma, J. K., et al. "An Outbreak of *Escherichia coli* O157 Infection Following Exposure to a Contaminated Building." *Journal of the American Medical Association*, Vol. 290, 2003, pp. 2709–2712.

Warner, M. "When It Comes to Meat, 'Natural' is a Vague Term." *New York Times*, 10 June 2006.

19

Coca-Cola and Polio

When it's hard to get started, start with a Coca-Cola.

—Coca-Cola advertising slogan (1934)

SUMMARY

In the 1940s and 1950s, many people believed that Coca-Cola and certain other sweetened beverages and foods caused children to develop polio—perhaps the most feared infectious disease of its time, but now largely forgotten in most developed nations. The scare appears to have resulted from a misinterpretation of the results of some early laboratory experiments on rabbits, combined with the dynamics of urban folklore and the desperate wish for a simple solution to polio and somebody to blame for the epidemic. The Coca-Cola scare decidedly fizzled in the light of common sense, even before the advent of the Salk and Sabin vaccines, but the story is instructive nonetheless. Dietary theories about polio have persisted to the present day in some countries and have interfered with vaccination campaigns.

SOURCE

The principal author of this health scare was Dr. Benjamin Sandler (1901–1979), a North Carolina physician who believed that the poliovirus caused illness only in people (usually children) whose blood sugar dropped below normal levels after a temporary increase resulting from consumption of Coca-Cola or other sweetened beverages and foods, such as ice cream. He drew this conclusion from questionable laboratory experiments involving rabbits, and also from the observation that polio outbreaks occurred in summer, when children increased their intake of soda and ice cream. In its early stages, this was not a bad hypothesis for its time; it just happened to be wrong, and nobody else succeeded in duplicating Dr. Sandler's results.

The Coca-Cola theory drew a great deal of publicity in the 1940s, when the poliovirus was sweeping North America, leaving dead or crippled children and devastated families in its wake. Some people, however, apparently interpreted Dr. Sandler's message to mean that sugar itself caused polio, and that the virus had nothing to do with it. As a result, when the vaccine came along in the 1950s, subscribers to the sugar theory did not believe that vaccination could help. Later variants of this idea, mostly confined to the fringe literature, became progressively stranger over the years.

SCIENCE

The agent of polio—also called poliomyelitis or infantile paralysis—is a virus that enters the body through the gastrointestinal tract and then destroys or damages motor nerve cells in the spinal cord. In countries where it still exists, it often spreads by contact with fecal matter or in contaminated food or water. Before the 1954 discovery of the Salk vaccine, there were large polio epidemics every summer. Some cases ended in paralysis or death; most infected children had either no symptoms or an acute illness with fever, headache, and sometimes meningitis. In 1952, for example, there were 58,000 reported cases of polio in the United States alone. About one-third had either permanent or temporary paralysis, and about 3,000 died.

Only humans normally get polio, but researchers can induce it in some laboratory animals by artificial means—for example, by injecting the virus into the brain. Dr. Sandler experimented with rabbits because he wanted to learn why they were resistant to the poliovirus. He noticed that a rabbit's blood sugar level is normally higher than that of (say) a rhesus monkey, which can contract polio under experimental conditions. So he exposed the rabbits to the poliovirus and then gave them a large dose of insulin to force their blood sugar to abnormally low levels. Lo and behold, the rabbits developed what appeared to be polio symptoms within a few hours, and died soon thereafter. But was the observed muscle weakness in these rabbits really an effect of the poliovirus, or was it the result of hypoglycemia or other effects of the insulin injections? Whatever happened, it appears that other researchers were unable to validate Dr. Sandler's findings.

It was common knowledge that most polio cases in temperate regions occurred in summer, but no one knew exactly why. Proposed explanations ranged from the abundance of flies, to the numbers of people in swimming pools, to the consistency of nasal secretions, to the ability of the virus to survive on environmental surfaces in warm, humid weather. But to Dr. Sandler, the reason was clear: children drank more Coca-Cola and ate more ice cream in summer, and the sugar in those foods caused their blood glucose levels to fluctuate, thus putting them at risk for polio. (Children probably ate more candy and cake during the winter holidays, but somehow those sources of sugar did not count.)

Although Dr. Sandler was wrong about polio, he was right about a number of other things. Americans clearly eat too much sugar, and this was already true in the 1940s. Without all that candy and soda, the controversial decision to protect children's teeth by fluoridating water (Chapter 26) might never have become necessary. Besides promoting tooth decay and making people fat, sugar may affect some people in exactly the way Dr. Sandler described: a large dose of sugar causes the blood glucose level to rise sharply and then to fall below normal, sometimes accompanied by mood changes. The classic (if unproven) example is the child who pigs out on candy on Halloween night and then runs screaming around the house for hours.

Not everyone responds to sugar in quite this way; the pancreas makes a hormone called insulin that is supposed to regulate the blood sugar level. But it is possible to overwhelm this process with an excess of sugar, and in people with diabetes—or those who are at risk for diabetes—insulin is either in short supply or cells do not respond properly to it. In other words, cutting down on sugar is such an excellent idea that we really hate to discourage it. But the apparent connection between blood sugar and polio was based on a mistake.

As we said, Dr. Sandler's original hypothesis was that low blood sugar could make a person or rabbit more susceptible to the poliovirus. From there, however, it was a natural step for some of his admirers to leave the virus out of the loop and claim that the low blood sugar itself, or dietary habits that resulted in low blood sugar, might be the direct cause of polio. And as this idea gained momentum, like a snowball rolling down a hill, other ideas stuck to it. Soon the sugar theory grew to encompass preexisting beliefs in the curative powers of vitamin C and honey and whole grains and kelp. Also, some people were reluctant to admit that their hero gave painful injections to poor innocent rabbits; so, in the improved version of the story, he induced polio by feeding sugar to the rabbits instead.

HISTORY

In the 1930s and 1940s, Americans were afraid of polio and would do almost anything to protect their children. During a local outbreak, communal gathering places such as schools, movie theaters, and public swimming pools were often closed. Polio outbreaks caused great fear, as a 1949 publication describes:

> The mass hysteria which affects the general public when an epidemic of poliomyelitis occurs, even nearby, gives the health officer a great deal of worry in advising and instituting any sort of reasonable, sane measures to combat the disease. As a matter of fact, the health officer spends more time trying to combat this reaction than he does in efforts and study to control the disease itself.[1]

According to a story that has improved over the years, Dr. Sandler went on the radio in North Carolina in the summer of 1948 and urged parents to stop giving their children so much sugar. By so doing, his supporters claim that he averted a polio epidemic; the number of reported local cases declined sharply between 1948 and 1949. But, the story continues, the Rockefeller Milk Trust or Coca-Cola or somebody filed a lawsuit (against the radio station?) and somehow forced families to resume their normal sugar-laden diet, and the incidence of polio increased again in 1950.

There are several obvious problems with this story. For one thing, a closer examination of the data shows that North Carolina had a sharp increase in polio cases in 1948, and the number returned to normal in 1949. The number of cases had always fluctuated from year to year. Also, polio diagnosis was not always accurate in those days, and the reported numbers might not be comparable. But even if a real decline occurred in 1949, there is no proof that it had anything to do with avoidance of sugar. Also, if parents believed in this preventive measure, why would they abandon it? Not even Big Food is powerful enough to force people to drink Coca-Cola and eat ice cream.

When the Salk vaccine became available in 1955, many people welcomed it as a miracle, but others were suspicious. The Coca-Cola theory of polio expanded to include the notion that the soda bottler was somehow in cahoots with the vaccine manufacturer. Fear makes people believe strange things. Of course, Coca-Cola was already a target of suspicion, because its beverages formerly contained the drug cocaine, and because it was a big, powerful company with lots of money. But if Coca-Cola was somehow in the business of promoting polio, would it not spare its own future CEO, the late J. Frank Harrison? He was one of several students at Baylor University who contracted polio in the fall of 1948. But he survived the disease, joined Coca-Cola in 1977, and served as its CEO until his death in 2002. During that time period, the company sponsored several major anti-polio drives in Third World countries.

The Salk vaccine is widely recognized as one of the greatest medical achievements of all time. But the public has a short memory, and by the late twentieth century, the anti-science movement claimed that polio vaccines were not only ineffective, but responsible for everything from the AIDS epidemic to developmental disorders in children. And in 2010, a major journal article about the history of polio repeatedly misspelled Dr. Salk's name as "Salt." *Sic transit gloria.*

CONSEQUENCES

In the early twenty-first century, the Coca-Cola Company continues its generous support of international campaigns to eradicate polio, but the world has not forgotten the rumors about its products that have circulated for over 60 years. In 2010, a number of Web sites continued to cite Dr. Sandler's work as gospel and to claim that sugar causes polio. One source even blames the disease on specific substances produced during the sugar refining process.

An even more complicated version of the Coca-Cola theory, published on an anti-vaccination Web site, claims that Coca-Cola syrup shipped to foreign countries causes polio because the local distributors mix it with pesticide-contaminated water. If the water is contaminated, it might cause neurological symptoms related to pesticide poisoning, but that has nothing to do with polio. Also, why would the water added to Coca-Cola syrup be more often contaminated than water used for drinking or other purposes?

Ironically, the notion that pesticides cause polio may have originated with a series of legitimate scientific experiments that Yale scientists conducted in the summer of 1945. In that study, pesticide spraying failed to stop (but did not start) a polio outbreak, so the researchers concluded that flies were not a significant vector (see Chapter 32). Some people apparently misunderstood the whole point of the experiment, and thought the scientists were asking if pesticides caused polio.

Now that wild poliovirus no longer exists in most developed nations, alternative practitioners have the luxury of claiming that it never existed in the first place. Some people continue to develop polio-like symptoms for a variety of reasons, including tick paralysis, West Nile encephalitis, ergot poisoning, and exposure to the pesticide parathion. These examples prove only that the human body has a limited bag of tricks, not that the polio vaccine was a waste of time.

WHAT WENT WRONG?

There are honest mistakes, based on a faulty step in reasoning, and there are dishonest mistakes, based on no reasoning. In the early days, polio researchers were often bombarded with suggestions from the general public, and they investigated any ideas that made sense. The honest mistakes often led to wrong turns and wasted resources. For example, one eminent researcher thought the poliovirus entered through the nose and went directly to the brain, so he assumed that a vaccine could never work, and that there was no point in trying to invent one. Dishonest mistakes, by contrast, often led their authors to patent medicines and lecture tours. It appears that the Coca-Cola theory was somewhere in between.

When parents see their children falling victim to something as terrible as polio, they look for a reason. The doctors who promoted the Coca-Cola theory and related dietary cures told the parents what they wanted to hear—that they were no longer powerless to protect their families. Adherence to a simple, harmless food taboo would fix everything. Medicine men (and women) have relied on that principle for thousands of years. A closely related problem appears to be a basic failure of evidence-based science education in the United States. A cause is not the same thing as a risk factor or correlate, and when two things happen at the same time, that fact does not prove that one thing "caused" the other. Instead of claiming that Coca-Cola caused polio, Dr. Sandler might just as well have concluded that polio made people drink Coca-Cola. In fact, that version makes slightly more sense, because caffeine can help relieve muscle pain and fatigue.

On a more positive note, it is possible that the Coca-Cola theory of polio saved some children from the ravages of obesity, cardiovascular disease, and adult-onset diabetes by persuading their parents to give them less sugar. If only the present generation of Americans were so easily scared, some of these epidemic health threats might be averted. Ironically, now that sugar has emerged as a real killer, nobody seems to be listening.

NOTE

1. J. W. R. Norton and C. P. Stevick, "Observations on the 1948 Poliomyelitis Epidemic in North Carolina" (*Southern Medical Journal*, May 1949).

REFERENCES AND RECOMMENDED READING

Ashlock, M. "High Protein Diet May Help Prevent Polio." *Cedar Rapids Gazette*, 30 July 1953.
Byrd, C. L. "The Survival of the Lansing Strain of the Poliomyelitis Virus in Ice Cream." *American Journal of Digestive Diseases*, Vol. 19, 1952, pp. 55–56.
"Continuing Mystery." *Time*, 2 January 1950.
Dillner, L. "A Case of Mass Hysteria." *The Guardian*, 6 July 1999.
"Doctor Asserts Controlled Diet Wards Off Infantile Paralysis." *United Press*, 6 August 1948.
Jette, A. M. "From the Brink of Scientific Failure." *Physical Therapy*, Vol. 85, 2005, pp. 486–488.

Manchester, W. "New Polio Vaccine Said to Show Great Promise." *Baltimore Evening Sun*, 21 October 1952.

Marks, H. M. "Dirt and Diseases: Polio before FDR, by Naomi Rogers (Review)." *Journal of Interdisciplinary History*, Vol. 26, 1995, pp. 154–156.

Marx, M. B. "Polio and High-Sulfate Diets." *Journal of the American Veterinary Medical Association*, Vol. 181, 1982, pp. 325, 328.

Meldrum, M. "A Calculated Risk: The Salk Polio Vaccine Field Trials of 1954." *British Medical Journal*, Vol. 317, 1998, pp. 1233–1236.

Meldrum, M. "The Historical Feud over Polio Vaccine: How Could a Killed Vaccine Contain a Natural Disease?" *Western Journal of Medicine*, Vol. 171, 1999, pp. 271–273.

Nathanson, N. "Eradication of Poliomyelitis in the United States." *Reviews of Infectious Diseases*, Vol. 4, 1982, pp. 940–950.

Oshinsky, D. "1954 Miracle Workers: More than a Million Children Participated in the Salk Poliomyelitis Vaccine Trials of 1954, the Largest Public Health Experiment in American History." *American Heritage*, Winter 2010, pp. 85+.

Richardson, M. W. "Recent Contributions to Our Knowledge Concerning Infantile Paralysis." *American Journal of Public Health*, Vol. 2, 1912, pp. 141–143.

Rogers, N. 1995. *Dirt and Disease: Polio before FDR*. New Brunswick, NJ: Rutgers University Press.

Rudloff, M. D. *A Vaccine Editorial*. Washington, MO: Washington Pediatric Associates, 2005.

Sandler, B. P. 1951. *Diet Prevents Polio*. Milwaukee: Lee Foundation for Nutritional Research.

Schachter, R. D., and C. R. Kenley. "Gaussian Influence Diagrams." *Management Science*, Vol. 35, 1989, pp. 527–550.

Shearer, J. "Baylor Class of '49 Remembers Tragedy of Polio." *Chattanoogan*, 2 October 2009.

Spetz, M. "Epidemicity of Poliomyelitis; Possible Role of Seasonal Variation in Food Quality." *California Medicine*, Vol. 81, 1954, pp. 409–411.

Van Meer, F. "Poliomyelitis: The Role of Diet in the Development of the Disease." *Medical Hypotheses*, Vol. 37, 1992, pp. 171–178.

Wrong, M. "Who Can Make Polio History?" *New Statesman*, 20 November 2006, pp. 26–27.

20

Fear of Foreign Cheese

Only peril can bring the French together. One can't impose unity out of the blue on a country that has 265 different kinds of cheese.

—Attributed to Charles de Gaulle (1890–1970)

SUMMARY

Every so often, American public health authorities trace an outbreak of listeriosis or another dangerous foodborne illness to a batch of soft cheese. In a highly publicized case in 1985, the offending cheese happened to be a Mexican product with a Mexican-sounding name. Xenophobic popular opinion focused immediately on "foreign" cheese made under supposedly unhygienic conditions in Mexico or France—even though, in the 1985 case, the manufacturing plant was in California. For a time, these health scares seriously impacted sales of imported cheese and other foods. The risk is higher for soft cheeses made from raw (unpasteurized) milk, but any food can become contaminated, regardless of the processing method or place of origin. The bacteria that cause listeriosis can even survive some forms of pasteurization. In recent years, saturation media coverage of numerous foodborne disease outbreaks (described in other chapters) may have contributed to the fizzling of food xenophobias in general.

SOURCE

Scientists have known about listeriosis since British microbiologist Everitt G. D. Murray (1890–1964) described it in 1926 as a disease of rabbits, but the general public heard little about it until 1952, when German doctors reported that listeriosis also caused serious illness in newborn infants. At first, this disease was not considered a threat to adults, except for those with compromised immune systems. A 1981 outbreak in Nova Scotia killed 18 people, mostly newborns and pregnant women, but the American press paid little attention, possibly because the outbreak was traced to cabbage contaminated with sheep manure—seemingly, an easy menace to avoid. In 1983, an outbreak in Massachusetts killed 14 of 49 victims, most of them with known risk factors.

The situation changed in 1985, when a large number of California residents, many of them pregnant women or mothers with infants, became ill after eating soft-ripened Mexican-style cheese made in Los Angeles. At least 142 people became sick enough to see a doctor, and 48 died, including 20 fetuses, 10 newborns, and 18 apparently healthy nonpregnant adults. There are many ways to die, but *Listeria* was more frightening than most because of its specific effect on babies. This bacterium often infects the placenta, causing spontaneous abortion (miscarriage), stillbirth, or severe meningitis.

Imported cheese suffered a double whammy a year later, in 1986, when the press trumpeted a series of government-enforced recalls of imported Brie and other French cheeses that were also found to harbor this bacterium. Thus, Americans learned to associate the fear of *Listeria* with foreign food, specifically cheese, although the bug occurs worldwide and holds no passport.

SCIENCE

The agent of listeriosis is a bacterium called *Listeria monocytogenes*. Although the disease itself is considered rare, the bacterium occurs on every continent, in soil, water, sewage, and the bodies of many wild and domesticated animals. A 1927 outbreak among gerbils near South Africa's Tiger River gave the infection its unofficial name, Tiger River disease.

The symptoms of listeriosis vary depending on the part of the body affected. When it causes meningoencephalitis, it may start with a sudden fever, intense headache, and nausea. More often, it is a less severe flu-like illness, but the hospitalization rate (over 90%) is higher than for any other known foodborne disease. The incubation period varies from three to 70 days, but is usually about a month. Antibiotic treatment often is effective, if started soon enough.

Listeriosis is not the only disease associated with dairy products. People have also contracted salmonellosis, E. coli O157:H7, brucellosis, bovine tuberculosis, toxoplasmosis, Q fever, diphtheria, typhoid fever, and possibly even polio from milk and cheese (see the sidebar, "Say Cheese"). This is why dairies need to keep their cows healthy and their equipment clean. Pasteurization—treatment with heat or radiation—can kill many of the microorganisms that raw milk contains, but not all. At least one major listeriosis outbreak in the U.S. was traced to cheese made from pasteurized milk. No food can be 100 percent safe, but pasteurization increases safety.

Say Cheese

In 2004, a medical journal[1] reported the unusual case of a 69-year-old man in Italy who developed fever and lower back pain a month after surgery for bladder cancer. His doctor naturally assumed that these symptoms were related to the cancer, but none of the standard treatments seemed to help. Then another clue appeared: the patient's wife, who did not have cancer, also developed fever and lower back pain. Further investigation revealed that the couple had contracted a serious bacterial disease called brucellosis by eating unpasteurized goat cheese about eight months earlier. Both the husband and wife recovered with appropriate antibiotic treatment. A third family member also ate the cheese and had a milder case of brucellosis, but recovered without treatment. Brucellosis is an ancient disease of goats and other livestock, but humans are rarely infected, except by close contact with animals or by consumption of unpasteurized dairy products.

Hard cheeses are generally considered safe to eat, because their low moisture content and relatively high acidity do not promote bacterial growth. Doctors often advise pregnant women not to eat soft-ripened cheeses, such as Brie, Camembert, Danish blue, Gorgonzola, and Stilton, especially if the cheese is made from raw (unpasteurized) milk. This warning should also be of interest to men and nonpregnant women, because listeriosis is potentially quite dangerous. About 2,500 Americans contract this disease in a typical year, and about 500 (20%) die. The risk may be highest for people with compromised immune systems, such as AIDS patients and organ transplant recipients. Infants, elderly people, and those with diabetes are also at increased risk. In 2000, listeriosis was added to the list of diseases that doctors are required to report to the CDC.

HISTORY

After listeriosis became famous in the mid-1980s, manufacturers responded by improving their quality control standards, but that was not the end of the story. Major listeriosis epidemics occurred in Great Britain in 1989, in France in 1992, and in the United States in 1995, 2006, and 2009. Numerous *Listeria*-related product recalls also occurred during the same time period. These facts do not, however, prove that the risk of contracting listeriosis is high. On the contrary, a 2004 risk assessment concluded that the expected number of severe listeriosis cases in a given year would be on the order of 0.002 cases per 17 million servings of Brie.

As the foreign cheese panic escalated during the late twentieth century, European cheesemakers complained that the listeriosis scare targeted their products unfairly and caused sales to drop, although cheese is not the only food that can harbor these bacteria. Nondairy foods that have caused listeriosis outbreaks include hot dogs, smoked fish products, and foie gras. In 2000, a major U.S. manufacturer recalled nearly 17 million pounds of turkey and chicken products with possible *Listeria* contamination. At one point, conspiracy theorists even claimed that American and Scandinavian interests were trying to force all cheesemakers to pasteurize their milk by imposing ever-tighter sanitary requirements. But why not pasteurize? This process reduces the risk of disease while yielding a perfectly edible product. People who believe otherwise can still buy raw milk (or a cow) and learn to make their own cheese, like the bathtub gin of Prohibition days.

Some government officials reportedly have asked if raw milk cheese might provide terrorists with a convenient vehicle for biological warfare. It is unclear why it would be easier to meddle with cheese than with other foods.

CONSEQUENCES

The push for pasteurization may have backfired by actually increasing demand for raw milk products. Although pasteurization was invented for good reasons, and it has saved many lives, it is not a cure-all. As noted above, pasteurized milk has even served as a vehicle for listeriosis. Many people have expressed a growing sense of frustration with the numerous government regulations that constrain our lives. Nearly everyone wants to protect children—but if the government can dictate what type of cheese a pregnant woman is allowed to eat, what else can it tell her to do?

Sellers of raw dairy products not only remain in business, but often charge a premium, claiming that their products have more complex flavors and contain more vitamins than the clean, impersonal foods sold in supermarkets. In fact, heating milk may destroy about 10 percent of its vitamin B_1 content, but this is not a significant loss; why not just drink 10 percent more milk? Some vendors take the argument a step further, and claim that people cannot be healthy without the "good" bacteria and enzymes that pasteurization destroys. This is misleading too, because adult humans before the domestication of animals did not have access to cheese or other milk products, raw or otherwise. Yet they must have been reasonably healthy, or we would not be here to debate the issue.

In 2000, two organizations called the American Cheese Society and the Old Ways Preservation and Trust Exchange got together and established the Cheese of Choice Coalition, which works with the U.S. Food and Drug Administration (FDA) and other government agencies to protect the industry's right to sell raw dairy products. As of 2009, 28 U.S. states allow the sale of raw milk, and the FDA allows the sale of raw milk cheese (domestic or imported) that has been aged for at least 60 days at 35°F (about 2°C). This aging process makes the cheese more acidic, thus killing many bacteria. Also, any remaining bacteria may form visible cultures during the aging period, and the cheese can then be discarded.

WHAT WENT WRONG?

Ambivalence about foreign foods and foreign people seems to be deeply entrenched in human nature. Most of the time, these fears stay more or less in balance with the opposing desire for novelty and exploration. But as soon as somebody gets sick, we tend to round up the least popular ethnic group. This was true when Americans blamed Haitians for AIDS in 1981 and when Europeans blamed Jewish people for the Black Death in 1349. We always seem to assume that foreigners will do weird things to our food and social institutions if left to their own devices. Numerous urban legends reinforce this idea, such as the story of the American couple who brought their dog to a Chinese restaurant and asked the waiter to feed it. The waiter disappeared into the kitchen leading the dog, and returned carrying it on a plate with sauce. But note that the couple had entered the restaurant voluntarily in the first place. The exotic food—most of it, anyway—was too delicious to resist.

NOTE

1. G. Taliani et al., "Lumbar Pain in a Married Couple who Likes Cheese: Brucella Strikes Again!" *Clinical and Experimental Rheumatology*, Vol. 22, 2004, pp. 477–480.

REFERENCES AND RECOMMENDED READING

Altekruse, S. F., et al. "Cheese-Associated Outbreaks of Human Illness in the United States, 1973 to 1992: Sanitary Manufacturing Practices Protect Consumers." *Journal of Food Protection*, Vol. 61, 1998, pp. 1405–1407.

Altman, L. K. "Cheese Microbe Underscores Mystery." *New York Times*, 2 July 1985.

"A Bad Bug." *Diabetes Forecast*, September 1999.

Bannister, B. A. "*Listeria monocytogenes* Meningitis Associated with Soft Cheese." *Journal of Infection*, Vol. 15, 1987, pp. 165–168.

Bemrah, N., et al. "Quantitative Risk Assessment of Human Listeriosis from Consumption of Soft Cheese Made from Raw Milk." *Preventive Veterinary Medicine*, Vol. 37, 1998, pp. 129–145.

"Big Stink over Smelly Cheese." *Time International*, 26 April 1999.

Bren, L. "Got Milk? Make Sure It's Pasteurized." *FDA Consumer*, September–October 2004.

"Canadian Health Officials Warn Against Raw Milk Cheese." *Dairy Foods*, August 2007.

De Buyser, M. L., et al. "Implication of Milk and Milk Products in Food-Borne Diseases in France and in Different Industrialised Countries." *International Journal of Food Microbiology*, Vol. 67, 2001, pp. 1–17.

Farber, J. M., and J. Z. Losos. "*Listeria monocytogenes*: A Foodborne Pathogen." *Canadian Medical Association Journal*, Vol. 138, 1988, pp. 413–418.

Farber, J. M., et al. "Health Risk Assessment of *Listeria monocytogenes* in Canada." *International Journal of Food Microbiology*, Vol. 30, 1996, pp. 145–156.

"FDA Warns of Contaminated Cheese." Associated Press, 15 August 1986.

Fleming, D. W., et al. "Pasteurized Milk as a Vehicle of Infection in an Outbreak of Listeriosis." *New England Journal of Medicine*, Vol. 31, 1985, pp. 404–407.

Halweil, B. "Setting the Cheese Whiz Standard." *WorldWatch*, November/December 2000.

James, S. M., et al. "Epidemiologic Notes and Reports: Listeriosis Outbreak Associated with Mexican-Style Cheese—California." *Morbidity and Mortality Weekly Report*, Vol. 34, 1985, pp. 357–359.

Jemmi, T., and R. Stephan. "*Listeria monocytogenes*: Food-Borne Pathogen and Hygiene Indicator." *Revue Scientifique et Technique*, Vol. 25, 2006, pp. 571–580.

Linnan, M. J., et al. "Epidemic Listeriosis Associated with Mexican-Style Cheese." *New England Journal of Medicine*, Vol. 319, 1988, pp. 823–828.

McLaughlin, L. "Off the Gourmet Shelves." *Time*, 20 September 2004.

Mellgren, J. "White Heat: Pasteurization vs. Raw-Milk Cheese." *Gourmet Retailer*, March 2005.

Park, A. "The Raw Deal." *Time*, 12 May 2008.

Pearson, L. J., and E. H. Marth. "*Listeria monocytogenes*—Threat to a Safe Food Supply." *Journal of Dairy Science*, Vol. 73, 1990, pp. 912–928.

Petrak, L. "Safety Locks: Foodborne Illness Rates Drop as Dairy Processors Continue to Implement Safety and Security Measures." *Dairy Field*, September 2005.

Planck, N. "The Raw Truth." *Bon Appetit*, May 2008.

"Rogue Creamery Makes Cheese History in Europe." *Dairy Foods*, December 2006.

Ryser, E. T., and E. H. Marth. " 'New' Food-Borne Pathogens of Public Health Significance." *Journal of the American Dietetic Association*, Vol. 89, 1989, pp. 948–954.

Saltijeral, J. A., et al. "Presence of Listeria in Mexican Cheeses." *Journal of Food Safety*, Vol. 19, 2007, pp. 241–247.

Sanaa, M., et al. "Risk Assessment of Listeriosis Linked to the Consumption of Two Soft Cheeses Made from Raw Milk: Camembert of Normandy and Brie of Meaux." *Risk Analysis*, Vol. 24, 2004, pp. 389–399.

Scholliers, P. "Defining Food Risks and Food Anxieties Throughout History." *Appetite*, Vol. 51, 2008, pp. 3–6.

Schwarzkopf, A. "*Listeria monocytogenes*—Aspects of Pathogenicity." *Pathologie-Biologie*, Vol. 44, 1996, pp. 769–774.

Vasavada, P. C. "Pathogenic Bacteria in Milk—A Review." *Journal of Dairy Science*, Vol. 71, 1988, pp. 2809–2816.

21

Fear of Mercury in Seafood

> Learning is like mercury, one of the most powerful and excellent things in the world in skillful hands; in unskillful, the most mischievous.
>
> —Alexander Pope, *Thoughts on Various Subjects* (1727)

SUMMARY

People have known for thousands of years that exposure to high levels of mercury can cause severe illness or death. Scientists have recently shown that mercury levels in human tissues are correlated with (among other things) consumption of tuna and certain other large fish. A compound called methylmercury is gradually building up in the oceans, probably as a result of industrial air and water pollution, and this chemical can accumulate in the bodies of fish. (It is not the same as the mercury compound in thimerosal, discussed in the vaccine chapters.) But are most American seafood consumers really exposed to dangerous levels of mercury? Probably not—yet—but consumers should heed EPA warnings. Since fish contains important nutrients that may outweigh the mercury risk, at least up to a poorly defined point, the fear of *not* eating fish has emerged as a secondary health scare. These issues have fizzled only in the sense that the level of risk is not fully understood, and multiple competing health scares and economic concerns have interfered with consumer response.

SOURCE

Most Americans probably heard about the tragic epidemic of mercury poisoning at Japan's Minamata Bay in the 1950s and 1960s (see Science), but it was far away and resulted from industrial pollution that seemed unlikely to occur in countries with more stringent environmental laws, such as the United States. Occasional outbreaks of mercury poisoning were reported in agricultural areas where mercury-based fungicides were used on crops, but ocean-caught fish seemed safe. By 1970, however, U.S. scientists were reporting unexpectedly high levels of mercury in American and Canadian rivers, and inevitably the oceans and their inhabitants were found to be polluted as well. Some scientists believed that the mercury found in tuna and other fish did not exceed safe levels; others disagreed, and the controversy has raged ever since.

We might have put this health scare in the section on chemical hazards instead, were it not for the fact that seafood and mercury are no longer separable. The hazard is the mercury, not the fish itself; but despite claims to the contrary, there is no known way to remove significant amounts of mercury from fish, or to prevent wild fish from accumulating mercury in their tissues. Eat large marine fish, and you eat mercury. Regulating factory waste might reduce the problem in specific locations and prevent a repeat of Minamata Bay, but no known precaution will stop the buildup of atmospheric mercury in the oceans. Also, since fish provide valuable nutrients, a diet without fish can also have negative health effects.

SCIENCE

Mercury (Hg) is a chemical element that has existed since the formation of the universe. The element itself is not a human invention, and the total amount of mercury present on Earth remains constant. Its distribution, however, changes as a result of both natural and industrial processes. Major sources of atmospheric mercury include volcanoes, coal-fired power plants, gold mine tailings, and municipal waste incinerators. Mercury levels in Earth's oceans and rivers appear to be increasing mainly as a result of deposition from the atmosphere. According to a 2009 study, methylmercury in the northern Pacific Ocean will reach twice its 1995 level by the year 2050. When that happens, it may become necessary to reevaluate the wisdom of eating tuna and other fish.

Methylmercury (CH_3Hg+) is an organic cation (positively charged molecule) that contains mercury. It is present not only in sea water but also in some manmade fungicides used on grain and other crops. Unlike most other mercury compounds, methylmercury can build up in living organisms—a process known as bioaccumulation—and some large ocean fish, such as tuna, contain significant amounts of this compound. It is unclear how many Americans develop low-level mercury poisoning each year as a result of eating ocean-caught fish. Estimates range from zero to thousands, depending on the source and the criteria for poisoning.

When people eat fish, contaminated grain, or other foods that contain very high levels of methylmercury, they may develop severe, incurable neurological problems, such as convulsions, lack of coordination, impaired vision and hearing, dementia, and coma. If the consumer is a pregnant woman, the fetus is also at risk. Mercury poisoning is sometimes called hydrargyria or mercurialism. Major outbreaks of methylmercury poisoning have occurred in Japan, the Middle East, Guatemala, and Ghana. The most notorious cases associated with seafood occurred between 1956 and 1965 in Japan, where the fish contained much higher than "normal" levels of methylmercury because factories had dumped chemical waste directly into coastal waters. The resulting condition, called Minamata disease, was eventually identified as severe mercury poisoning.

Lower levels of mercury poisoning are not always apparent, and sources do not agree as to what constitutes an acceptable level. Studies of the effects of mercury from seafood have also yielded inconsistent results. For example, in one 2008 study, pregnant women who ate fish actually had babies with *higher* developmental scores than those who did not eat fish. Of course, this result does not imply that mercury is good for the fetus; it proves only that more than one variable was in play. Women who ate low to moderate levels of fish had healthier babies (on average) than those who ate no fish, because fish contains nutrients called omega-3 fatty acids, which promote brain development. But women who ate a great deal of fish had slightly less healthy babies than those who ate no fish, because the harmful effects of the mercury outweighed the beneficial effects of the omega-3 fatty acids.

HISTORY

In 210 B.C., the Chinese emperor Qin Shi Huang reportedly went insane and then died after his doctors gave him mercury pills that were intended to make him immortal. In a sense, they succeeded; certainly his legend will live forever. His tomb (not yet excavated as of 2010) reportedly contained elaborate defenses, including rivers of flowing mercury and carvings made from cinnabar, a toxic mercury ore.

The ancient Egyptians, Greeks, and Romans also recognized the power of mercury and used it in a wide range of drugs and cosmetics. Medieval alchemists believed that mercury was the key to transforming base metals into gold, if only they could get the formula just right. In Victorian England, long before the invention of antibiotics, doctors used a mercury compound called calomel (Hg_2Cl_2) to treat syphilis and other sexually transmitted diseases. That quaint custom was the basis of the saying "A night with Venus [the goddess of love], a lifetime with Mercury." When the patient began to salivate and urinate to excess, losing his teeth and hair and eventually his mind, the doctors knew this powerful drug must be working to expel bad stuff from his body. It is unclear if calomel could actually cure syphilis or any other disease. At one point, patent medicine dealers sold tomato pills as a substitute (Chapter 16). Mercury was also used in the manufacture of hats in the same era, and personal protective equipment was not yet in general use, so the "mad hatter" became a familiar figure—although medical historians have recently argued that the *Alice in Wonderland* character of that name showed symptoms that were inconsistent with mercury poisoning.

In other words, doctors and scientists were aware of the toxicity of mercury long before the twentieth century, and it is unclear how the tragedy at Minamata Bay ever took place. The factories that reportedly dumped mercury waste into waters where people caught fish, and the government that failed to stop them, have paid damages to survivors for decades.

As recently as the 1960s, children's chemistry sets and "mercury mazes" sold in the United States contained small amounts of liquid metallic mercury, and it was really fun to handle. Less obvious exposures also occur; for example, in 2004, a day-care center in New Jersey occupied a contaminated building that was formerly a thermometer factory. Many children were exposed to elemental mercury and required medical evaluation.

CONSEQUENCES

Not everyone agrees that environmental mercury is a disaster in progress, and the debate has inspired both sides to make exaggerated claims. For example, one source has claimed that the alleged architects of this health scare—environmental scientists and activists—are responsible for limiting the intellectual capacity of an entire generation of low-income children, thus making it harder than ever for them to break the cycle of poverty. The reasoning here is that the mercury in tuna was never harmful in the first place, but that canned tuna is the only food rich in omega-3 fatty acids that low-income families can afford. In other words, since omega-3 fatty acids are good for brain development, succumbing to political pressure by *not* eating tuna supposedly makes people less intelligent.

Anyone who took this accusation seriously might feel insulted by it: the low-income children, their parents struggling to feed them, the dastardly environmentalists, or all the people who simply do not like tuna. We considered adding another chapter entitled "Fear of Not Eating Tuna," but it sounded too ridiculous. Yes, fish contains important nutrients, but humans are highly adaptable omnivores. A child can grow up in poverty (or in a vegetarian household) with no tuna or sushi and still accomplish great things.

At the other extreme, some sources have blamed even low-level methylmercury exposure for a wide range of health problems, including autism. As also discussed in several other chapters, autism is such a devastating condition that nearly everything has been blamed for it: bad parenting, measles, the vaccine used to prevent measles, bottle feeding, pesticides, ultraviolet light, magnetic fields, monosodium glutamate—the list is endless. Everybody wants to find the evil and banish it. The problem with the bandwagon approach, however, is that it may interfere with more objective study. Making parents afraid of everything, or eroding their ability to distinguish fact from fiction, cannot be good for their children either.

Another consequence of the mercury health scare is increased consumer demand for test kits that measure the level of mercury in human body fluids or in seafood. It is unclear how accurate these tests are, or what action is appropriate if they detect mercury. Contaminated fish can be thrown away, fed to the cat, or returned to the store; but what about mercury in our own bodies? Naturally, health food stores and Web sites that sell the test kits also sell antioxidants and herbal potions that are supposed to flush the body of excess mercury. According to these vendors, such vague symptoms as headache, fatigue, perspiration, or a runny nose all point to mercury poisoning. One such Web site claims that even a single atom of mercury in the body is harmful. That is ridiculous. Doctors sometimes treat severe mercury poisoning with drugs called chelating agents, but their use is controversial and not something to experiment with at home.

In 2008, American actor Jeremy Piven reportedly developed symptoms of mercury poisoning after consuming large amounts of fish for 20 years, and the incident set off a prolonged media debate.

WHAT WENT WRONG?

Mercury contamination is an extremely complicated problem, both for scientists and for the news media. Telling people that tuna and other large fish contain potentially toxic levels of mercury, but then telling them to eat it anyway because they need the omega-3 fatty acids, is a compromise that appears to have backfired. Meanwhile, people must eat something, and with so many health scares involving so many foods, it is hard to know which warnings to take seriously.

REFERENCES AND RECOMMENDED READING

Berman, R. "The Unintended Consequences of the Activist-Driven Mercury Scare Hurt the Public, and Kids in Particular." *Nation's Restaurant News*, 29 September 2008.

Burger, J., et al. "Do Scientists and Fishermen Collect the Same Size Fish? Possible Implications for Exposure Assessment." *Environmental Research*, Vol. 101, 2006, pp. 34–41.

Chen, C. Y., et al. "Methylmercury in Marine Ecosystems—from Sources to Seafood Consumers." *Environmental Health Perspectives*, Vol. 116, 2008, pp. 1706–1712.

Chick, N. H. "I'll Miss You Tuna." *Useless Knowledge*, 9 August 2004.

Choi, A. L., et al. "Negative Confounding in the Evaluation of Toxicity: The Case of Methylmercury in Fish and Seafood." *Critical Reviews in Toxicology*, Vol. 38, 2008, pp. 877–893.

Choi, A. L., et al. "Methylmercury Exposure and Adverse Cardiovascular Events in Faroese Whaling Men." *Environmental Health Perspectives*, Vol. 117, 2009, pp. 367–372.

Clarkson, T. W. "The Three Modern Faces of Mercury." *Environmental Health Perspectives*, Vol. 110 (Suppl. 1), 2002, pp. 11–23.

Clifton, J. C. "Mercury Exposure and Public Health." *Pediatric Clinics of North America*, Vol. 54, 2007, pp. 237–269.

Díez, S. "Human Health Effects of Methylmercury Exposure." *Reviews of Environmental Contamination and Toxicology*, Vol. 198, 2009, pp. 111–132.

Eyl, T. "Tempest in a Teapot." *American Journal of Clinical Nutrition*, Vol. 24, 1971, pp. 1199–1203.

Fineberg, H. V. "Balancing the Scales of Health: The Science Behind Eating Seafood." *Medscape General Medicine*, Vol. 9, 2007, p. 34.

Foley, D. "Healthy . . . or Harmful?" *Prevention*, October 2006.

Geier, D. A., et al. "A Comprehensive Review of Mercury Provoked Autism." *Indian Journal of Medical Research*, Vol. 128, 2008, pp. 383–411.

Grandjean, P., et al. "Human Milk as a Source of Methylmercury Exposure in Infants." *Environmental Health Perspectives*, Vol. 102, 1994, pp. 74–77.

Hertz-Picciotto, I., et al. "Blood Mercury Concentrations in CHARGE Study Children with and without Autism." *Environmental Health Perspectives*, 19 October 2009.

Hughner, R. S., et al. "Review of Food Policy and Consumer Issues of Mercury in Fish." *Journal of the American College of Nutrition*, Vol. 27, 2008, pp. 185–194.

Lederman, S. A., et al. "Relation between Cord Blood Mercury Levels and Early Child Development in a World Trade Center Cohort." *Environmental Health Perspectives*, Vol. 116, 2008, pp. 1085–1091.

Lite, J. "What is Mercury Poisoning?" *Scientific American*, 19 December 2008.

Lumière, E. "Fish: Healthy or Toxic?" *Harper's Bazaar*, May 2004, p. 86.

"Mercury Poisoning—Not Just Another Scare." *United Press International*, 29 November 1970.

Mozaffarian, D. "Fish, Mercury, Selenium and Cardiovascular Risk: Current Evidence and Unanswered Questions." *International Journal of Environmental Research and Public Health*, Vol. 6, 2009, pp. 1894–1916.

Mozaffarian, D., and E. B. Rimm. "Fish Intake, Contaminants, and Human Health: Evaluating the Risks and the Benefits." *Journal of the American Medical Association*, Vol. 296, 2006, pp. 1885–1899.

Neth, M. "Danger in the Daily Diet." *Stars and Stripes*, 23 April 1982.

Oken, E., and D. C. Bellinger. "Fish Consumption, Methylmercury and Child Neurodevelopment." *Current Opinion in Pediatrics*, Vol. 20, 2008, pp. 178–183.

"Poisoning Suit Ends with Big Settlement." Associated Press, 3 February 1976.

Saldana, M., et al. "Diet-Related Mercury Poisoning Resulting in Visual Loss." *British Journal of Ophthalmology*, Vol. 90, 2006, pp. 1432–1434.

Sunderland, E. M., et al. "Mercury Sources, Distribution, and Bioavailability in the North Pacific Ocean: Insights from Data and Models." *Global Biogeochemical Cycles*, 1 May 2009.

U.S. Environmental Protection Agency. Mercury Study Report to Congress, Volume I: Executive Summary. EPA-452/R-97-003, December 1997.

Wobeser, G. "Mercury Poisoning from Fish." *Canadian Medical Association Journal*, Vol. 102, 1970, p. 1209.

22

Java Madness

May God deprive of this drink the foolish man who condemns it with incurable obstinacy.
—Abd-al-Kadir ibn Mohammed, *In Praise of Coffee* (1511)

SUMMARY

Although coffee is one of the world's most popular beverages and the object of extravagant claims, people keep finding things wrong with it. At various times in history, doctors, journalists, religious leaders, and sellers of competing beverages have blamed coffee for heart disease, stroke, high blood pressure, birth defects, miscarriage, stomach ulcers, menstrual cramps, impotence, nervous irritability, immoral conduct, and cancers of the throat, stomach, pancreas, and bladder. At the time this book was written, the consensus appeared to be that coffee and other caffeinated drinks are harmless when consumed in moderation, and may even confer some (limited) health benefits. In other words, this health scare appears to be in a temporary state of fizzle, analogous to that of a volcano that may be either dormant or dead.

SOURCE

Coffee in something like its present form has existed for centuries, and it would be impossible to say when someone first started worrying about its health effects. In fact, to the extent that caffeine heightens the capacity for critical thinking or jangles the nerves, the chemical itself might promote such concerns. As early as the sixteenth century, religious leaders in the Ottoman Empire voiced some concerns about coffee and the ideologically liberated places where people drank it. By tradition, Muslims do not use intoxicants, but the effects of caffeine were quite unlike those of alcohol, and coffee quickly caught on throughout the Muslim world. The Catholic Church also disapproved of coffee on moral grounds, until Pope Clement VIII (1536–1605) tried it and liked it.

Since then, the story of coffee has been one of nervous fretting rather than outright persecution. The Church of Jesus Christ of Latter-Day Saints (LDS) discourages its members from drinking hot beverages, including hot coffee. LDS further advises its members to avoid anything that is not "wholesome and prudent," including anything that contains caffeine. The Seventh-Day Adventists also discourage the use of coffee, not because of its temperature, but for the specific reason that caffeine is a stimulant.

Some diet doctors and health-food practitioners take a third tack, advising people to avoid all cooked or processed foods and beverages, including coffee. So there are at least three philosophical reasons for avoiding coffee, but they are all somewhat vague. If hot drinks are bad, what about soup? If coffee contains more antioxidants than grape juice, why is it not wholesome? If stimulants are bad, what about ginseng? And if all processed food is bad, what about yogurt?

SCIENCE

Long ago, on an Ethiopian hillside, there lived a plant (*Coffea arabica* and related species) that would one day change the world. According to a popular legend, the culture bearer who first recognized the true nature of this wondrous plant was a young goatherd named Kaldi in the ninth century A.D., who noticed that his goats stayed awake all night after munching some of the cherry-like fruit of a certain bush—what we now call coffee beans. This is a cute story with the ring of fakelore; more likely, people in that region had known the properties of coffee and other local plants for thousands of years. Cacao, tea, and some other plants also provide caffeine, but none with quite the bada-bing of coffee.

About 55 percent of the U.S. population drinks coffee every day, and an estimated 90 percent of the global population uses caffeine in some form. Studies appear to show that caffeine sharpens the intellect, heightens creativity, deadens pain, obviates the need for sleep, and reduces the risk of many diseases—liver cancer, alcohol-related cirrhosis of the liver, diabetes, gout, cataracts, and even Alzheimer's disease. Perhaps best of all, caffeine gives people something relatively harmless to argue about: is coffee bad for us, or not? And which coffee is best, Starbucks or Dunkin' Donuts or Kopi Luwak?

Coffee has been called the "beverage of truth," but the reason is unclear. Studies of caffeine, like those of alcohol and tobacco, are often poorly designed, strongly biased, and inconclusive. It's an old story; scientists who publish their research findings in peer-reviewed journals are often required to disclose any potential conflicts of interest—for example, if they use the product they are studying, or own stock in the company that makes it. But who among us can claim to be unbiased on the subject of caffeine?

That said, we will examine some recent studies and issues related to this controversial subject:

- Does caffeine cause high blood pressure? Some sources say yes, others say no. Finally, a 2008 study appears to provide the answer. yes *and* no. When the investigators drew a graph of caffeine consumption against blood pressure, they did not get a straight line, but an inverse U shape (∩). In other words, BP was elevated in some people who drank only one or two cups of coffee per day, but it was normal in those who drank more than six cups per day.
- Does caffeine cause heart failure? Some older studies appear to show that people who drank at least 5 cups of coffee every day—that is, the equivalent of about 10 bottles of caffeinated soda—had increased risk of heart failure. However, a 2009 study of over 37,000 Swedish men found no such effect.
- Does coffee cause breast cancer? Some early studies raised that possibility, but in 2009, doctors released the results of a 10-year study involving some 38,000 women.

There was no evidence that even hardcore coffee drinkers were at increased risk for breast cancer.

- Does coffee cause other forms of cancer? Not as far as we can tell. On the contrary, a recent study claims that coffee drinking reduces the risk of head and neck cancer by 39 percent.
- Does coffee cause headaches, or does it cure them? Yes, both.
- Does coffee cause bone loss? Yes, but the loss is measurable only in people who take in at least 400 mg of caffeine per day, or about six 8-ounce cups of coffee.
- Does coffee make people crazy? Sources vary, but it appears that coffee may worsen symptoms of existing schizophrenia. Also, in at least one reported case, a high dose of caffeine caused temporary psychosis in an otherwise healthy man.
- Does coffee increase the risk of rheumatoid arthritis? Yes, according to a 2002 study of 31,000 people. No, according to a 2005 study of 57,000 people.
- Is coffee devoid of valuable nutrients? No, not quite. A 2006 study showed that a typical serving of coffee contains more antioxidants than a serving of grape juice, blueberries, raspberries, or oranges. Who knew?

HISTORY

Not all the historic opposition to coffee has been medical or religious in nature. For centuries, coffeehouses have been known as places where buzzed-up intellectuals assemble to drink coffee, play chess, and plan to overthrow the existing social order. The first serious centers of coffee drinking apparently were in fifteenth-century Yemen and Saudi Arabia, and the custom and the plant soon spread from there to Europe, Southeast Asia, and the Americas. The Dutch grew coffee in greenhouses and later in their colonies, particularly in Java, a name that is now synonymous with coffee.

Once large-scale coffee plantations appeared in Brazil in the early nineteenth century, coffee ceased to be an elitist luxury and became the drink of the common people. The early history of coffee was inextricably bound to that of slavery, as the European growers tended to enlist and exploit local people to work in the fields. In the late nineteenth century, Brazilian coffee plants finally circled the globe and reached east Africa, not far from their place of origin.

In the mid-to-late twentieth century, coffee houses in the San Francisco Bay area helped launch the beatnik and hippie movements that would transform American culture. More recently, upscale cappuccino and espresso bars have become so popular that fast-food restaurants have begun to offer more or less equivalent products. For many, coffee is not only a favorite topic of conversation but the basis of existence. For Internet users and texters, perhaps the ultimate statement of moral outrage or blindsiding is the Unix expression C|N>K, which means "coffee through nose into keyboard."

Coffee preparation methods have also evolved over the years. According to some sources, the coffee delivery system of choice in ancient Ethiopia was a ball of ground seeds mixed with animal fat, suitable for chewing on long journeys. Sometimes the raw seeds were also boiled to make a medicinal drink similar to tea. By the late fifteenth century, people were roasting and crushing the seeds and extracting their essence with hot water, as we do today. Instant and freeze-dried forms of coffee did not become widely available until the mid-twentieth century. Suffice it to say that each preparation method and each brand of coffee has its opponents and associated health scares. For example, some studies appear to show that drinking brewed coffee (but not instant coffee) may increase the serum cholesterol level, and purveyors of urban legend claim that one specific brand of coffee contains dangerous levels of nicotine, which, of course, it does not.

CONSEQUENCES

The American coffee vendor Dunkin' Donuts reportedly sells nearly 1 billion cups of coffee per year, or 30 cups of coffee every second. Global coffee production for 2010 is estimated at 7 million metric tons. Kaldi the goatherd would be astonished. Yet despite the popularity and alleged benefits of coffee, people often express the wish or intention to drink less of it. Many a broken New Year's resolution has reflected this theme. If coffee is such great stuff, why quit?

According to the 2009 National Coffee Drinking Trends survey, coffee is one institution that appears to be largely recession-proof. People still spend their money on this seemingly unnecessary beverage. During the economic recession of 2009, nearly everything else went out the window—jobs, education, social programs, faith in government—but not coffee. Kaldi the goatherd is no doubt smiling down on us, or, more likely, laughing at us.

WHAT WENT WRONG?

Anything that is powerful can be turned to the dark side. Coffee clearly is powerful, since the majority of people on Earth drink it and many claim to be dependent on it. But despite years of research, we still do not know for certain if coffee has any harmful effects. In a long-term prospective study, unlike a well-controlled clinical trial of a drug, the researchers must rely on self-reported data that may be highly inaccurate. People do not always remember or admit exactly what they ate, drank, or did. Also, caffeine content varies greatly from one brand or batch of coffee to another, so even if people accurately report how many cups they drink, their caffeine intake may be hard to estimate. Thus, it seems likely that the quest for the truth about coffee will continue, and that new discoveries await researchers in this recession-proof field of endeavor.

REFERENCES AND RECOMMENDED READING

Ahmed, H. N., et al. "Coffee Consumption and Risk of Heart Failure in Men: An Analysis from the Cohort of Swedish Men." *American Heart Journal*, Vol. 158, 2009, pp. 667–672.

Alpert, J. S. "Hey, Doc, Is It OK for Me to Drink Coffee?" *American Journal of Medicine*, Vol. 122, 2009, pp. 597–598.

Bakalar, N. "Coffee as a Health Drink? Studies Find Some Benefits." *New York Times*, 15 August 2006.

Broderick, P., and A. B. Benjamin. "Caffeine and Psychiatric Symptoms: A Review." *Journal of the Oklahoma State Medical Association*, Vol. 97, 2004, pp. 538–542.

"Coffee Linked to Less Liver Fibrosis." United Press International, 5 January 2010.

Foley, D. "Healthy . . . or Harmful?" *Prevention*, October 2006.

Galeone, C., et al. "Coffee and Tea Intake and Risk of Head and Neck Cancer." *Cancer Epidemiology*, Biomarkers and Prevention, Vol. 19, 2010, pp. 1723–1736.

Geleijnse, J. M. "Habitual Coffee Consumption and Blood Pressure: An Epidemiological Perspective." *Vascular Health and Risk Management*, Vol. 4, 2008, pp. 963–970.

Greenberg, J. A. "Coffee, Diabetes, and Weight Control." *American Journal of Clinical Nutrition*, Vol. 84, 2006, pp. 682–693.

"Headaches and Coffee." *British Medical Journal*, Vol. 2, 1977, p. 284.

Hedges, D. W., et al. "Caffeine-Induced Psychosis." *CNS Spectrums*, Vol. 14, 2009, pp. 127–129.

Lopez-Garcia, E., et al. "The Relationship of Coffee Consumption with Mortality." *Annals of Internal Medicine*, Vol. 148, 2008, pp. 904–914.

Lopez-Garcia, E., et al. "Coffee Consumption and Risk of Stroke in Women." *Circulation*, Vol. 119, 2009, pp. 1116–1123.

Lozano R., P., et al. "Caffeine: A Nutrient, a Drug or a Drug of Abuse." *Adicciones*, Vol. 19, 2007, pp. 225–238. [Spanish]

Luciano, M., et al. " 'No Thanks, It Keeps Me Awake': The Genetics of Coffee-Attributed Sleep Disturbance." *Sleep*, Vol. 30, 2007, pp. 1378–1386.

Mikuls, T. R., et al. "Coffee, Tea, and Caffeine Consumption and Risk of Rheumatoid Arthritis: Results from the Iowa Women's Health Study." *Arthritis and Rheumatism*, Vol. 46, 2002, pp. 83–91.

Muncie, H. L. "The Safety of Caffeine Consumption." *American Family Physician*, Vol. 76, 2007, pp. 1285–1286.

Pendergrast, Mark. 1999. *Uncommon Grounds*. New York: Basic Books.

Reissig, C. J., et al. "Caffeinated Energy Drinks—A Growing Problem." *Drug and Alcohol Dependence*, Vol. 99, 2009, pp. 1–10.

Shils, M. E., and M. G. Hermann. "Unproved Dietary Claims in the Treatment of Patients with Cancer." *Bulletin of the New York Academy of Medicine*, Vol. 58, 1982, pp. 323–340.

van Dam, R. M. "Coffee Consumption and Coronary Heart Disease: Paradoxical Effects on Biological Risk Factors versus Disease Incidence." *Clinical Chemistry*, Vol. 54, 2008, pp. 1489–1496.

Varma, S. D., et al. "UV-B-Induced Damage to the Lens in Vitro: Prevention by Caffeine." *Journal of Ocular Pharmacology and Therapeutics*, Vol. 24, 2008, pp. 439–444.

Vlachopoulos, C., et al. "Chronic Coffee Consumption has a Detrimental Effect on Aortic Stiffness and Wave Reflections." *American Journal of Clinical Nutrition*, Vol. 81, 2005, pp. 1307–1312.

23

Fear of *Salmonella*

I aimed at the public's heart, and by accident I hit it in the stomach.
                                         —Upton Sinclair, on his novel *The Jungle* (1906)

SUMMARY

Manufacturers and regulatory agencies recall foods and other consumer products for many reasons. One of the most frequent is known or suspected contamination with non-typhoidal *Salmonella* bacteria. The resulting gastrointestinal upset, called salmonellosis, usually does not exceed the proverbial Montezuma's Revenge, but it often causes large outbreaks and occasionally becomes more serious. Salmonellosis affects an estimated 1 to 2 million people every year in the United States alone, and it is a reliable source of highly publicized class action lawsuits. Other food recalls have involved *E. coli* (Chapter 18), *Listeria* (Chapter 20), and other pathogenic bacteria, but this chapter will focus on *Salmonella* alone. Although deaths from foodborne illness are relatively infrequent in the United States, the total economic impact of these outbreaks and recalls is substantial—an estimated $152 billion per year as of 2010. The problem itself will never fizzle, but consumer perception of death lurking in every head of lettuce may be on the wane.

SOURCE

The United States has experienced numerous multistate or nationwide outbreaks of food poisoning in recent years (Table 23.1)All these outbreaks have much in common, as illustrated by the three examples in the History section:

- The cantaloupe recall of 2007
- The tomato recall of 2008
- The peanut recall of 2009

Although salmonellosis is rarely fatal, it is one of many diseases that healthcare providers are required to report to the U.S. Centers for Disease Control and Prevention (CDC). The CDC compiles the resulting data, investigates the outbreaks, and publishes its findings in *Morbidity and Mortality Weekly Reports* (MMWR) and other periodicals.

Table 23.1. **Examples of Recent Food Recalls due to** *Salmonella*

Date	Location	Food	Volume	Cases
Sept 2005	U.S.	Orange juice		0
Oct 2005	U.S.	Clam meat		0
Dec 2005	U.S. & Canada	Anchovies		2+
Mar 2006	Minnesota	Chicken	75,000+ lb.	>1 [USDA/FSIS]
June 2006	U.S. & Canada	Fruit salad		41
July 2006	U.S & Canada	Salad mix		0(?)
Aug 2006	Florida	Alfalfa sprouts		[See FDA]
Nov 2006	U.S. (4+ states)	Cantaloupe	504 cartons	n/a
Nov 2006	U.S. & Canada	Dessert topping		
Feb 2007	Western U.S.	Cantaloupe		0
Mar 2007	California	Fruit trays	1,000+ lb	0
Mar 2007	New Jersey	Dog food		0
Apr 2007	U.S.	Dog food		0
June 2007	U.S. (17 states)	Veggie snacks		51+
Oct 2007	Hawaii	Frozen tuna	5,452 lb.	>1 (check)
Oct 2007	U.S. (35 states)	Pot pies		272+
Nov 2007	U.S. (5+ states)	Ground beef	alert only	[USDA]
Mar 2008	U.S. & Canada	Cantaloupe	n/a	50+
Mar 2008	U.S. (6+ states)	Alfalfa sprouts		
Apr 2008	U.S.	Puffed cereals		21+
May 2008	Florida	Pork cracklings	1,100 lb.	0
June 2008	U.S. & Canada	Jalapeño		1200+
July 2008	U.S. (3+ states)	Basil		0 (?)
Aug 2008	California & Nevada	Dog food		0
Oct 2008	U.S. (15 states)	Cat food		0
Jan 2009	U.S. (40+ states)	Peanut butter		600+
Mar 2009	Nebraska	Alfalfa sprouts		228+
Apr 2009	U.S. (3 states)	Mayonnaise		0
Apr 2009	U.S. (5+ states)	Spices		90+
Apr 2009	U.S.	Pistachio nuts	1 million lb+	>1 (check)
May 2009	U.S. (3+ states)	Cantaloupe	n/a	n/a
June 2009	U.S. (11+ states)	Ground beef	825,000+ lb.	40+
July 2009	Texas	Cilantro	104 crates	0
Aug 2009	Michigan	Alfalfa sprouts	n/a	12+
Aug 2009	U.S. (9+ states)	Green onions	3,360 boxes	0
Sep 2009	Texas & Louisiana	Red pepper		0
Sep 2009	U.S. & Canada	Spinach	1,715 boxes	0
Sep 2009	U.S.	Tahini	840 cases	0
Nov 2009	U.S. (10 states)	Cantaloupes		0

Unusual outbreaks often attract the attention of the news media, and all outbreaks attract the attention of law firms that specialize in personal injury litigation.

Depending on the type of food and the circumstances of the outbreak, a government agency such as the Food and Drug Administration (FDA) or the U.S. Department of Agriculture (USDA) may request a product recall and notify the public. In some cases, the outbreak is not foodborne, and there is nothing to recall. For example, in 1996, at least 50 people contracted salmonellosis from contact with a fence surrounding a zoo exhibit of Komodo dragons, which have messy personal habits. In other cases, the outbreak results from a single contaminated batch of food that is gone by the time people start getting sick. A recall is helpful only if the problem is ongoing and likely to put others at risk.

A health scare can be "real" without being serious, and it can fizzle silently. Salmonellosis outbreaks are so frequent that they overlap in time like the shingles on a roof, and the moment when each related health scare starts or fizzles may be hard to identify. It might be the time when sales of the recalled or maligned product return to normal, or when the media start reporting the next outbreak.

SCIENCE

Nontyphoidal salmonellosis—acute diarrhea caused by *Salmonella* bacteria other than the ones that cause typhoid or paratyphoid fever—is extremely common in the United States and in the rest of the world. Its agent is a bacterium called *Salmonella enterica*, which exists in several different forms, or serovars. The disease causes profuse watery diarrhea, sometimes with vomiting, headache, and abdominal pain.

There are about 18 reported outbreaks and 40,000 to 100,000 reported cases of salmonellosis in the United States in a typical year, plus an estimated 38 unreported mild cases for every one reported. Thus, the actual number of U.S. cases per year may exceed 2 million, but very few people see their doctors and demand laboratory tests every time they have an upset stomach. The percentage of reported cases probably rises during a product recall, because mild illness suddenly takes on a new meaning. The death rate for uncomplicated salmonellosis is very low, usually on the order of 1 in every 2,000 to 3,000 untreated cases. The usual treatment is nothing more than rest and rehydration. Antibiotics may be needed, but like many bacteria, salmonellae have begun to show resistance.

Anyone who handles raw meat, owns a pet, eats raw vegetables or fruit, visits a zoo, or does practically anything else is at some risk for salmonellosis. But so what? This disease normally causes a mild case of diarrhea that lasts a couple of days, with the attendant discomfort and laundry problems. For most people, the only real danger is dehydration, so it is important to drink enough to replace lost fluid and electrolytes. The idea of being terrified of fresh spinach or other produce because of the possibility of contracting salmonellosis is absurd, except for people at high risk for complications, such as those with compromised immune systems. Some studies have shown that *Salmonella* bacteria may cause arthritis years after the initial infection; but since most people are exposed to salmonellosis, and most people also develop arthritis if they live long enough, it is hard to establish a connection.

HISTORY

The name of the bacterial genus *Salmonella* is a patronymic to honor American veterinary pathologist Daniel Elmer Salmon (1850–1914), the administrator of a USDA program that first discovered a form of salmonellosis in swine in 1885. In 1888, German microbiologist August Anton Hieronymus Gaertner (1848–1934), identified a related bacterium as the cause of a food poisoning epidemic in Germany. It soon became apparent that *Salmonella* was a major cause of food poisoning in humans.

In recent years, three typical salmonellosis outbreaks unfolded as follows:

The cantaloupe recall of 2007 started small. In February of that year, a wholesale produce importer announced that it was recalling some 2,560 cartons of cantaloupes that had been shipped to grocery stores in California. The FDA had tested the fruit and detected *Salmonella*, the importer advertised the recall, and that was that. Few, if any, illnesses were reported. But as the year progressed, at least five other importers encountered similar problems and ended up recalling a total of more than 700,000 potentially contaminated cantaloupes, most of them grown in Mexico or Costa Rica. The FDA is responsible for inspections of most foods other than meat and poultry, and as food imports have increased over the years, the understaffed agency has reportedly found it hard to keep up.

The tomato recall of 2008 was somewhat more serious. In May, the New Mexico Department of Health notified the CDC of several salmonellosis cases that appeared to be associated with raw produce. This outbreak soon expanded to include thousands of cases in at least 43 states, including two possibly related deaths. Meanwhile, the FDA identified the source of the outbreak more specifically as tomatoes and jalapeño peppers imported from Mexico. The CDC and the FDA issued nationwide public advisories, and the tomato industry had a black eye until the next product recall diverted public attention elsewhere. The CDC's conclusion was that enhanced food safety measures were needed.

The great peanut scandal of 2009 actually started in 2004, when a worker at a peanut butter processing plant in Georgia notified FDA of unsanitary conditions and *Salmonella* contamination. FDA investigated, but when the company refused to hand over its records, the matter was put on hold for three years and the whistleblower reportedly lost his job. (Or maybe not; accounts vary.) In 2007, FDA finally demanded the records, but agreed not to make them public. Even after the whistleblower's claims were verified, and hundreds of people had gotten sick, no action was taken other than a voluntary cleanup at the processing plant. Similar conditions existed at nearby facilities, but FDA did not have enough contract inspectors to keep track of all of them.

In January 2009, another peanut product manufacturer in Georgia announced the voluntary recall of a wide range of products that it had made during the previous six months. FDA inspectors reported that this firm had knowingly shipped peanut products contaminated with *Salmonella* on at least twelve occasions during the previous two years. The report further stated that there were large leaks in the roof directly above open product containers; that the same sink was used to wash hands, utensils, and mops; that raw and finished products were not adequately separated; and that a storage area was coated with "a slimy, black-brown residue."

In February 2010, "Goobergate" took a giant step forward when U.S. Federal Bureau of Investigation (FBI) agents raided one of the Georgia peanut butter processing plants in connection with the FDA's criminal investigation. As of that date, the outbreak had sickened somewhere between 600 and 19,000 people, depending on the source. At the time this book was written, the case was ongoing.

CONSEQUENCES

A milestone in the history of the salmonella health scare came in 2010, when an AirTran Airways flight attendant stopped a plane on the runway because a passenger had a small turtle in a cage. (Close contact with turtles may transmit salmonellosis.)

Frequent recalls of contaminated produce may lead the public to doubt the safety of raw fruits and vegetables. This perception may adversely affect public health if it drives more people to packaged junk food and microwaveable meals. Also, it is virtually impossible to keep track of all these alerts and recalls, so if a really serious one comes along, will anybody listen? Recalls of foods and other products have become so commonplace that some retail chain stores reportedly use customer loyalty cards to send automated recall announcements.

According to a 2007 Gallup poll, 71 percent of Americans had reacted to at least one food scare during the previous year, either by avoiding or discarding certain foods or by worrying about something they had eaten. A 2008 survey by the Rutgers Food Policy Institute showed that most Americans took food recalls seriously, but the survey also detected widespread misunderstanding of the government's role in the food recall process. For example, less than 10 percent of the sample realized that the government has no authority to force companies to recall products (other than baby formula).

People who will pay alternative practitioners good money to evacuate their colons by artificial means (Chapter 46) shudder at the thought of bacteria doing the same job for free. There are now *Salmonella* support groups—no, we are not kidding—and some law firms have Web sites that list all recent food recalls related to salmonella outbreaks or potential contamination, inviting victims to review their recent bathroom habits and sign up for a piece of the action. Online vendors are also doing a brisk business in home test kits for *Salmonella*.

In 2010, the FDA announced that it was in the process of drafting the first nationwide safety standards for the growing, harvesting, and packing of fresh produce.

WHAT WENT WRONG?

Since nobody likes the idea of getting sick from contaminated food or water, outbreaks of salmonellosis and other forms of food poisoning offer a reliable source of public outrage on a slow news day. Another problem is the prevailing view that the government must protect its citizens from every possible hazard, even a minor upset stomach from inadequately washed vegetables. Federal and state agencies simply are not adequately funded to provide this level of oversight.

Some outbreaks have even served to reinforce popular fears of bioterrorism. The world has not forgotten the obscure Oregon cult that spiked a salad bar with *Salmonella* in 1984, giving 751 people diarrhea. Had the terrorists used botulin toxin instead, half of those 751 people might have died. Why didn't somebody stop them? Mainly, because that would require intolerable security measures at every salad bar.

REFERENCES AND RECOMMENDED READING

Barak, J. D., et al. "Differential Attachment to and Subsequent Contamination of Agricultural Crops by *Salmonella enterica*." *Applied and Environmental Microbiology*, Vol. 74, 2008, pp. 5568–5570.

Brumback, K. "Tiny Caged Turtle Causes Taxiing AirTran Plane to Return to Gate." Associated Press, 25 June 2010.

Cronquist, A., et al. "Multistate Outbreak of *Salmonella typhimurium* Infections Associated with Eating Ground Beef—United States, 2004." *Morbidity and Mortality Weekly Reports*, 24 February 2006.

Cuite, C. L., et al. "Public Response to the Contaminated Spinach Recall of 2006." Rutgers University, Food Policy Institute, 5 February 2007.

Cuite, C. L., and W. K. Hallman. "Public Response to Large-Scale Produce Contamination." *Choices*, Vol. 24, 2009, pp. 21–25.

Darby, J., and H. Sheorey. "Searching for Salmonella." *Australian Family Physician*, Vol. 37, 2008, pp. 806–810.

Hallman, W. K., et al. "Consumer Responses to Food Recalls: 2008 National Survey Report." Rutgers University, Food Policy Institute, 14 April 2009.

Hanning, I. B., et al. "Salmonellosis Outbreaks in the United States due to Fresh Produce: Sources and Potential Intervention Measures." *Foodborne Pathogens and Disease*, Vol. 6, 2009, pp. 635–648.

Harrington, R. "Nationwide Food Recall System Unveiled in U.S." *Food Production Daily*, 23 September 2009.

Harris, G. "U.S. Food Safety No Longer Improving." *New York Times*, 10 April 2009.

Heilman, D. "A Full Plate: Growth in Foodborne Illness Cases Gives Lawyers Handling Them a Lot to Chew On." *Minnesota Lawyer*, 28 July 2008.

Herikstad, H., et al. "Emerging Quinolone-Resistant Salmonella in the United States." *Emerging Infectious Diseases*, Vol. 3, 1997, pp. 371–372.

Martin, A., and G. Harris. "Outbreaks Put Worry on the Table." *New York Times*, 11 May 2009.

Medus, C., et al. "Multistate Outbreak of Salmonella Infections Associated with Peanut Butter and Peanut Butter-Containing Products—United States, 2008–2009." *Morbidity and Mortality Weekly Reports*, Vol. 58, 2009, pp. 85–90.

Moss, M. "Peanut Case Shows Holes in Safety Net." *New York Times*, 9 February 2009.

Rabin, R. C. "Many Americans Unaware of Food Recalls, Survey Finds." *New York Times*, 14 February 2009.

Roberts, J. A. "Economic Aspects of Food-Borne Outbreaks and their Control." *British Medical Bulletin*, Vol. 56, 2000, pp. 133–141.

Roberts, T. "Salmonellosis Control: Estimated Economic Costs." *Poultry Science*, Vol. 67, 1988, pp. 936–943.

Ryser, E. T., and E. H. Marth. "'New' Food-Borne Pathogens of Public Health Significance." *Journal of the American Dietetic Association*, Vol. 89, 1989, pp. 948–954.

Scholliers, P. "Defining Food Risks and Food Anxieties Throughout History." *Appetite*, Vol. 51, 2008, pp. 3–6.

Trevejo, R. T., et al. "Epidemiology of Salmonellosis in California, 1990–1999: Morbidity, Mortality, and Hospitalization Costs." *American Journal of Epidemiology*, Vol. 157, 2003, pp. 48–57.

Vij, V., et al. "Recalls of Spices due to Bacterial Contamination Monitored by the U.S. Food and Drug Administration: The Predominance of Salmonellae." *Journal of Food Protection*, Vol. 69, 2006, pp. 233–237.

Weise, E., and J. Schmit. "Spinach Recall: 5 Faces, 5 Agonizing Deaths, 1 Year Later." *USA Today*, 20 September 2007.

Part Four

Additives in Foods and Beverages

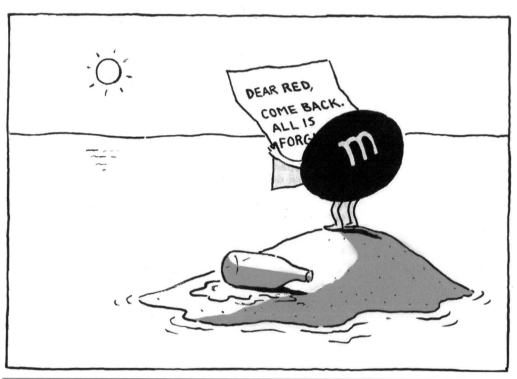

Figure 4   Between 1976 and 1986, the Mars Company stopped making red M&M'S candies due to rumors about their contents.
(*Source:* Copyright Nurit Karlin, 1988, originally published in *The Atlantic Monthly* magazine.)

24

Fear of Red Dye

Be cautious. You are holding the bad color.

—Lucius Hunt in *The Village* (2004)

SUMMARY

In 1976, the candy manufacturer Mars Inc. decided to stop producing red M&M'S candies. To this day, nobody seems to know why. The U.S. Food and Drug Administration (FDA) banned two food colorings called Red No. 2 and Red No. 4 as suspected human carcinogens in 1976, after earlier restrictions on their use; but M&M'S candies contained Red No. 3. At the time, the official reason for the manufacturer's decision was "to avoid any consumer confusion and concern." Rumors about red dyes were running wild, and it was deemed best to err on the side of caution. Red food colorings are among the many food additives that some groups have blamed not only for major diseases such as cancer but also for hyperactivity in children, thin eggshells and tongue tumors in hummingbirds, and a host of other problems, both real and apocryphal. After a promotional trial run, red M&M'S returned to the market in 1987 (see Figure 4) with a new red dye—Red No. 40, which was promptly banned in Europe on the basis of the same data that exonerated it here. It seems that safe red chemicals are hard to make. As of 2010, this health scare has largely fizzled, but the review process continues.

SOURCE

The specific event that precipitated the M&M'S health scare was the January 1976 FDA ban on a food coloring called Red No. 2, followed by a ban on Red No. 4 that went into effect the same year. The dye used in red M&M'S candies was actually Red No. 3, but apparently that was close enough to cause public alarm. (The use of Red No. 3 was also restricted, but not until 1990.)

Rumors spread, and the manufacturer stopped making red M&M'S between 1976 and 1987, except for a holiday promotion in 1985. The FDA is always banning or restricting the use of something, but the public might have taken these events more seriously than usual because of the color red and the fact that children eat candy. People have always assigned magical properties to colors, and red seems to be the universal attention-getter. The controversy has continued to some extent, because Red No. 40

(which largely replaced the other red food colorings) also has some possible health effects, as discussed below.

SCIENCE

A list of players in this melodrama may shed some light on the confusion, or possibly make it worse. (The abbreviation FD&C stands for the U.S. Food, Drug, and Cosmetic Act of 1938.)

- FD&C Red No. 2, also called E123, Amaranth, E123, C.I. Food Red 9, Acid Red 27, Azorubin S, or C.I. 16185. The CAS (Chemical Abstracts Service) number for this red dye is 915-67-3. Before 1976, when the FDA banned this chemical as an additive in any food intended for human consumption, it was the main source of red color in maraschino cherries and certain other foods—*not* including red M&M'S. Animal studies showed that it might cause cancer.
- FD&C Red No. 3, also called E127 or erythrosine (CAS 16423-68-0). FDA restricted its use in 1990, because it can release iodide when it degrades in heat. Very high doses may also cause cancer in laboratory animals. FDA did not totally ban this dye, however, and some red foods still contain it. According to unverifiable sources, Red No. 3 was the dye in red M&M'S sold before 1976.
- FD&C Red No. 4, also called E124, Ponceaux 4R, or Food Red 1 (CAS 4548-53-2). FDA first banned the use of this dye in any human food in 1964, then allowed its use in maraschino cherries, and finally banned it again in 1976. It is still an ingredient in some mouthwashes and other products. Sometimes this dye is called Cochineal Red A, although it is synthetic in origin (see below). Animal studies have shown that it might cause cancer.
- FD&C Red No. 40, also called E129, Food Red 17, or Allura Red AC (CAS 25956-17-6). This dye and Red No. 40 Lake (insoluble in water) are the synthetic dyes now used in red M&M'S and some other foods in the United States. In Europe, however, Red No. 40 is not considered fit for human consumption, so M&M'S in some European countries contain a red dye called cochineal or carmine, instead.
- Cochineal Extract, also called E120, Natural Red 4, Carmine, or Crimson Lake (CAS 1260-17-9). This widely used red dye is extracted from the crushed bodies of female cochineal bugs (*Dactylopius coccus*), which live on prickly pear cactuses. About 70,000 of these dead insects yield one pound of dye.

If all these red dyes sound unappetizing or dangerous in one way or another, remember that people consume them in very small quantities. There is just one maraschino cherry on the average ice cream sundae, not 50 of them. Would that cherry taste as good if it were pale beige?

HISTORY

We will not review the entire history of plain and peanut M&M'S in war and peace, or the colors available in specific years. As far as we can determine, bags of Mars plain

M&M'S candies sold between 1949 and 1976 contained a mixture of six colors: brown, yellow, orange, red, green, and tan. (The blue ones did not appear until 1995.) Early in the history of this product, red was the rarest color, with between one and three (occasionally zero or four) red pieces per bag. The often-quoted statement that red M&M'S first appeared in 1960 refers to the peanut variety.

The event that precipitated this food scare—the FDA ban on Red No. 2—caused a great deal of confusion and paranoia that spilled over to any product with a similar name and color. The schoolyard rumors that green M&M'S were aphrodisiacs and yellow ones caused polio were bad enough without a cancer scare, so Mars temporarily stopped making the red ones until 1987. Some wags claimed that glasnost and the perceived fall of communism made the world safe for red M&M'S; according to others, the ban on Red No. 2 resulted largely from a series of laboratory mistakes that should never have happened. A 1976 *Science* article claims that the study was not properly supervised, that dead rats were often not retrieved from cages in time for a valid necropsy, and that the experimental and control groups of rats were sometimes returned to the wrong cages, so that the results did not lend themselves to a proper analysis. Also, some scientists have asked if Red No. 40 was really any safer than its banned predecessors.

In 1982, a student named Paul Hethmon at the University of Tennessee founded the Society for the Restoration and Preservation of Red M&M'S and enlisted some 500 members to bombard Mars Inc. with letters. In 1987, on the occasion of his victory, Mr. Hethmon reportedly told the press: "Somebody else can fight for blue and purple M&Ms, but not me."[1]

Every so often, Red No. 2 still turns up on an FDA list of product recalls. In 1999, for example, an Ohio distributor recalled a batch of Life Savers that contained Red No. 2 and other uncertified or unapproved colors. The candy apparently was manufactured in Canada, where Red No. 2 was not banned. Again, it is unclear if this dye really poses a health threat or not.

In July 2009, news magazines and Web sites ran assorted permutations of the following headline: "Blue M&M'S May Help People Recover from Spinal Injuries." Although this sounds like an obvious urban legend, it turns out to be true, sort of. Researchers studying spinal injuries in rats reported that the same blue dye found in blue M&M'S, called Brilliant Blue G, seemed to reduce nerve damage when injected near the site of the injury.

CONSEQUENCES

At present, we regret to report that *no* available red food coloring seems entirely safe by any universally accepted criteria. The Cold War mantra "Better dead than red" (or was it "Better red than dead"?) has taken on a new meaning. Some of these dyes are potential carcinogens, if consumed at unrealistically huge doses. Others are made from squashed insects that not only sound icky, but may cause hyperactivity or allergic reactions in some children. Some religions forbid consumption of anything that contains insects; others frown on the sacrifice of living animals as food.

Even hummingbirds are no longer considered safe from the red syrup that traditionally fills their outdoor feeders. According to a widespread urban legend that has started near-fistfights in pet stores, an unidentified red dye can give these little birds tumors or thin eggshells. A company that sells hummingbird products recently offered a $100 reward for a copy of any scientific paper supporting this assertion, but nobody to date has collected. That company succeeded in tracing the rumor to a 1990 hoax published in a Connecticut newspaper, but even hoaxsters have motives, and this one is elusive. The hummingbird story hit the big time in the summer of 1998, when someone sent a frantic letter to the internationally syndicated "Dear Abby" column, warning readers that red dye in feeders would cause tumors to grow on hummingbirds' tongues. Although Abby responded properly with a brief rebuttal, scary stories are often more exciting than facts, and the rumor has persisted. There are a lot of people out there who really hate red food coloring and think the manufacturers are evil.

One thing is certain: anyone who feels guilty about giving red food coloring to a hummingbird should think twice before feeding it to children. Are the products bad, or is the state of knowledge bad? One argument in favor of the latter is the fact that different countries allow the use of different red dyes. In other words, everybody seems to be interpreting the same data differently. But there are some safe blue food colors on the market, so why can't we simply take all the maraschino cherries and red candies and dye them bright blue instead? Consumers would adapt in time. It seems that humanity has more urgent problems to solve than this.

WHAT WENT WRONG?

As noted above, some of the laboratory studies that led to the banning of Red No. 2 may have been substandard. Otherwise, nothing really went wrong. The FDA is supposed to protect people from exposure to chemicals that might cause cancer or other health hazards, and the agency made a judgment call. But when it banned both Red No. 2 and Red No. 4 in the same year, consumers apparently split the difference and thought Red No. 3 must be dangerous too. The rules of chemical nomenclature are enough to confuse anybody. Finally, the manufacturer of M&M'S made another judgment call and suspended the product for 11 years, although the factors underlying corporate decisions are seldom made public. Overall, this health scare actually went fairly well, except for one nagging problem: are we any better off with Red No. 40 than we were with Red No. 2?

NOTE

1. J. Ehmann, "Battle Waged, Battle Won" (*Post-Standard* [Syracuse, NY], 20 January 1987).

REFERENCES AND RECOMMENDED READING

Ballentine, R. "Cancerphobia—or Whatever Happened to Red M&Ms?" *Drug Intelligence and Clinical Pharmacy*, Vol. 16, 1982, pp. 60–61.
Bateman, B., et al. "The Effects of a Double Blind, Placebo Controlled, Artificial Food Colourings and Benzoate Preservative Challenge." *Archives of Disease in Childhood*, Vol. 89, 2004, pp. 506–511.

Boffey, P. M. "Color Additives: Botched Experiment Leads to Banning of Red Dye No. 2." *Science*, Vol. 191, 1976, pp. 450–451.

Boffey, P. M. "Color Additives: Is Successor to Red Dye No. 2 Any Safer?" *Science*, Vol. 191, 1976, pp. 832–834.

Center for Science in the Public Interest. "CSPI Urges FDA to Ban Artificial Food Dyes Linked to Behavior Problems." Press release, 2 June 2008.

Comarow, A. "Less-than-Scary Health Scares." *U.S. News and World Report*, Vol. 129, 2000, p. 70.

Drummond, H. "Add Poison for Flavor & Freshness." *Mother Jones*, April 1977, pp. 13–14.

"FDA Sued Over Red Dye No. 3." *Washington Post*, 29 September 1989.

"FDA Limits Red Dye No. 3." *New York Times*, 30 January 1990.

Feord, J. "Food Colours and the Law." *International Food Ingredients*, April–May 2003.

Finkel, A. "Rodent Tests Continue to Save Human Lives." *Insight on the News*, 12 December 1994.

Gladwell, M. "FDA: Red Dye's Reluctant Regulator." *Washington Post*, 7 February 1990.

Holson, J. F., et al. "Teratological Evaluation of FD&C Red No. 2—A Collaborative Government-Industry Study. V. Combined Findings and Discussion." *Journal of Toxicology and Environmental Health*, Vol. 1, 1976, pp. 875–885.

"Many Manufacturers Have Stopped Use of Red Dye No. 2." *United Press International*, 21 January 1976.

Mills, B. "FDA Told to Ban Last of Red Dyes." Ottaway News Service, 8 December 1976.

Owen, D. "Seeing Red: The Mysterious Moves of a Nationally Prominent Candy Manufacturer." *The Atlantic*, October 1988.

Penman, K. G., et al. "Bilberry Adulteration Using the Food Dye Amaranth." *Journal of Agricultural and Food Chemistry*, Vol. 54, 2006, pp. 7378–7382.

Pollock, I., and J. O. Warner. "Effect of Artificial Food Colours on Childhood Behaviour." *Archives of Disease in Childhood*, Vol. 65, 1990, pp. 74–77.

Radomski, J. L. "Toxicology of Food Colors." *Annual Review of Pharmacology*, Vol. 14, 1974, pp. 127–137.

"The Red Dye Dodge." *Washington Post*, 20 July 1989.

"Regulation: Death of a Dye." *Time*, 2 February 1976.

Shenk, J. W. "True Colors." *U.S. News and World Report*, 24 March 1997.

Strickland, E. "Blue Food Dye Helps Rats with Spinal Injuries." *Discover*, 28 July 2009.

Weisburger, J. H. "Social and Ethical Implications of Claims for Cancer Hazards." *Medical and Pediatric Oncology*, Vol. 3, 1977, pp. 137–140.

Weiss, B. "Food Additives and Hyperactivity." *Environmental Health Perspectives*, Vol. 116, 2008, pp. A240–A241.

Whelan, E. M. "Stop Banning Products at the Drop of a Rat." *Insight on the News*, 12 December 1994.

Winter, C. "Color It Orange May Be the Answer." Knight News Service, 18 November 1976.

25

Fear of Artificial Sweeteners

As a surfeit of the sweetest things
The deepest loathing to the stomach brings.

—William Shakespeare, *A Midsummer Night's Dream* (1596)

SUMMARY

Artificial sweeteners—saccharin, cyclamate, aspartame, and other sugar substitutes—are popular because they help people cut down on sugar and total caloric intake. Yet ever since the U.S. Food and Drug Administration (FDA) banned cyclamate as a possible human carcinogen in 1969, all artificial sweeteners have been the target of exaggerated claims, rumors, and urban legends. "Natural" sugar substitutes, such as the plant extract stevia, are also controversial. No sweetener (or any other food or additive) is entirely safe; honey is the most frequent vehicle of infant botulism. In 1985, the U.S. National Academy of Sciences reviewed available data and concluded that cyclamate is not a carcinogen, except under unusual circumstances that result in its conversion to a more toxic chemical. As of 2010, the FDA ban on cyclamate remains in effect, although many European and Asian countries continue to use this chemical as a food additive. The health scare has slowly fizzled as the use of artificial sweeteners has increased.

SOURCE

In 1937, a graduate student at the University of Illinois discovered the artificial sweetener sodium cyclamate. The product was a great success at first, because it tasted better than an older sweetener called saccharin (of which more later). In 1969, however, laboratory studies showed that rats developed bladder cancer after ingesting cyclamate—at a dosage that, according to some sources, was equivalent to about 350 cans of diet soda per day in a human. In fact, direct comparisons such as this may be inappropriate, both because of allometry (scaling problems) and because a rat's metabolism is not the same as ours. But the word "cancer" trumps other considerations, and this finding received a great deal of publicity in the late 1960s, when health scares were not yet routine.

According to some studies, cyclamate also caused developmental defects when injected into chicken eggs. Again, it is unclear if this approach has direct relevance to humans, but caution was in order. The manufacturer of cyclamate, Abbott Laboratories, immediately reported these adverse findings to FDA. Although some researchers doubted that cyclamate was really a health hazard, the Delaney Clause in the 1958 Food, Drug, and Cosmetic Act forced the FDA to prohibit the use of this chemical as a food additive.

In October 1969, the news media jumped on cyclamate and stayed there, while those of us who had confidently guzzled diet soda for years discovered our inner activist. At one point, an FDA scientist "carried a grossly deformed chicken through the administrative offices of the FDA so the Commissioner and his various assistants could see for themselves what Americans were drinking in larger and larger quantities."[1] Food and beverage manufacturers scrambled to find a substitute sweetener on short notice, despite suspicions that the risk was overstated. Whether the FDA's action was warranted or not, the American public definitely listened.

SCIENCE

The sweetener known as cyclamate is the water-soluble sodium or calcium salt of a chemical called cyclamic acid. As a result, many sources refer to the product as sodium cyclamate or calcium cyclamate. Before the FDA banned cyclamate in 1969, food manufacturers often used it in combination with saccharin to achieve optimum sweetness and balance. As discussed earlier, exposure to high levels of cyclamate appeared to cause cancers in rats and malformations in chickens, but it was unclear if these results applied to humans. Also, in some early studies, cyclamate appeared to shrink the testes of male rodents and other mammals—a finding that might not apply to humans either, but was unlikely to enhance the chemical's image.

Although the literature is inconsistent, and some early studies could not be replicated, it appears that cyclamate itself is not the main problem. As with many potentially harmful chemicals, the damage is associated with breakdown products, which may vary from one species or individual to another. In a small percentage of people (reportedly less than 5%), bacteria in the gastrointestinal tract can convert cyclamate to a more toxic, possibly carcinogenic chemical called cyclohexylamine. Despite this finding, cyclamate does not appear to qualify as a carcinogen by present-day standards.

In 1973, Abbott petitioned the FDA to reverse the cyclamate ban, but the petition was denied in 1980. The FDA's own Cancer Assessment Committee determined in 1983 that cyclamate did not cause cancer, and the U.S. National Academy of Sciences added its vote of confidence in 1985. As of 2010, however, the use of cyclamate as an additive in human food remained illegal in the United States. It is possible that, even if FDA lifted the ban tomorrow, consumer acceptance of cyclamate would be low because of all the years of adverse publicity.

Other artificial sweeteners and sugar substitutes currently approved for use in the United States include the following:

- Saccharin. The first widely used artificial sweetener, invented in 1878, was extremely sweet but had a strange aftertaste that not everyone liked. Some early reports also claimed a link to bladder cancer, aphthous ulcers, or other health problems. As a result, it was often used in combination with cyclamate or another sweetener. Sweet'N Low and some other products still contain saccharin, a water-soluble sodium salt of a chemical called benzoic sulfimide.

- Aspartame. This chemical is related to the amino acid phenylalanine, so people with the rare genetic disorder phenylketonuria (PKU) must avoid it. Otherwise, available data (vs. rumors and hoaxes) indicate that it is safe in moderation. Familiar brand names of products containing aspartame include NutraSweet, Canderel, and Equal.
- Sucralose. A British scientist discovered this sweetener in 1976, allegedly as a result of one of those dry British jokes. His colleague asked him to *test* the chemical, but it sounded like he said *taste* it. Many chemical discoveries have had similar origins, a testimony to the trust among chemists. Sucralose is sold in the United States as Splenda.
- Acesulfame potassium ("ace-K"). Brand names for this chemical in Europe include Sunett and Sweet One. The FDA has also approved it for use in the U.S., but critics claim that laboratory testing has been inadequate. Ace-K is the potassium (K) salt of a chemical known as 6-methyl-1,2,3- oxathiazine-4 (*3H*)-one 2,2-dioxide.
- Alitame. This sweetener sounds great on paper, and it is available (as Aclame) in several countries, but at present it does not have FDA approval. It is chemically similar to aspartame, but sweeter, more heat-resistant, and not harmful to people with PKU. The pharmaceutical giant Pfizer developed it in 1979.
- Neotame. As its name suggests, this sweetener is chemically similar to alitame and aspartame. Neotame received FDA approval in 2002, over the protests of activists, but it is not yet widely available in the United States.
- Stevia. This sweetener is not exactly artificial, because it comes from a flowering plant (*Stevia rebaudiana*) rather than a laboratory. Some stevia products are approved for use in the United States. Despite the appeal of the word "natural," however, the origin of this chemical does not automatically make it any safer than cyclamate. For those who claim that anything hard to pronounce should not be eaten, the stevia sweetener actually consists of 13-[(2-O-β–D-glucopyranosyl-β–D-glucopyranosyl)oxy] kaur-16-en-18-oic acid, β-D-glucopyranosyl ester, or stevioside for short.

HISTORY

The quest for sweetness has probably been a human priority ever since the first hominids broke open a beehive, but the origin of this custom is lost in time. Cave paintings and archaeological finds show that people have gathered wild honey and refined the art of beekeeping for at least 10,000 years. These are not exclusively human concerns; certain birds in Africa, called honeyguides, have trained people to break open beehives for them (although the people may not see it that way).

Inevitably, humans figured out at some point that an excess of honey or sugar could make them fat, rot their teeth, and put them at risk for diabetes. Thus, chemists started looking for substances that tasted sweet, but yielded less (or no) energy and did not over-tax the pancreas. The first widely used artificial sweetener was saccharin, first synthesized in 1878. It is unclear if its discovery was accidental or not; various urban legends hold that nearly all artificial sweeteners were invented as a result of laboratory mistakes involving pesticides gone wrong, or careless investigators licking their hands.

The 1965 discovery of aspartame, followed by its FDA approval in 1980, seemed to fill the gap created by the 1969 exodus of cyclamate. In recent years, however, a number of bizarre urban legends and email hoaxes have targeted aspartame. Many people blame it for a list of health problems that should be familiar by now: chronic fatigue syndrome, fibromyalgia, attention deficit disorder, epileptic seizures, headaches, memory loss, depression, insomnia, weight gain—and, of course, autism and multiple sclerosis. There are entire Web sites that promise *the truth* about aspartame. One such Web site lists 61 diseases or symptoms that aspartame allegedly causes, and 13 diseases that it mimics or makes worse.

CONSEQUENCES

As of 2009, an estimated 15 percent of the American population over age 2 uses aspartame or other non-nutritive sweeteners. But as the use of these products increases, so does the prevalence of obesity and the volume of literature claiming that these products are harmful. Some sources claim that artificial sweeteners directly promote weight gain, whereas others claim that already-obese people turn to artificial sweeteners in an effort to lose weight (see also Chapter 48).

With all the negative press on cane sugar (sucrose) and artificial sweeteners, the popularity of honey has increased. Unfortunately, honey is not much of an improvement over sugar, because the chemicals that make honey sweet (fructose and glucose) are the same ones that result from the enzymatic breakdown of sucrose in the human body. Also, raw honey often contains *Clostridium botulinum* spores, which pose a threat to infants, as explained in Chapter 13. As a result, some health-oriented product manufacturers have gone back to sucrose derived from sugar cane—in other words, ordinary table sugar—by renaming it "evaporated organic cane juice."

A more favorable consequence of cyclamate paranoia was that it prompted FDA to take a second look at saccharin, monosodium glutamate (MSG), and other GRAS (generally recognized as safe) food additives. Retesting is not a bad idea, but doing it right in the first place is even better.

WHAT WENT WRONG?

It is hard to find artificial sugar substitutes that are both demonstrably safe and capable of fooling the brain into thinking they are sugar. FDA approval is a hellish process under the best of conditions, and some harmful chemicals may slip through the cracks. But these facts alone do not fully explain the passionate dedication of some anti-aspartame activists. Only a few other products, such as fluoridated tap water (Chapter 26), have elicited such fury for so long.

Why do so many people hate aspartame? Do they believe it is just another cyclamate waiting to happen? As discussed above, not even cyclamate itself was another cyclamate waiting to happen. No known epidemic of cancer or anything else has resulted from consumption of either of these sweeteners. (As always, this statement might become obsolete with tomorrow's news.)

NOTE

1. H. Drummond, "Add Poison for Flavor and Freshness" (*Mother Jones*, April 1977).

REFERENCES AND RECOMMENDED READING

Ahmed, F. E., and D. B. Thomas. "Assessment of the Carcinogenicity of the Nonnutritive Sweetener Cyclamate." *Critical Reviews in Toxicology*, Vol. 22, 1992, pp. 81–118.

Andreatta, M. M., et al. "Artificial Sweetener Consumption and Urinary Tract Tumors in Cordoba, Argentina." *Preventive Medicine*, Vol. 47, 2008, pp. 136–139.

Arnold, D. L. "Toxicology of Saccharin." *Fundamentals of Applied Toxicology*, Vol. 4, 1984, pp. 674–685.

Brusick, D. J. "A Critical Review of the Genetic Toxicity of Steviol and Steviol Glycosides." *Food and Chemical Toxicology*, Vol. 46 (Suppl. 7), 2008, pp. S83–S91.

Chan, J. M., et al. "Sweets, Sweetened Beverages, and Risk of Pancreatic Cancer in a Large Population-Based Case Control Study." *Cancer Causes and Control*, Vol. 20, 2009, pp. 835–846.

Christoffel, T. "Fluorides, Facts, and Fanatics: Public Health Advocacy Shouldn't Stop at the Courthouse Door." *American Journal of Public Health*, Vol. 75, 1985, pp. 888–891.

Comarow, A. "Less-than-Scary Health Scares." *U.S. News and World Report*, Vol. 129, 2000, p. 70.

Cordle, F., and S. A. Miller. "Using Epidemiology to Regulate Food Additives: Saccharin Case-Control Studies." *Public Health Reports*, Vol. 99, 1984, pp. 365–369.

Craig, W. J. "Sweet, Sweet Stevia." *Vibrant Life*, March-April 2009.

Crampton, R. F. "Problems of Food Additives, with Special Reference to Cyclamates." *British Medical Bulletin*, Vol. 26, 1970, pp. 222–227.

"Current Attitudes about Sweetener Use." *Beverage World*, 15 April 2008.

"The Cyclamate Story Unfolds." *Food and Cosmetics Toxicology*, Vol. 8, 1970, pp. 563–565.

"Cyclamates." *IARC Monographs on the Evaluation of Carcinogenic Risks to Humans*, Vol. 73, 1999, pp. 195–222.

"Cyclamate's Reapproval Expected in Due Course." *Chemical Marketing Reporter*, 22 May 1989.

"Cyclamates' Sour Aftertaste." *Time*, 31 October 1969.

Drummond, H. "Add Poison for Flavor & Freshness." *Mother Jones*, April 1977, pp. 13–14.

Greeley, A. "Not Only Sugar is Sweet." *FDA Consumer*, April 1992.

Jeffrey, A. M., and G. M. Williams. "Lack of DNA-Damaging Activity of Five Non-Nutritive Sweeteners in the Rat Hepatocyte/DNA Repair Assay." *Food and Chemical Toxicology*, Vol. 38, 2000, pp. 335–338.

Lecos, C. W. "Sweeteners Minus Calories = Controversy." *FDA Consumer*, February 1985.

Magnuson, B., and G. M. Williams. "Carcinogenicity of Aspartame in Rats Not Proven." *Environmental Health Perspectives*, Vol. 116, 2008, pp. A239–A240.

Mattes, R. D., and B. M. Popkin. "Nonnutritive Sweetener Consumption in Humans: Effects on Appetite and Food Intake and their Putative Mechanisms." *American Journal of Clinical Nutrition*, Vol. 89, 2009, pp. 1–14.

Renwick, A. G. "The Intake of Intense Sweeteners—An Update Review." *Food Additives and Contaminants*, Vol. 23, pp. 327–338.

Shaw, J. H. "Sweeteners—An Overview. Part I." *Dental Abstracts*, Vol. 26, 1981, pp. 116–120.

Shaw, J. H. "Sweeteners—An Overview. Part II." *Dental Abstracts*, Vol. 26, 1981, pp. 172–175.

Soffritti, M., et al. "Life-Span Exposure to Low Doses of Aspartame Beginning during Prenatal Life Increases Cancer Effects in Rats." *Environmental Health Perspectives*, Vol. 115, 2007, pp. 1293–1297.

Soffritti, M. "Carcinogenicity of Aspartame: Soffritti Responds." *Environmental Health Perspectives*, Vol. 116, 2008, p. A240.

U.S. Food and Drug Administration. "Guidance for Industry: Ingredients Declared as Evaporated Cane Juice." Draft, October 2009.

Weihrauch, M. R., and V. Diehl. "Artificial Sweeteners—Do They Bear a Carcinogenic Risk?" *Annals of Oncology*, Vol. 15, 2004, pp. 1460–1465.

Whelan, E. M. "Stop Banning Products at the Drop of a Rat." *Insight on the News*, 12 December 1994.

26

Fear of Fluoridation and Chlorination

Whiskey is for drinking. Water is for fighting over.
—Attributed to Mark Twain (who probably did not say it)

SUMMARY

Anti-fluoridation rhetoric has plagued municipal water districts for over 60 years, ever since many American cities made the controversial decision to improve dental health by adding fluoride to tap water. Three generations of zealots have insisted that the real purpose of fluoridation is to make people sick or subservient. During the Cold War, the rumor spread that the Soviets gave fluoride to gulag prisoners as a mind-control device, and of course free Americans would never submit to a similar fate. But if that was the intended purpose of fluoride, it does not seem to be working here, if rates of crime and social upheaval during the past half-century are any indication. Smaller numbers of people also object to the use of chlorine or any other chemicals for water treatment. These concerns show signs of fizzling in recent years, as the last holdouts begin to understand that dosage is everything. Also, the people who object to fluoridation often are the same ones who can afford bottled water and dental care. For lower-income people with no insurance, fluoridated water (like enriched flour and fortified milk) looks more like a free preventive health measure that a few elitists are trying to take away.

SOURCE

When the first American cities started adding fluoride to tap water between 1945 and 1950, most governments in the developed world were already treating water with chlorine or other chemicals to prevent waterborne disease outbreaks. Few people objected to that practice, because nobody really liked typhoid or cholera. Water treatment was one of the great benefits of civilization. Even for those who rejected the germ theory of disease, the idea of drinking water contaminated with sewage was not aesthetically appealing.

Fluoride was a different matter, because the connection between fluoridation and dental health was far less obvious. Not everyone who drank fluoridated water ended up with good teeth; not everyone who avoided it had bad teeth. To see improvement, it was necessary to monitor the dental health of entire populations for years and compare the overall results.

Worse, the proponents of fluoridation tended to make fun of the opposition instead of taking their concerns seriously. In the hilarious 1964 Cold War satire *Dr. Strangelove*, for example, a character with obvious mental problems refers to fluoridation as a communist conspiracy. Where were the censors when we needed them? That motion picture, and its enthusiastic reception, woke some Americans to the realization that power brokers in smoke-filled rooms were not only putting what seemed to be poison in their drinking water—yes, fluoride can be a poison at much higher doses—but adding insult to injury by making a joke of it.

SCIENCE

Fluorine (F) is a chemical element, and fluoride is its reduced form (F^-). Fluoride occurs naturally in surface water and groundwater, but the concentration varies from one place and source to another. When the fluoride level is somewhere between 0.7 and 1.2 milligrams per liter (mg/L), people who drink the water on a daily basis tend to have less tooth decay than people who drink unfluoridated water. The maximum safe level is somewhere between 1.5 and 2.0 mg/L; higher levels than that can cause pitted teeth, nausea, or more severe symptoms, up to and including death in rare cases. Natural well water in some parts of the world already contains the right amount of fluoride. In other places, where it contains too little or too much, public health agencies may intervene by adding or removing fluoride.

As the famous Swiss alchemist Paracelsus (1493–1541) pointed out long ago, every substance is a poison if the dose is high enough. A recent incident at a northern California trailer park provides an example. In 2003, park residents learned that their drinking water had contained harmful levels of fluoride since 1995, yet neither the park owners nor the county health agency had thought to notify them. It is unclear if any of the residents suffered physical injuries, but they might have, because they were exposed to fluoride at three to four times the maximum safe level for over eight years. So, doesn't this case prove that meddling with water can have deadly consequences? No, it proves that *not* meddling with water can be even worse. People at that trailer park were at risk because the natural, untreated well water contained high levels of fluoride.

Anti-fluoridation activists claim that even low fluoride levels can cause numerous diseases, including (but not limited to) cancer, heart disease, high cholesterol, autism, multiple sclerosis, Parkinson's disease, Alzheimer's disease, Down's syndrome, chronic fatigue syndrome, fibromyalgia, hypothyroidism, and obesity. They support these statements with anecdotal evidence, very old studies, or quotations from the recent scientific literature taken out of context. It is true that the majority of people who drink fluoridated water will eventually suffer from at least one of these common disorders—but so will those who do not drink fluoridated water. Besides, even if the government wanted to wreck everybody's health (thereby reducing its own tax base and making its soldiers less effective), how could one chemical do all these things?

Chlorine (Cl) is another controversial chemical element. People who oppose the chlorination of tap water, and those who sell products to remove chlorine from water, are just as creative as the anti-fluoridation activists when interpreting scientific data. For example, some Web sites claim that taking a shower in chlorinated water is just like being exposed to chlorine gas on the battlefields of World War I. Again, there is that small matter of dosage. The same chemicals that are demonstrably harmful at high levels can be harmless or beneficial at low levels.

HISTORY

There is ample precedent for the belief that Big Brother controls hapless enslaved populations by putting something in their water or food. Generations of sailors believed or joked that their respective navies fed them saltpeter (potassium nitrate) to suppress their sexual drive and maintain proper discipline on long sea voyages. According to urban legend, crime rates are low in some parts of the United States because the drinking water contains high levels of lithium (naturally occurring or otherwise). And during the Cold War, an Air Force officer supposedly told Congress that the Russians gave fluoridated water to prisoners to keep them docile and subservient. But even if that officer existed, and even if he saw the Russians putting fluoride in the water, and even if the Russians said "Da, this is to make prisoners docile"—that does not mean it *worked*. There is no scientific evidence that fluoride makes people docile. During World War II, the Germans supposedly gave fluoride to their prisoners to make them sterile. It can do just about everything, can't it?

On occasion, anti-fluoridation activists have deliberately misquoted scientific studies or historic fact. This seems to be a standard tactic for the leaders of any crusade. Being privy to a higher truth, these people have the right—nay, the obligation—to persuade others by any means necessary. In 2004, for example, an Australian study confirmed that fluoridation reduced dental caries in children; but a group that opposes fluoridation claimed that the study reached the opposite conclusion. Did they misunderstand it, or did they even read it? Similarly, these crusaders often claim that the fluoride added to drinking water is a waste product of the aluminum or fertilizer industry, or some other big business in cahoots with government. The phrase "waste product" has connotations of garbage or sewage, but fluoride is simply a chemical, regardless of where it comes from.

While some scientists and journalists continue to praise fluoridation, others suggest that this practice may have outlived its usefulness. In 2011, the U.S. Department of Health and Human Services advised communities to make a slight reduction in the amount of fluoride added to drinking water, to compensate for other sources such as fluoride toothpaste. In an earlier era, it made sense to add many things to food and water—for example, niacin to flour and cornmeal to prevent pellagra, vitamin D to milk and butter to prevent rickets, and iodine to table salt to prevent goiter. These measures represented a public health victory that improved quality of life for millions. But now that vitamin pills are cheap, and low-income people no longer must live on salt pork and cornbread, the need for this approach is unclear. Also, to stay current with the surging tide of recent nutritional claims and counter-claims, it would be necessary to add numerous vitamins and minerals and other nutrients to foods and beverages, while also adjusting the content of salt and trans fat and sugar and fiber. Some public figures are trying to do exactly that, but it is a losing battle. People want to choose what they put in their bodies.

Chlorination of drinking water is a different matter, because some form of treatment is necessary to prevent waterborne disease outbreaks. Yet even that point is controversial. For nearly two decades, some authors have claimed that the South American cholera epidemic of 1991 resulted from Peru's decision to stop chlorinating its drinking water, while others have claimed that the story is nothing more than a politically motivated urban legend. As it turns out, the truth is somewhere in between. The cholera epidemic was real enough; about 1 million people contracted the disease, and at least 13,000 died. But was unchlorinated water responsible? Yes, according to studies published in the journals *Nature* and *Lancet*. The unresolved question is whether the Peruvian government decided to stop chlorinating for political and/or environmental reasons, or whether the water treatment system simply deteriorated or was inadequate in the first place.

CONSEQUENCES

Growing numbers of Americans question the safety of municipal tap water, with some justification. Fluoride is not the only issue; many cities issue routine annual notifications of excess nitrates, turbidity, or other water quality problems. The bottled water industry and manufacturers of home water filters have certainly benefited, but incredible numbers of plastic bottles are accumulating in landfills—this despite the fact that most bottled water contains fluoride, and most affordable water filters do not claim to remove it. Thus, a number of mainstream scientists and dentists have proposed that maybe it is time for fluoridation to end. The federal government has already taken away some public health services (such as free dental care for Medicaid patients) as a cost-cutting measure, and municipal governments are not exactly rolling in cash these days either. But if cities stop fluoridating, will people then turn around and sue them for causing tooth decay?

Another consequence of the long fluoridation battle is that some mainstream agencies, such as the American Dental Association, have adopted some of the same tactics as their opponents. For example, many people who are looking for the anti-fluoridation Web site www.fluoridealert.org probably type the wrong extension by mistake, such as www.fluoridealert.com or www.fluoridealert.net. Either typo (as of 2010) will take these pilgrims to a Web site of the American Dental Association, which acquired the two domain names in 2001. This is like digging a hole in the middle of a game trail and then lecturing whatever unsuspecting prey falls in.

WHAT WENT WRONG?

Why do people rebel when a government agency adds fluoride to water, but not when it adds (or requires others to add) vitamins to flour and dairy products, or iodine to salt? The history and motivation of all these practices are similar, so what is the difference? Maybe the problem is that fluoride sounds dangerous and nutrients don't. It is human nature to rebel against any authority that tries to make us do virtually anything, and there is something vaguely creepy about the idea of the government adding potentially toxic chemicals to drinking water. Accepting this practice means trusting public health officials to add (or subtract) the right amount, and trusting scientists to draw the right conclusions from studies. Granted, trust does not come easily in today's world, but it is pointless for anti-fluoridation activists to insist that doctors and researchers are motivated by sheer mindless evil. We drink the water too.

REFERENCES AND RECOMMENDED READING

Allolio, B., and R. Lehmann. "Drinking Water Fluoridation and Bone." *Experimental and Clinical Endocrinology & Diabetes*, Vol. 107, 1999, pp. 12–20.

Anderson, C. "Cholera Epidemic Traced to Risk Miscalculation." *Nature*, 28 November 1991, p. 255.

Armfield, J. M. "When Public Action Undermines Public Health: A Critical Examination of Antifluoridationist Literature." *Australia and New Zealand Health Policy*, Vol. 4, 2007, p. 25.

Challacombe, S. J. "Does Fluoridation Harm Immune Function?" *Community Dental Health*, Vol. 13 (Suppl. 2), 1996, pp. 69–71.

Christoffel, T. "Fluorides, Facts and Fanatics: Public Health Advocacy Shouldn't Stop at the Courthouse Door." *American Journal of Public Health*, Vol. 75, 1985, pp. 888–891.

Christoffel, T. "Fluoridation: Legal and Political Issues." *Journal of the American College of Dentists*, Vol. 59, 1992, pp. 8–13.

Clarkson, J. J., and J. McLoughlin. "Role of Fluoride in Oral Health Promotion." *International Dental Journal*, Vol. 50, 2000, pp. 119–128.

Diesendorf, M., et al. "New Evidence on Fluoridation." *Australian and New Zealand Journal of Public Health*, Vol. 21, 1997, pp. 187–190.

Kassirer, B. "The Fluoridation Controversy: A Debate. Part II: The Pros of Fluoridation." *Ontario Dentist*, Vol. 71, 1994, pp. 31–32.

König, K. G. "Clinical Manifestations and Treatment of Caries from 1953 to Global Changes in the 20th Century." *Caries Research*, Vol. 38, 2004 pp. 168–172.

Kumar, J. V. "Is Water Fluoridation Still Necessary?" *Advances in Dental Research*, Vol. 20, 2008, pp. 8–12.

Lewis, C. W., et al. "Fluoride." *Pediatrics in Review*, Vol. 24, 2003, pp. 327–336.

Li, Y. "Fluoride: Safety Issues." *Journal of the Indiana Dental Association*, Vol. 72, 1993, pp. 22–26.

Loh, T. "Thirty-Eight Years of Water Fluoridation—The Singapore Scenario." *Community Dental Health*, Vol. 13 (Suppl. 2), 1996, pp. 47–50.

McDonagh, M. S., et al. "Systematic Review of Water Fluoridation." *British Medical Journal*, Vol. 321, 2000, pp. 855–859.

Newbrun, E. "The Fluoridation War: A Scientific Dispute or a Religious Argument?" *Journal of Public Health Dentistry*, Vol. 56 (5 Spec No.), 1996, pp. 246–252.

Newbrun, E., and H. Horowitz "Why We Have Not Changed Our Minds about the Safety and Efficacy of Water Fluoridation." *Perspectives in Biology and Medicine*, Vol. 42, 1999, pp. 526–543.

"Position of the American Dietetic Association: The Impact of Fluoride on Health." *Journal of the American Dietetic Association*, Vol. 100, 2000, pp. 1208–1213.

Ripa, L. W. "A Half-Century of Community Water Fluoridation in the United States: Review and Commentary." *Journal of Public Health Dentistry*, Vol. 53, 1993, pp. 17–44.

Simko, L. C. "Water Fluoridation: Time to Reexamine the Issue." *Pediatric Nursing*, Vol. 23, 1997, pp. 155–159.

Whelton, H. P., et al. "A Review of Fluorosis in the European Union: Prevalence, Risk Factors and Aesthetic Issues." *Community Dental and Oral Epidemiology*, Vol. 32 (Suppl. 1), 2004, pp. 9–18.

Whiting, P., et al. "Association of Down's Syndrome and Water Fluoride Level: A Systematic Review of the Evidence." *BMC Public Health*, 24 July 2001.

Whyte, M. P., et al. "Skeletal Fluorosis from Instant Tea." *Journal of Bone and Mineral Research*, Vol. 23, 2008, pp. 759–769.

Yeung, C. A. "A Systematic Review of the Efficacy and Safety of Fluoridation." *Evidence Based Dentistry*, Vol. 9, 2008, pp. 39–43.

Zettle, K. "The Fluoridation Controversy: A Debate. Part I: The Cons of Fluoridation." *Ontario Dentist*, Vol. 71, 1994, pp. 27–28.

27

Fear of MSG

God sends meat, and the Devil sends cooks.

—John Taylor, *Works* (1630)

SUMMARY

Monosodium glutamate (MSG) is a chemical used as a flavor enhancer in many processed foods. It is the sodium salt of a natural amino acid and is usually prepared from corn, seaweed, or other plants. Manufacturers add it to many foods, and it also occurs naturally in some fermented sauces and other foods. Some people claim that MSG causes headaches, flushing, rapid heartbeat, increased appetite, or other symptoms, but as of 2010, most studies have shown that the substance is harmless when used in moderation. Most doctors and nutritionists have accepted this conclusion. Until recently, anyone who believed otherwise could avoid MSG simply by reading product labels or preparing meals from scratch. Now, however, anti-MSG activists claim that many unrelated food ingredients are really the same thing as MSG, and that the food industry has conspired to hide this chemical in its products for the apparent purpose of making people sick and fat. Hailed as a culinary miracle in the 1950s and 1960s, MSG has evolved into a full-blown health scare that shows recent signs of fizzling.

SOURCE

Most American consumers first learned about MSG in 1947, when a Japanese manufacturer marketed the chemical in this country as Ac'cent flavor enhancer. This product was quite popular here at first, and did not begin the long slide toward health scare status until 1968, when an article in the *New England Journal of Medicine* proposed that MSG might be responsible for a possibly apocryphal condition known as "Chinese restaurant syndrome," in which a few people reported vague symptoms after eating Chinese food. Again, MSG was originally a Japanese product, but it found its way into many American and Chinese foods. By the time the television news program *60 Minutes* ran a controversial segment on MSG in 1991, the health scare was in full tilt.

Numerous studies over the years have failed to prove that MSG causes any serious health problems, but some of these studies yielded equivocal findings, and research continues. Meanwhile, MSG is in so many foods that consumers find it hard to avoid.

As of 2010, some food manufacturers report that they have stopped using MSG, while others use it without apology, presumably because their customers like it.

SCIENCE

Monosodium glutamate (MSG) is the sodium salt form of a common amino acid called glutamic acid. It is chemically similar to the L-glutamic acid sold as a dietary supplement in health food stores. Japanese cooks extracted a flavor enhancer from seaweed and added it to various dishes long before a Japanese chemist isolated the chemical in 1908 and defined its flavor as *umami*, or "savory." Other sources claim that MSG has no flavor of its own, but merely enhances the flavor of meat and other foods. A 1929 newspaper article, published before most Americans were familiar with this product, described MSG somewhat confusingly as "salt that tastes like meat."[1] Umami is now widely regarded (by those who can taste it) as "the fifth flavor," the first four traditional flavors being sweet, sour, bitter, and salty. Specific receptors on the tongue are believed to detect these flavors or combinations.

Despite its unnatural-sounding chemical name, most monosodium glutamate is the product of old-fashioned bacterial fermentation of plant products such as wheat gluten, corn, soybeans, sugar beets, and certain seaweeds. As a byproduct of the beet sugar manufacturing process, MSG production even qualifies as an efficient use of natural resources. The U.S. Food and Drug Administration (FDA) classifies MSG under the catch-all acronym GRAS, or "generally recognized as safe." Although this flavor extender has retained its popularity in the United States, and is present in a wide range of prepared foods, some people may have allergic reactions to it and others question its safety, as further discussed under History.

MSG and glutamic acid belong to a controversial class of chemicals known as excitotoxins. At high levels—much higher levels than would normally be present in any food, processed or otherwise—excitotoxins can damage the central nervous system. Scientists first described this phenomenon in about 1970, and consumer activists have argued about it ever since. Some sources claim that MSG can cause depression and suicidal thoughts in susceptible individuals. The so-called Chinese restaurant syndrome may result from sensitivity to low levels of MSG, but serious or irreversible injury is another matter. As with several chemicals discussed in this book, and many others that are not, the difference between a beneficial effect and death is often a matter of dosage. Apparently there are no confirmed records of anyone dying, suffering brain damage, or becoming seriously ill from an overdose of MSG.

In 1980 and again in 1995, the FDA commissioned the Federation of American Societies for Experimental Biology (FASEB) to review the safety of monosodium glutamate. Both reports concluded that MSG was safe for most people at normal levels of use, but that some individuals reported symptoms such as headache, nausea, rapid heartbeat, or a sensation of warmth. A 2000 double-blind study found that a large dose of MSG, if given without food, caused more symptoms than a placebo in people who believed they were sensitive to MSG. The investigators noted, however, that the results were inconsistent and not reproducible, and that the symptoms did not occur when the MSG was given with food.

Unfortunately, these studies have done little to relieve public concern about MSG. In 2010, one typical consumer-oriented Web site described MSG as "a silent killer that's worse than alcohol, nicotine and drugs." Alternative health practitioners now blame this chemical for obesity, diabetes, heart disease, cancer, stroke, insomnia, epilepsy, autism, attention deficit disorder, fibromyalgia, depression, brain tumors, migraine, Alzheimer's, and dozens of other medical conditions—the same list, in fact, that others attribute to vaccines, Lyme disease, aspartame, or fluoridated tap water.

MSG is not an essential nutrient, and there is some evidence that it might cause temporary discomfort in a few individuals. It increases the sodium content of food, and we already get plenty. So, why put it in food? There can be only one reason. People like it, and they buy the products that contain it.

HISTORY

Some early advertisements for MSG made claims that went far beyond the mystique of the Far East or the promise of transcendent stuffing for the reader's Thanksgiving turkey. In the 1940s, some of these ads claimed that MSG improved concentration or simply was "good for you" in some undefined way. Stranger still, some newspaper medical columns reported that developmentally disabled children living in institutions were being treated successfully with a combination of monosodium glutamate and B complex vitamins. These supplements allegedly made the children more alert and intelligent. It is not clear what really happened, but perhaps the MSG simply made their food taste better and relieved the boredom of hospital life. In any case, here is yet another example of a theme that appears throughout this book: the power of the dark side. Any substance that somebody thinks is dangerous will eventually turn out to have magical powers, and vice versa.

As we have said, American consumers loved MSG at first, but it aroused some suspicions in the 1960s, and by 1991 the honeymoon was definitely over. That year, CBS News ran a somewhat exaggerated (not to say alarmist) *60 Minutes* segment on MSG. For example, the narrator claimed that "millions are suffering a host of symptoms and some get violently sick" as a result of exposure to this common flavor enhancer. The script largely brushed aside the FDA's conclusions about MSG, focusing instead on the anecdotal reports and fears of consumer activists. It also failed to mention that glutamate occurs naturally in some foods.

CONSEQUENCES

The MSG controversy seems to have started two opposing trends. On the one hand, some food manufacturers have made public announcements to the effect that they are removing all MSG from their products. Swanson and Progresso soups are among the best-known recent examples. Baby food manufacturers stopped using MSG in the 1970s. On the other hand, there has been a sharp increase in the number of processed foods that still contain MSG, but list it under other names (such as glutamate, free glutamic acid, autolyzed yeast, or "natural flavor"). In response, some activists have posted lists of alleged MSG synonyms on their Web sites, but some of this information is highly misleading. For example, several sources claim that the common food ingredient maltodextrin is just another name for MSG, but that is false, as anyone with access to a chemical dictionary can easily verify. Maltodextrin is a type of carbohydrate called a polysaccharide.

Perhaps the saddest consequence of the MSG scare involves an American legend. At least two popular books have "outed" Colonel Sanders (in 1983 and 2009, respectively) by claiming that MSG is one of the secret spices in the original Kentucky Fried Chicken coating. If this is true, why have so many people eaten KFC without developing the symptoms of Chinese restaurant syndrome? Maybe some people did have such symptoms, but since they did not know the chicken contained MSG, they wrote off the occasional headache or hot flash as a random event.

WHAT WENT WRONG?

Just the name "monosodium glutamate" might be enough to arouse suspicion in some consumers. After all, we do not sprinkle sodium chloride on the food; we sprinkle salt, a much more comfortable word. By analogy, most readers have probably heard about practical jokes involving an allegedly dangerous chemical called dihydrogen monoxide, which is known to cause thousands of deaths every year. At least one city government in California was on the verge of banning the stuff when the joker 'fessed up. "Dihydrogen monoxide" is simply water. More recently, a high school student reportedly did a science fair project on the dangers of dihydrogen monoxide and won a trophy—or maybe that is an urban legend. Our point is that things with long chemical names sound scary to some people.

The foreign origin of MSG might not have helped either. The Japanese manufacturer brought this product to the United States just two years after the end of World War II, when Japan's popular image was not at an all-time high, but an effective advertising campaign did the trick. Newspaper food sections in that era were filled with delicious-sounding recipes that included MSG, and columnists predicted that soon it would be customary to have three shakers on the table: salt, pepper, and MSG. It is not clear how many Americans even knew MSG was a Japanese product, because Chinese cooks used it too, and there were more Chinese restaurants in the United States than Japanese ones; but in the 1950s, everything Chinese or Japanese was in vogue, and there was no obvious reason to suspect a product that made food taste better. But when the first reports of possible allergic reactions appeared, note that the new malady was promptly labeled "Chinese restaurant syndrome," not "Colonel Sanders' complaint."

NOTE

1. "Salt that Tastes like Meat" (*Zanesville Signal*, 29 December 1929).

REFERENCES AND RECOMMENDED READING

Beyreuther, K., et al. "Consensus Meeting: Monosodium Glutamate—An Update." *European Journal of Clinical Nutrition*, Vol. 61, 2007, pp. 304–313.
CBS News. "No MSG." *60 Minutes* broadcast, November 1991.

Compton, D. "As-Salt on Science." *New York Post*, 13 January 2010.

Freeman, M. "Reconsidering the Effects of Monosodium Glutamate: A Literature Review." *Journal of the American Academy of Nurse Practitioners*, Vol. 18, 2006, pp. 482–486.

Geha, R. S., et al. "Review of Alleged Reaction to Monosodium Glutamate and Outcome of a Multicenter Double-Blind Placebo-Controlled Study." *Journal of Nutrition*, Vol. 130, 2000, pp. 1058S–1062S.

Kwok, R. H. M. "Chinese Restaurant Syndrome." *New England Journal of Medicine*, Vol. 18, 1968, p. 796.

Lecos, C. "New Regulation to Help Sodium-Conscious Consumers." *FDA Consumer*, May 1986.

Mallick, H. N. "Understanding Safety of Glutamate in Food and Brain." *Indian Journal of Physiology and Pharmacology*, Vol. 51, 2007, pp. 216–234.

Meadows, M. "MSG: A Common Flavor Enhancer." *FDA Consumer*, January–February 2003.

Moskin, J. "Yes, MSG, the Secret Behind the Savor." *New York Times*, 5 March 2008.

Rubini, M. E. "The Many-Faceted Mystique of Monosodium Glutamate." *American Journal of Clinical Nutrition*, Vol. 24, 1971, pp. 169–171.

"Salt that Tastes like Meat." *Zanesville Signal*, 29 December 1929.

Sand, J. "A Short History of MSG: Good Science, Bad Science, and Taste Cultures." *Gastronomica*, Vol. 5, 2005, pp. 38–49.

Sano, C. "History of Glutamate Production." *American Journal of Clinical Nutrition*, Vol. 90, 2009, pp. 728S–732S.

Schaumburg, H. H., et al. "Monosodium L-Glutamate: Its Pharmacology and Role in the Chinese Restaurant Syndrome." *Science*, Vol. 163, 1969, pp. 826–828.

Settipane, G. A. "The Restaurant Syndromes." *New England and Regional Allergy Proceedings*, Vol. 8, 1987, pp. 39–46.

Simon, R. A. "Adverse Reactions to Food Additives." *New England and Regional Allergy Proceedings*, Vol. 7, 1986, pp. 533–542.

Stevenson, D. D. "Monosodium Glutamate and Asthma." *Journal of Nutrition*, Vol. 130 (4S Suppl.), 2000, pp. 1067S–1073S.

Strong, F. C. "Why Do Some Dietary Migraine Patients Claim They Get Headaches from Placebos?" *Clinical and Experimental Allergy*, Vol. 30, 2000, pp. 739–743.

Tarasoff, L., and M. F. Kelly. "Monosodium L-Glutamate: A Double-Blind Study and Review." *Food and Chemical Toxicology*, Vol. 31, 1993, pp. 1019–1035.

Walker, R., and J. R. Lupien. "The Safety Evaluation of Monosodium Glutamate." *Journal of Nutrition*, Vol. 130 (4S Suppl.), 2000, pp. 1049S–1052S.

Wallis, C. "Salt: A New Villain?" *Time*, 15 March 1982.

Williams, A. N., and K. M. Woessner. "Monosodium Glutamate 'Allergy': Menace or Myth?" *Clinical and Experimental Allergy*, Vol. 39, 2009, pp. 640–646.

Yamamoto, S., et al. "Can Dietary Supplementation of Monosodium Glutamate Improve the Health of the Elderly?" *American Journal of Clinical Nutrition*, Vol. 90, 2009, pp. 844S–849S.

Yang, W. H., et al. "The Monosodium Glutamate Symptom Complex: Assessment in a Double-Blind, Placebo-Controlled, Randomized Study." *Journal of Allergy and Clinical Immunology*, Vol. 99, 1997, pp. 757–762.

Zautcke, J. L., et al. "Chinese Restaurant Syndrome: A Review." *Annals of Emergency Medicine*, Vol. 15, 1986, pp. 1210–1213.

28

Fear of Other Additives and Preservatives

> All substances are poisonous, there is none that is not a poison; the right dose differentiates a poison from a remedy.
>
> —Philippus Aureolus Paracelsus (1538)

SUMMARY

Additives are chemicals that manufacturers add to foods to improve their taste or appearance. Preservatives are chemicals that prevent food spoilage or deterioration. All foods (and all consumers) consist entirely of chemicals, and many additives and preservatives are of natural origin, yet there is an apparently widespread belief that food additives and preservatives are artificial and harmful. Some consumer groups oppose all food processing on principle, whereas others focus on specific chemicals and their alleged links to various health problems. As specific health scares in this category fizzle, new ones take their place, because there are so many additives and preservatives to choose from. Manufacturers keep inventing new ones, while researchers make new discoveries about old ones. It is important to remember that these chemicals were invented for a specific purpose—not to poison people, but to keep food palatable and nutritious far beyond its time and place of origin. As the global population becomes larger and increasingly urbanized, additives and preservatives will be hard to avoid. The chapter focuses mainly on two common additives (lecithin and maltodextrin) and two preservatives (sodium benzoate and sodium bisulfite).

SOURCE

The origin and story arc of this health scare have much in common with those of many other health scares. First came the problem: spoiled, discolored, or unappetizing food, which nobody likes. Then came the solution: a modern miracle, in the form of an arsenal of chemicals that kept food from spoiling, improved its appearance, or made it taste better. And then came the inevitable realization that no solution is perfect, that some chemicals are safer than others, and that some people are allergic or sensitive to substances that are safe for the majority.

For more than a century, some scientists have wondered if new food additives might cause cancer—an idea that reached a larger audience in the 1940s, when a graduate nutritionist named Adelle Davis (1904–1974) published the first in a series of increasingly unconventional books on diet and its relationship to health. Some of her ideas turned out to be correct; others did not. These concerns came to a head in about 1950, thus paving the way for the 1958 Delaney Amendment to the U.S. Food, Drug, and Cosmetic Act, which prohibited FDA approval of any food additive that caused cancer (at any dosage) in laboratory animals.

In the late 1960s, the Love Generation embraced the notion that food additives were not only poisonous and unnecessary, but actually represented a form of government mind control. These beliefs persisted into the 1970s, together with claims that food colors and other additives caused hyperactivity and other behavioral problems in children. As of 2010, variations on all these themes are alive and well and circulating via the Internet.

SCIENCE

Processed foods contain many controversial additives, such as emulsifiers, stabilizers, and acids, in addition to food colorings (Chapter 24), artificial sweeteners (Chapter 25), and flavor enhancers (Chapter 27). Vitamins and minerals added to foods also qualify as additives, but people rarely seem to worry about them, although high doses of some vitamins (such as excess niacin in bread) can cause discomfort. Enriched foods contain added nutrients that were lost during processing, whereas fortified foods contain nutrients that were not present in the original product. Widely used preservatives include antimicrobials, such as nitrites and sulfites, and antioxidants, such as BHA and BHT. The definitions of additives and preservatives overlap somewhat; salt, for example, can be either or both.

Food additives and preservatives can cause unintended harm in several ways. Prolonged or high-level exposure to some of these chemicals may cause cancer or other diseases. For example, the declining incidence of stomach cancer in the United States since the 1930s may be partly a consequence of refrigeration and the decreasing use of preserved meats, which are high in nitrosamines and other carcinogens. One hopes that all such chemicals will eventually be eliminated from today's food supply as a result of appropriate safety testing. Some other food additives and preservatives cause allergic reactions in a few people, and it may be impossible to ban every such chemical. An example is cochineal red dye (Chapter 24). Then there is a grab bag of indirect hazards that are harder to classify. MSG (Chapter 27) and other flavor enhancers may induce some people to overeat, for the simple reason that it makes food taste better. The results may include obesity, type 2 diabetes, and associated diseases of excess.

There are so many controversial food additives and preservatives that an entire book could scarcely do justice to all of them, but four examples will suffice:

- Soy lecithin is an emulsifier—a chemical that helps to prevent mixtures from settling out, by dispersing one substance as small droplets within another substance. For example, candy makers put it in chocolate bars to keep the cocoa fraction mixed with the cocoa butter. Unlike some emulsifiers, soy lecithin is completely metabolized in the human body and is considered nontoxic. This chemical is used not only as a food additive but also for treatment of high serum cholesterol. Some food Web sites, however, describe lecithin as a toxic waste product that is full of pesticides and has an unpleasant sticky appearance.

- Maltodextrin is a natural polysaccharide that is prepared by breaking down starch molecules into shorter chains. The usual source of the starch is corn or wheat, and at first glance, it is hard to see why this common food additive should be controversial. For some reason, however, a number of health food advocates have recently claimed that maltodextrin is just another name for monosodium glutamate (Chapter 27), an unrelated additive that some people consider harmful.
- Sodium benzoate is a preservative used in many processed foods and soft drinks. Some studies suggest that this chemical may form benzene, a known carcinogen, when combined with vitamin C. There is also some evidence that sodium benzoate may trigger hyperactive behavior in susceptible children, particularly in combination with certain food colorings. Although these studies are not conclusive, Coca-Cola recently stopped adding sodium benzoate (E211) to Diet Coke because of consumer concerns, and other manufacturers may follow its example. However, some diet sodas have simply switched to another preservative called potassium benzoate, which has similar properties.
- Sulfite salts (sodium bisulfite and others) are chemical preservatives that are often used to prevent dried fruit from losing its color. Sulfites also turn up in wines, dried potato products, and a number of other beverages and foods. In 1986, FDA banned the use of sulfites on raw fruits and vegetables or on meat. An estimated 1 percent of the U.S. population reacts to sulfites by rapidly developing symptoms, including severe asthma or hives. These chemicals may be hard to avoid, because the declaration requirements are somewhat complex, and not all products list sulfites on the label. Food recalls sometimes result from the discovery of undeclared sulfites.

HISTORY

Contrary to popular opinion, there is no evidence that people in ancient times used spices to disguise the odor and taste of rotten meat. What they really needed was some way to keep meat and other foods fresh without refrigeration. Various forms of salt have been used to preserve meat for thousands of years, but this method has certain disadvantages, including the formation of carcinogenic or toxic chemicals. Inventions such as refrigeration and canning (Chapter 13) have made it possible to reduce dependence on preserved meat, but the search for safe preservatives continues.

In 1904, Dr. William Frear (1860–1922) of Pennsylvania State College summarized medical opinion on the subject of food preservatives in a *New York Times* interview. More than a century later, we cannot improve on his statement, which applies equally to other food additives:

The best opinion seems to be against the use of preservatives as a general proposition as injurious, but, on the other hand, it is argued that the quantity used is so small as to be harmless in the products in which they are most necessary. The manufacturers seem to believe that it ought to be enough if all goods containing preservatives were plainly labeled, so that the consumer could see for himself, and take the responsibility for what he is taking into his stomach.[1]

In 1971, *Mad Magazine* published a sendup of the TV series *Sesame Street* (called "Reality Street"), in which a character called Cake Monster developed abdominal pain after eating a snack cake that contained a long list of chemical additives. The cartoon was a fair statement of public sentiment, then and now.

CONSEQUENCES

The backlash against additives has fueled demand for so-called health foods. People are willing to pay extra for foods advertised as free of artificial or nonorganic ingredients. This trend has expanded to include eggs laid by free-roaming chickens and milk from happy cows. As others have pointed out, however, the recent epidemic of obesity and type 2 diabetes in the United States suggests either that most people are not sticking to a health food diet, or that it is not working.

When famed nutritionist Adelle Davis was dying of bone cancer in 1974, a somewhat blunt interviewer asked how she accounted for her condition, when she had always claimed that an organic diet would prevent disease. She insisted that her theory was correct, blaming her cancer on the additives in junk food that she ate temporarily while attending college.[2] Nobody can be right about everything, but many of her ideas helped promote good health, by making food manufacturers accountable for their products and by introducing consumers to the principles of good nutrition. Sadly, those principles may be honored more in the breach than in the observance.

WHAT WENT WRONG?

Most doctors would probably agree that fresh vegetables, whole grains, and other "natural" foods are nutritionally superior to the usual western diet of greasy hamburgers and french fries. That does not, however, mean that a health food diet without artificial additives or preservatives will automatically prevent all cancers and other diseases. It is also important to remember why additives and preservatives were invented in the first place, and why it would be expensive and risky to stop using them. Most food travels a long distance or spends time in storage before reaching the consumer, who expects it to look and taste fresh and to be free of dangerous bacteria and fungi. These chemicals achieve the desired result, sometimes at a cost.

NOTES

1. "Use of Food Preservatives" (*New York Times*, 5 June 1904).
2. "Adelle Davis, Organic Food Advocate, Dies." UPI, 1 June 1974.

REFERENCES AND RECOMMENDED READING

Barrett, J. R. "Diet and Nutrition: Hyperactive Ingredients?" *Environmental Health Perspectives*, Vol. 115, 2007, p. A578.

Burros, M. "U.S. Food Regulation: Tales from a Twilight Zone." *New York Times*, 10 June 1987.

Cormier, E. and J. H. Elder. "Diet and Child Behavior Problems: Fact or Fiction?" *Pediatric Nursing*, Vol. 33, 2007, pp. 138–143.

Drummond, H. "Add Poison for Flavor & Freshness." *Mother Jones*, April 1977, pp. 13–14.

Eckardt, R. E. "Experimental Carcinogenesis and the Problem of Food Additives." *American Journal of Public Health*, Vol. 50, 1960, pp. 1488–1492.

Ehrenfeld, T. "Five Controversial Food Additives." *Newsweek*, 13 March 2008.

Foulke, J. E. "A Fresh Look at Food Preservatives." *FDA Consumer*, October 1993.

Gilbert, R. P., et al. "Greater Awareness of Sulfite Allergy Needed." *Western Journal of Medicine*, Vol. 146, 1987, p. 236.

Jian, L., et al. "Do Preserved Foods Increase Prostate Cancer Risk?" *British Journal of Cancer*, Vol. 90, 2004, pp. 1792–1795.

Jiang, R., et al. "Consumption of Cured Meats and Prospective Risk of Chronic Obstructive Pulmonary Disease in Women." *American Journal of Clinical Nutrition*, Vol. 87, 2008, pp. 1002–1008.

Khan, A., et al. "Deadly Meatballs—A Near Fatal Case of Methaemoglobinaemia." *New Zealand Medical Journal*, Vol. 119, 2006, p. U2107.

McCann, D., et al. "Food Additives and Hyperactive Behaviour in 3-Year-Old and 8/9-Year-Old Children in the Community: A Randomised, Double-Blinded, Placebo-Controlled Trial." *Lancet*, Vol. 370, 2007, pp. 1560–1567.

Paik, D. C., et al. "The Epidemiological Enigma of Gastric Cancer Rates in the U.S.: Was Grandmother's Sausage the Cause?" *International Journal of Epidemiology*, Vol. 30, 2001, pp. 181–182.

Polônio, M. L., and F. Peres. "Food Additive Intake and Health Effects: Public Health Challenges in Brazil." *Cadernos de Saúde Pública*, Vol. 25, 2009, pp. 1653–1666.

Rosenthal, E. "Some Food Additives Raise Hyperactivity, Study Finds." *New York Times*, 6 September 2007.

Settipane, G. A. "The Restaurant Syndromes." *New England and Regional Allergy Proceedings*, Vol. 8, 1987, pp. 39–46.

Simon, R. A. "Adverse Reactions to Food Additives." *New England and Regional Allergy Proceedings*, Vol. 7, 1986, pp. 533–542.

"Use of Food Preservatives." *New York Times*, 5 June 1904.

Varraso, R., et al. "Prospective Study of Cured Meats Consumption and Risk of Chronic Obstructive Pulmonary Disease in Men." *American Journal of Epidemiology*, Vol. 166, 2007, pp. 1438–1445.

Wallis, C. "Hyper Kids? Check their Diet. Research Confirms a Long-Suspected Link between Hyperactivity and Food Additives." *Time*, 24 September 2007.

Weiss, B. "Food Additives as a Source of Behavioral Disturbances in Children." *Neurotoxicology*, Vol. 7, 1986, pp. 197–208.

Weiss, B. "Food Additives and Hyperactivity." *Environmental Health Perspectives*, Vol. 116, 2008, pp. A240–A241.

Wiles, N. J. " 'Junk Food' Diet and Childhood Behavioural Problems: Results from the ALSPAC Cohort." *European Journal of Clinical Nutrition*, Vol. 63, 2009, pp. 491–498.

Wilson, B. G., and S. L. Bahna. "Adverse Reactions to Food Additives." *Annals of Allergy, Asthma and Immunology*, Vol. 95, 2005, pp. 499–506.

Wilson, J. "Steady Progress in Cancer Battle." *Reuters*, 22 August 1954.

Part Five

Other Biological Hazards

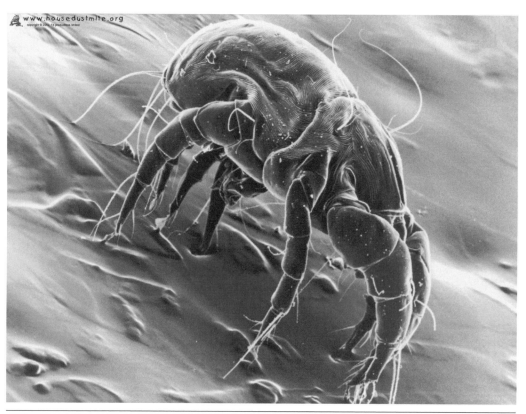

Figure 5   House dust mite.
(*Source:* www.HouseDustMite.org. Courtesy of Electron Microscopy and Audio Visual Unit, London School of Hygiene and Tropical Medicine.)

29

Fear of Mites

Now they knew that she was a real princess because she had felt the pea right through the twenty mattresses and the twenty eider-down beds. Nobody but a real princess could be as sensitive as that.

—Hans Christian Andersen, *The Princess and the Pea* (1835)

SUMMARY

Tiny animals called house dust mites, and their dead friends and droppings, are present in most house dust and also tend to accumulate in upholstered furniture and bedding after years of use. Tiny animals called follicle mites live in eyelash follicles and other locations on the human face. Cable mites, by contrast, are not real animals but mythic creatures that once formed the basis of practical jokes in offices. Tiny, creepy animals in general make fine health scares on slow news days, and several television documentaries and popular books in the 1970s and 1980s exploited this theme. House dust mites and follicle mites are not only remarkably unattractive by human standards (when highly magnified), but also cause allergic reactions in some people. By the early twenty-first century, however, the topic of invisible creepy-crawlies had largely fizzled in favor of a host of scarier issues, until the recent economic recession or some invisible force prompted mattress manufacturers to revive urban legends about dust mites and other microscopic horrors.

SOURCE

By about 1971, newspapers had embraced dust mites as a reliable filler topic of the "believe it or not" variety. When scanning electron microscopy became widely available in the 1970s, the general public saw many small creatures up close and personal for the first time (Figure 5). Many remarked that these animals looked like outer-space aliens, when in fact it was the other way around. Science fiction writers and artists have no idea what real aliens look like, but they know what is scary here on Earth. Dust mites and follicle mites starred in the 1996 PBS documentary "The Unknown World," and in the words of a *New York Times* reviewer, these images were "enough to make a person scratch." Finally, in 2000, the usually reliable *Wall Street Journal* ran a poorly researched article that appeared to validate a circulating rumor:

the accumulation of dead dust mites and their feces can double the weight of a mattress in just ten years!

Scientists first discovered follicle mites (*Demodex*) in the mid-nineteenth century, but until recently everyone assumed they were harmless. These little creatures became well-known at about the same time as dust mites, and for the same reason: TV documentaries and tabloids wanted everybody to see them. Unlike dust mites, follicle mites did not appear to cause asthma or other serious illness. But nobody really liked the idea of tiny upside-down animals, harmless or not, living in their eyelash and nose follicles.

The mythical beings known as cable mites or paper mites—not to be confused with genuine insects called book lice—originated in 1966, when workers at an American laboratory complained about tiny airborne particles that caused itching sensations after recent installation of overhead cables. Exterminators could find nothing, but the highly quotable term "cable mites" caught on and spread to other labs, offices, and factories. The phenomenon peaked in the 1970s and 1980s. At some point, itching sensations associated with "cable mites" apparently merged with sick building syndrome, the fear of toxic mold, and illusory parasitosis to create a headache for middle management and a minor gold rush for the pest control industry.

SCIENCE

Mites are tiny, usually eight-legged animals that are related to spiders. Many mite species live as pests in stored food, whereas others are parasites on living animals or plants. If dead skin cells shed by humans are food, house dust mites are in the first category. The generic name of the most famous house dust mite, *Dermatophagoides*, means literally "skin eater." These mites commonly live in mattresses and pillows, a fact that the bedding and vacuum cleaner industries exploit to good advantage.

It might seem like a good idea to have these mites patrolling our beds like tiny housekeepers, cleaning up the refuse that we leave behind. Unfortunately, the mites simply convert the dead human skin cells to mite feces, which contain proteins that can trigger asthma or allergic rhinitis attacks in susceptible people. Asthma has reached epidemic proportions in the industrialized world, and some scientists have proposed that increasing numbers of dust mites may be a contributing factor. But people cannot be shedding more skin cells or keeping their beds dirtier on average than at earlier times in history, so the reason for this proliferation is unclear. Maybe we have inadvertently destroyed or altered something that formerly kept the dust mites in check.

The two most common house dust mite species, *Dermatophagoides farinae* and *D. pteronyssinus*, occur in America and Europe, respectively. Another house dust mite that may prefer more humid parts of the world is called *Euroglyphus maynei*. Many other dust mites have similar habits, but this brief introduction should suffice.

Follicle mites (*Demodex folliculorum* and *D. brevis*) live on people's faces, particularly in the skin follicles of the nose, eyelashes, and eyebrows, where they spend most of their lives upside down. Until recently, most doctors believed these mites were harmless. It turns out that some people, particularly (but not exclusively) those with suppressed immune systems, harbor follicle mites in great numbers and suffer from related skin diseases, such as acne rosacea and inflammation of the eyelids. Older people are also more likely than younger ones to be infested with follicle mites. Now that an increasing percentage of the human population is either elderly or immunologically compromised, follicle mites have emerged as a minor but noteworthy health scare.

A 1983 journal article actually advised dermatologists not to tell their patients if they were infested with follicle mites, for fear of triggering an attack of symbiophobia (defined as "fear of intimate association with another life form") or delusory parasitosis. But a more recent study published in 2009 presented these ancient passengers in a more favorable light, by suggesting that follicle mites in healthy people could actually play a role in the skin's defense against disease-causing bacteria, such as *Staphylococcus* and *Streptococcus*. Acne, like asthma, has become prevalent in modern societies, and in both cases mites are implicated. Perhaps the problem is not too many mites, or too few, but mites struggling to cope with disturbed ecosystems.

The word *mite* does not always mean a tiny arachnid; it can also refer to any small object, living or not. Cable mites originated as nothing more sinister than fragments of rockwool or foam insulation dislodged from ceilings when new cables were installed in offices. Foam fragments, in particular, have a disconcerting tendency to become charged with static electricity and jump from the floor to people's socks. Other cable mite outbreaks apparently resulted from small slivers of irritating paper or other material associated with computer cable insulation or old-fashioned keypunch machines. Some offices even assigned new employees to track down the resident cable mites, in a rite of passage comparable to the time-honored snipe hunt.

According to some authorities, however, a more serious investment in cable mites could be a sign of illusory or delusory parasitosis. Illusory parasitosis means the sensation of being bitten by tiny creatures, when in fact something else is causing the sensation, such as dry skin, allergies, static electricity, or restless leg syndrome. It may progress to delusory parasitosis, or the unshakable belief that one is infested with harmful parasites, irrespective of evidence.

HISTORY

It has been common knowledge at least since the 1920s—more likely for centuries—that house dust causes some people to sneeze, or even to develop symptoms of asthma. The specific reason remained elusive until about 1964, when Japanese and Dutch researchers determined that house dust mites (*Dermatophagoides*) were the most important allergenic component in house dust. Over the next several years, scientists in other countries confirmed their findings.

Before long, the general public or the mattress industry figured out that dust contained dust mites and that mattresses contained dust, and a new urban legend was born. It held that, after 8 (or 10) years, the weight of a mattress would increase by 50 percent (or 10%) due to the accumulation of dust mites feeding on skin cells and defecating and dying, mere inches from our sleeping bodies and those of our innocent children. (In 2010, TV mattress salesmen continued to make similar claims.) As noted above, the prestigious *Wall Street Journal* did the world a disservice in 2000 by lending its support to this farce without checking the facts carefully.

But what are the facts? Dust mites do live in mattresses, and they multiply and defecate and die like everyone else, but can they really be that heavy? We found some legitimate statistics on this subject, and discovered the likely origin of the urban legend, to wit:

1. According to one published study, a typical used mattress of unknown age contains somewhere between 100,000 and 10 million dust mites. (We will assume the higher number.)
2. According to another published study, 1 gram of house dust contains up to 1,000 dust mites. Thus, if dust contained *only* dust mites, it would be fair to say that 1,000 dust mites weigh 1 gram.
3. If 1,000 dust mites weighed 1 gram, then the 10 million dust mites in the mattress would weigh 10,000 grams, or about 22 pounds—just about 50 percent of the weight of an average new twin-sized mattress! But in fact, this conclusion is false. The weight of 1,000 dust mites is *not* 1 gram, but a tiny fraction of a gram.
4. The problem was in Step 2. That gram of dust contains many other materials in addition to dust mites, such as pollen, fungi, and mineral soil. The soil accounts for nearly all the weight in most samples.

The sidebar ("The Author Weighs Her Mattress") presents further refutation of the mattress industry's claims. The respective histories of the follicle mite and "cable mite" health scares are short, and they are adequately summarized in the preceding sections.

The Author Weighs Her Mattress

There are only a few tasks more awkward than weighing a king-sized mattress, and one of those tasks is determining how much that mattress weighed when it was new. Hardly anyone routinely weighs a mattress upon bringing it home, and, contrary to rumor, the tag does not disclose the original weight of the mattress itself—only the weight of filler material.

In 2009, while writing this book, the author decided to put a common advertising claim to the test. Does the weight of a mattress really increase by 50 percent in 8 years (or by 100% in 10 years) due to the accumulation of dead dust mites and their waste products?

The author's mattress was made and purchased in 2003. When contacted in 2009, the manufacturer stated that the weight of the specific model at the time of manufacture was 75 pounds—near the low end of the known range for a king-sized mattress. In 2010, the mattress had not yet reached the eight-year cutoff point, but the book deadline loomed. Thus, the author weighed the mattress on a properly calibrated balance scale. The result: Seven years after purchase, it still weighed 75 pounds.

In conclusion, either (a) advertising claims about dust mites are bogus, or (b) mite buildup is punctuated rather than gradual, and in 2011 the weight of the mattress will suddenly increase by about 37 pounds. A future edition will present the sequel.

CONSEQUENCES

It is unclear if dust mite anxiety has had any net effect on mattress and box spring sales. This health scare might have persuaded Americans to buy new mattresses more often, but box springs have declined in popularity as more people discover the advantages of platform beds, which provide excellent back support and are easier to keep clean. Manufacturers of high-end air filters and vacuum cleaners have probably benefited from publicity about dust mites.

Follicle mites have not inspired the same level of health scare, probably because their impact (if any) is limited to cosmetic problems. In 2000, a photograph in one of our favorite New Age product catalogs portrayed a man whose nose resembled a large dill pickle, allegedly as a result of infestation with follicle mites. In the "after" photograph, after using the advertised herbal product, the man had a small nose and was smiling again.

WHAT WENT WRONG?

Quotable numbers can live forever in popular culture, even if they are based on faulty arithmetic and make no intuitive sense. We will never know who first misread those numbers about the weight of dust mites in mattresses, but it is unlikely that he or she anticipated that a respected magazine like the *Wall Street Journal* would publish the result as gospel, and perpetuate an urban legend, without ever checking the arithmetic or stopping to consider if such a thing is possible. Science writers and their editors should be more careful.

What we would really like to know is this: How can manufacturers and retailers offer a 20- or 30-year warranty on a mattress, while at the same time claiming that every mattress requires replacement after 8 years of use due to the unavoidable buildup of dust mites?

REFERENCES AND RECOMMENDED READING

"Attack of the Microcritters." *Current Events*, 13 March 1995.

Bodanis, D. 1986. *The Secret House*. NY: Simon and Schuster.

Brunton, S. A., and R. L. Saphir. "Dust Mites and Asthma." *Hospital Practice*, Vol. 34, 1999, pp. 67–68, 71–72, 75–76.

Burns, D. A. "Follicle Mites and their Role in Disease." *Clinical and Experimental Dermatology*, Vol. 17, 1992, pp. 152–155.

de Boer, R., and K. Kuller. "Mattresses as a Winter Refuge for House-Dust Mite Populations." *Allergy*, Vol. 52, 1997, pp. 299–305.

"Dust Mites Found in Many Homes." Associated Press, 20 June 1971.

Fernández-Caldas, E., and V. Iraola Calvo. "Mite Allergens." *Current Allergy and Asthma Reports*, Vol. 5, 2005, pp. 402–410.

Flora, C. "Cult of Clean." *Psychology Today*, September–October 2008.

Forton, F. "Demodex-Associated Folliculitis." *American Journal of Dermatopathology*, Vol. 20, 1998, pp. 536–537.

Gøtzsche, P. C., and H. K. Johansen. "House Dust Mite Control Measures for Asthma: Systematic Review." *Allergy*, Vol. 63, 2008, pp. 646–659.

Hambling, D. "Scratching the Surface." *The Guardian*, 28 November 2002.

Hill, M. R. "Quantification of House Dust Mite Populations." *Allergy*, Vol. 53, 1998, pp. 18–23.

Hinkle, N. "Ekbom Syndrome: The Challenge of 'Invisible Bug' Infestations." *Annual Review of Entomology*, Vol. 55, 10 August 2009.

Kemp, T. J. "House Dust Mite Allergen in Pillows." *British Medical Journal*, Vol. 313, 1996, pp. 916–919.

Layton, D. W., and P. I. Beamer. "Migration of Contaminated Soil and Airborne Particulates to Indoor Dust." *Environmental Science and Technology*, Vol. 43, 2009, pp. 8199–8205.

Nadchatram, M. "House Dust Mites, Our Intimate Associates." *Tropical Biomedicine*, Vol. 22, 2005, pp. 23–37.

Namazi, M. R. "A Possible Role for Human Follicle Mites in Skin's Defense Against Bacteria." *Indian Journal of Dermatology, Venereology and Leprology*, Vol. 73, 2007, p. 270.

Norn, M. S. "Incidence of *Demodex folliculorum* on Skin of Lids and Nose." *Acta Ophthalmologica*, Vol. 60, 1982, pp. 575–583.

Nutting, W. B. "Hair Follicle Mites (Acari: Demodicidae) of Man." *International Journal of Dermatology*, Vol. 15, 1976, pp. 79–98.

Nutting, W. B., and H. Beerman. "Demodicosis and Symbiophobic Status, Terminology, and Treatments." *International Journal of Dermatology*, Vol. 22, 1983, pp. 13–17.

Parker-Pope, T. "Those Costly Weapons Against Dust Mites May Not Be Worth It." *Wall Street Journal*, 18 February 2000.

Powell, F. C. "Rosacea and the Pilosebaceous Follicle." *Cutis*, Vol. 74, 2004, pp. 32–34.

Rufli, T., and Y. Mumcuoglu. "The Hair Follicle Mites *Demodex folliculorum* and *Demodex brevis*: Biology and Medical Importance. A Review." *Dermatologica*, Vol. 162, 1981, pp. 1–11.

Ryan, P. "Mite Mystery: Critters Have UTMB Employees Itching." *Galveston Daily News*, 11 May 1983.

Schei, M. A., et al. "House-Dust Mites and Mattresses." *Allergy*, Vol. 57, 2002, pp. 538–542.

Solarz, K. "Risk of Exposure to House Dust Pyroglyphid Mites in Poland." *Annals of Agricultural and Environmental Medicine*, Vol. 8, 2001, pp. 11–24.

Spieksma, F. T. "House Dust Mites: Introduction." *Experimental and Applied Acarology*, Vol. 16, 1992, pp. ix–xiii.

Thomas, W. R., et al. "The Allergenic Specificities of the House Dust Mite." *Chang Gung Medical Journal*, Vol. 27, 2004, pp. 563–569.

Vollmer, R. T. "*Demodex*-Associated Folliculitis." *American Journal of Dermatopathology*, Vol. 18, 1996, pp. 589–591.

Voorhorst, R. "Housedust, a Source of Allergens and of Misunderstanding." *Nederlands Tijdschrift voor Geneeskunde*, Vol. 110, 1966, pp. 46–48. [Dutch]

30

Fear of Toxic Mold

It became necessary to destroy the town to save it.
            —Peter Arnett (Associated Press, 10 February 1968)

SUMMARY

The fungus *Stachybotrys chartarum*, sometimes called Stacky or Mojo Mold, is one of several common greenish-black molds that often grow on wood or paper surfaces that have been exposed to water for several days or longer, such as paper-covered sheetrock walls in basements after flooding or stored piles of damp newspapers. It does not grow on concrete, linoleum, or tile surfaces. The news media, some researchers, and toxic mold support groups have blamed *Stachybotrys* for a bewildering range of health problems, including lung hemorrhages, liver disease, seizures, depression, fatigue, headaches, memory loss, and personality change—and, of course, hyperactivity and attention deficit disorder in children. Most studies have failed to support these conclusions, although this fungus (and others) can produce harmful mycotoxins, and its spores may trigger allergic reactions. In the past 15 years, Mojo Mold has become a key player in the lore and literature of "sick building syndrome." This health scare has fizzled in the sense that scientists and the media no longer take it very seriously, but it remains a hot topic for contractors, attorneys, and the insurance industry.

SOURCE

Between 1993 and 1994, 10 infants in Cleveland, Ohio had lung hemorrhages for unknown reasons, and one of those children died. Scientists from the U.S. Centers for Disease Control and Prevention (CDC) investigated the outbreak, and their preliminary finding was that the cluster of hemorrhages resulted from exposure to the *Stachybotrys* fungus growing in the basements of the children's homes. The news media, the legal profession, and the real estate, construction, insurance, and environmental consulting industries all promptly went wild, each in its own way. The "new" fungus became not only the alleged killer of Ed McMahon's dog Muffin, but also the subject of some unusual documentaries and lifestyle choices, as further discussed later in the chapter. The CDC retracted its original conclusion about the Cleveland outbreak in 2000, citing major errors in the 1994 investigation, but the damage was done. During the intervening six years, the mold crisis had acquired a cult following and taken on a life of its own. As so often happens, the original report received extensive media coverage, but apparently the retraction was considered less newsworthy.

SCIENCE AND HISTORY

Mold is a fuzzy growth that some fungi produce, usually on damp surfaces. Molds of many different species produce mycotoxins (toxic chemicals), as well as spores that can cause allergic reactions in some people. A common fungus called *Aspergillus flavus*, for example, produces a mycotoxin known as aflatoxin, which contaminates some stored foods and appears to be a risk factor for cancer. Yet this dangerous fungus is not nearly as famous as the unrelated "toxic mold" that threatened to engulf the insurance industry near the turn of the twenty-first century. This greenish-black fungus, sometimes called Stacky or Mojo Mold in popular accounts, has the scientific name *Stachybotrys chartarum*, which means something like "grapes on a stick with an affinity for paper." August Carl Joseph Corda (1809–1849), a European physician and mycologist, first discovered this fungus growing on the damp wall of a house in Prague in 1837.

There is no doubt that some people are allergic to this fungus, but in most homes the spores do not exist in sufficient numbers to cause a reaction. *Stachybotrys* spores, unlike those of some fungi, are relatively large and do not remain airborne for long. People cleaning moldy surfaces in basements or other enclosed spaces should wear protective masks to avoid inhaling fungal spores—or other harmful materials found in similar places, such as dust or rodent droppings. People with compromised immune systems should minimize their exposure to molds in general.

Stachybotrys and other fungi also produce toxic chemicals called mycotoxins under some growth conditions. In Ukraine in the 1930s, horses and cows showed signs of nervous disorders and internal hemorrhages after eating large quantities of damp, moldy straw contaminated with this fungus. People who handled the straw also reported headaches and nosebleeds, probably as a result of inhaling mycotoxins that became airborne on spores or other particulates. Well-documented modern examples are hard to find, but it is clearly a good idea to clean up any visible mold in homes and offices.

And that is where the controversy begins. Is it possible to remove toxic black mold from a contaminated house, just by airing it out and washing discolored surfaces? Or is it necessary (as some consultants claim) to burn or bulldoze the house and everything in it?

The immediate aftermath of the 1994 Cleveland outbreak gave little hint of the pandemonium that would follow. The investigators soon suspected *Stachybotrys*, apparently because of the hemorrhagic symptoms reported in the Ukraine. There was one previous report of this fungus apparently making an American family sick (in Chicago in 1986); pulmonary hemorrhages were not among the reported symptoms in that case, but it was still a reasonable hypothesis. At that stage, CDC experts advised the public that the toxic mold, if found, was fairly easy to remove from walls using a solution of chlorine bleach. As of 1997, the official report on the Cleveland incident stated that ten infants became sick and one of them died.

At that stage, Mojo Mold had already captured the public imagination and displayed powers that its discoverer could not have foreseen. According to the news media and popular opinion, exposure to this fungus could cause memory loss, personality change, attention deficit disorder, brain lesions, liver failure, premature aging, arthritis—you name it, Stacky could do it—and *nothing* short of fire and money could stop it, neither chlorine bleach nor the Roman rite of exorcism.

Several families in Arizona and Texas reported that the toxic black mold had invaded their homes, and one family's 1999 experience became the focus of a truly strange 2000 television documentary. Both husband and wife reported coughing up blood clots, feeling dizzy, undergoing personality changes, and eventually losing the ability to concentrate; their young son also developed asthma. The husband's boss stated that the *Stachybotrys* fungus had turned his employee into a "nincompoop" (his word, not ours). On the advice of consultants, the family had their beautiful 22-room house and all its contents demolished, even china and glassware that should have been easy to clean.

A press release about another family's toxic mold experience was even stranger, alleging that the family fled their Arizona home "when a garden of fluorescent mushrooms and molds were found growing in the walls."[1] Wait a minute—fluorescent mushrooms? Many fungi grow in buildings, and some common mushrooms are fluorescent, but what has this to do with the toxic black mold *Stachybotrys?*

In 2000, at the peak of toxic mold hysteria, the CDC reexamined its data and retracted its original conclusions, citing "serious shortcomings" in the 1994–1997 investigation. The pulmonary hemorrhages in Cleveland were not related to *Stachybotrys* after all. That retraction should have marked a turning point in public opinion of toxic mold, but in fact the scare took a few more years to wind down. Meanwhile, remediation or replacement of each mold-infested house might cost several hundred thousand dollars, and the homeowner's insurance industry was beside itself. In 2003, the media reported that talk-show host Johnny Carson's former sidekick Ed McMahon accepted a $7 million settlement in a toxic mold case that centered on the death of his dog.

In other words, the Mold Rush that started in modest homes in Cleveland had somehow migrated to high-end suburban houses in the Southwest. We do not doubt that many of the people in question felt sick and had moldy houses. Before fizzling, however, the phenomenon reportedly grew to include families who were facing foreclosure or had no medical insurance. For increasing numbers of homeowners, toxic mold beckoned like the American dream. By about 2005, it seemed that the tide of public opinion shifted, as juries began to scratch their heads in response to a sudden proliferation of similar cases. It soon became clear that the majority of houses, if searched carefully enough, contained at least a few *Stachybotrys* spores and at least one person with medical issues.

In the aftermath of Hurricane Katrina, *Stachybotrys* and other molds grew in many water-damaged homes, but the larger problems facing New Orleans tended to dwarf the issue of mycotoxins.

CONSEQUENCES

The Mold Rush has created or benefited a number of related industries. Some mycologists inspect homes and offices for the presence of toxic mold and give expert testimony for one side or the other in related lawsuits. The International Association of Mold Remediation

Specialists, founded in 2001, offers a Master Certified Remediation program and a Certified Mold Worker program. Some attorneys and physicians also specialize in such cases. Several companies do a brisk business in antifungal coatings, products for removal of mold from surfaces, and home test kits for identification of fungi. The homeowner's insurance industry coped with the crisis by raising premiums and adding mold exclusions and limits to most policies.

But was the original question ever answered? Can *Stachybotrys* cause babies to have fatal pulmonary hemorrhages? The possibility cannot be ruled out, but as of 2009, no other reported clusters of similar symptoms have been clearly associated with water damage. The 1994 Cleveland outbreak remains unexplained, and yet the media and the public have exaggerated it beyond recognition. It was tragic enough for 10 babies to become sick and for 1 to die—but by 2007, several Web sites claimed that the 1994 Cleveland outbreak involved 45 babies, of whom 16 died. In fact, those numbers refer to all unexplained cases of pulmonary hemorrhage in infants in Cleveland between 1993 and 2000. At this rate, future generations will speak in hushed tones of the Plague of Cleveland.

WHAT WENT WRONG?

It would be unfair to accuse the CDC of leaping to a premature conclusion, when in fact they spent nearly three years analyzing the Cleveland data before deciding—incorrectly, as it turned out—that mycotoxins made the infants sick. Mistakes are impossible to avoid, but this one had unforeseen consequences. Virtually all houses contain mold spores, not usually at harmful levels, and the construction defects litigation industry is always in the market for new material.

The Mold Rush was the next logical step after "sick building syndrome," a vaguely defined illness that first gained media attention in the 1970s and now strikes an estimated 10 to 25 million office workers each year in the United States alone. Both phenomena are based partly on fact and partly on the ancient motif of the haunted house. When people go inside certain houses (or caves), they feel uneasy or hear strange noises. Mold, or evil spirits? Perhaps mycotoxins make people believe that a house is haunted, or enable them to see what others cannot. But the opposite interpretation seems equally valid. Those who truly believe in the possibility of a haunted house may also be ready to accept a quick answer to all their health problems.

NOTE

1. "Moldy Homes Making Arizonans Ill" (Associated Press, 14 December 1999).

REFERENCES AND RECOMMENDED READING

Bowers, B. "Mixing—and Separating—Mold and Myth." *Best's Review*, February 2003.

Campbell, G. "Opportunism in the Golden Age of Irresponsibility." *Walls and Ceilings*, October 2001.

Chapman, J. A., et al. "Toxic Mold: Phantom Risk vs. Science." *Annals of Allergy, Asthma & Immunology*, Vol. 91, 2003, pp. 222–232.

Clepper, I. "The Ultimate Cure for Sick Building: Level It, Says Minnesota Governor." *Air Conditioning, Heating and Refrigeration News*, 4 May 1998.

Dearborn, D. G., et al. "Acute Pulmonary Hemorrhage/Hemosiderosis among Infants—Cleveland, January 1993–November 1994." *Morbidity and Mortality Weekly Report*, 9 December 1994.

Egan, M. E. "The Fungus that Ate Sacramento." *Forbes*, 21 January 2002.

"The Fire Cure." *People Weekly*, 9 July 2001.

Fung, F., et al. "*Stachybotrys*, a Mycotoxin-Producing Fungus of Increasing Toxicologic Importance." *Journal of Toxicology, Clinical Toxicology*, Vol. 36, 1998, pp. 79–86.

Gots, R. E. "Mold Claims: Recognizing what is Real." *Claims*, August 2002.

Heimpel, D. "The Toxic Mold Rush: California Mom Helps Fuel an Obsession." *Los Angeles Weekly*, 24 July 2008.

Hossain, M. A., et al. "Attributes of *Stachybotrys chartarum* and its Association with Human Disease." *Journal of Allergy and Clinical Immunology*, Vol. 113, 2004, pp. 200–208.

"An Insidious Mold." CBS News, 2 December 2000.

Jarvis, B. B., and J. D. Miller. "Mycotoxins as Harmful Indoor Air Contaminants." *Applied Microbiology and Biotechnology*, Vol. 66, 2005, pp. 367–372.

Khalili, B., et al. "Inhalational Mold Toxicity: Fact or Fiction? A Clinical Review of 50 Cases." *Annals of Allergy, Asthma & Immunology*, Vol. 95, 2005, pp. 239–246.

Kirn, T. F. "Concern about Risks from *Stachybotrys* Mold Unwarranted." *Family Practice News*, 1 February 2001.

Levine, H. "It's Invisible. It's Deadly. And It's in Your Home." *Redbook*, April 2004.

Levy, M. B., and J. N. Fink. "Toxic Mold Syndrome." *Advances in Applied Microbiology*, Vol. 55, 2004, pp. 275–288.

McCarthy, M. "Mold Puts Apartment Sale on Hold." *Sacramento Business Journal*, 4 September 1998.

Miller, J. D., et al. "*Stachybotrys chartarum*: Cause of Human Disease or Media Darling?" *Medical Mycology*, Vol. 41, 2003, pp. 271–291.

"Moldy Homes Making Arizonans Ill," Associated Press, 14 December 1999.

Page, E. H., and D. B. Trout. "The Role of *Stachybotrys* Mycotoxins in Building-Related Illness." *American Industrial Hygiene Association Journal*, Vol. 62, 2001, pp. 644–648.

Pestka, J. J., et al. "*Stachybotrys chartarum*, Trichothecene Mycotoxins, and Damp Building-Related Illness: New Insights into a Public Health Enigma." *Toxicological Sciences*, Vol. 104, 2008, pp. 4–26.

Skaer, M. "Protect Your Business against Mold Litigation." *Air Conditioning, Heating and Refrigeration News*, 5 June 2006.

Terr, A. I. "Are Indoor Molds Causing a New Disease?" *Journal of Allergy and Clinical Immunology*, Vol. 113, 2004, pp. 221–226.

U.S. Centers for Disease Control and Prevention, Office of the Director. "Update: Pulmonary Hemorrhage/Hemosiderosis among Infants—Cleveland, Ohio, 1993–1996." *Morbidity and Mortality Weekly Report*, Vol. 49, 2000, pp. 180–184.

Wakefield, J. "A Killer Smell: Mold Toxin Destroys Olfactory Cells in Mice." *Environmental Health Perspectives*, Vol. 114, 2006, p. A428.

Zalma, B. "Mold Isn't Gold: Texas Supreme Court Concludes Mold Claims Not Covered." *Claims*, March 2007.

31

The Cell from Hell

And the fish that was in the river died, and the river stank, and the Egyptians could not drink of the water of the river.

—King James Bible, Exodus 7:18

SUMMARY

Pfiesteria piscicida and related dinoflagellates are single-celled marine organisms that live in tidal rivers and estuaries. Some studies appear to show that *Pfiesteria* releases toxins that can cause large-scale fish kills as well as severe human health problems, including short-term memory loss and personality change. Other studies, however, have failed to confirm the human health hazard. When *Pfiesteria* first made headlines in 1995, the news media tended to sensationalize its effects and started assigning it cute names, such as the Cell from Hell or the Blob. The fact that the name of this organism rhymes with the word "hysteria" did not help matters either. Some officials even vilified the North Carolina researchers and environmental activists who first publicized the problem, accusing them of hurting the state's economy and discouraging tourism. This health scare has fizzled in the sense that the media and the public have apparently lost interest in it, but the organism itself still exists, and research continues.

SOURCE

Before the mid-1990s, the only people who had ever heard of *Pfiesteria* were a few biologists who specialized in the study of plankton. Starting in 1995, a series of highly publicized reports claimed that this organism had not only produced lethal bloody sores on billions of fish but had also released a neurotoxin with unusual effects on humans, including frightening symptoms such as short-term memory loss, outbursts of temper, and other personality changes. Some researchers reported becoming sick from handling infected fish or contaminated aquarium water. According to some studies, even staying out of the water was not a sufficient precaution, because the toxin could become airborne and affect people who inhaled it.

The media knew a good thing when they saw it, and soon the Cell from Hell joined Mojo Mold and Bat Boy on the front pages of supermarket tabloids. A new health scare was born, but in the process, the investigators who first reported the effects of *Pfiesteria* soon found themselves under fire. There is no question that some dinoflagellates produce dangerous toxins, or that the researchers who study these organisms may put themselves at risk. Most of the controversy focuses on the extent to which these toxins pose a threat to the general pubic or to commercial fishing. Inevitably, people also want to know whether *Pfiesteria* has really become more abundant in recent years, perhaps as a result of sewage runoff from farms along the Atlantic coast, or whether it has been there all along and nobody noticed.

SCIENCE

Pfiesteria and other dinoflagellates are members of the phytoplankton, a group of single-celled organisms that drift with the ocean currents and obtain energy from sunlight by photosynthesis. Some older sources refer to dinoflagellates as algae, or even classify them as plants, but most biologists now assign them to a loose grouping of unrelated organisms called Protista, which are neither plants nor animals. Some dinoflagellates are important components of "red tides," large algal blooms that sometimes discolor the surface water in coastal areas and produce neurotoxins that cause fish to die in large numbers. The water may appear reddish or brown, depending on the color of the species causing the bloom. However, some dinoflagellates also release such toxins without this warning coloration. *Pfiesteria* apparently releases its toxins only in the presence of large numbers of fish.

Researchers at North Carolina State University discovered this new dinoflagellate genus in 1988 and named it after algae researcher Lois Ann Pfiester (1936–1992). In a 1992 paper, the investigators described this dinoflagellate as a "phantom" because it disappeared into the mud of coastal estuaries after killing fish. The species name *piscicida* ("fish killer") is appropriate, as this organism has reportedly killed enormous numbers of fish in coastal waters from Delaware to Alabama. Nutrient runoff from coastal development, including poultry and hog farms, seems to promote its growth. The 1997 outbreak alone killed an estimated 1 billion fish and cost about $60 million in lost fisheries and tourism. A closely related dinoflagellate, discovered in 2000, was named *Pfiesteria shumwayae* in honor of marine biologist Sandra Shumway. Several other, less famous dinoflagellates resemble *Pfiesteria* and produce similar toxins, including species in the genera *Cryptoperidiniopsis*, *Luciella*, and *Karlodinium*.

Pfiesteria toxin causes skin lesions on fish and possibly also on humans who handle contaminated fish or water. The fish develop bleeding sores and often die, typically in huge numbers. For example, one outbreak in the late 1990s killed an estimated 1 billion fish off the Atlantic coast. Humans exposed to the toxin have reported itching, diarrhea, and other nonspecific symptoms. The most alarming effects of this toxin, however, are subjective changes that cannot be measured directly in fish, such as dizziness and loss of short-term memory.

Some other dinoflagellate toxins are known to cause paralysis, including a form of poisoning called ciguatera, which reportedly causes the sensation of loose teeth in the lower jaw—strange, but not terrifying. A different group of algae called diatoms can produce a toxin (domoic acid) that causes memory problems or abnormal behavior, but only after ingestion of a large dose in contaminated fish or shellfish. Early reports of *Pfiesteria* toxin suggested that it was far more insidious than any of the others, even sneaking up on people who got a small amount of contaminated water in their eyes. Dozens of people who were exposed to *Pfiesteria* during the mid-1990s reported such symptoms, including some of the biologists who discovered the organism. In 1994, at least one laboratory worker in North Carolina reportedly received a large Worker's Compensation settlement for injuries resulting from *Pfiesteria* exposure, but long-term injuries appear to be rare.

HISTORY

To a large extent, the history of this organism is also the history of Dr. JoAnn M. Burkholder, professor of aquatic ecology at North Carolina State University and a leading authority on toxic algae blooms. As the co-discoverer of *Pfiesteria piscicida*, Dr. Burkholder has worked for many years to determine how its growth is stimulated by nutrient enrichment, and how it affects commercially important finfish and shellfish in North Carolina estuaries and aquaculture farms. In recent years, harmful marine microalgae and dinoflagellates have caused worldwide increases in death and disease of coastal fishes, so it is important to separate the real biological threat from the media hype.

Dr. Burkholder's early efforts reportedly drew some unfavorable reactions from special interest groups. Farmers resented the implication that coastal pollution was related to farm wastes, and state officials feared that her findings might discourage tourism. According to one report, angry state officials and hog farmers challenged her methods and even attacked her personal character. Some scientific colleagues were also skeptical, because the reported effects of the toxin were unusual, and some reported observations were hard to duplicate. She persevered, however, and in 1997 succeeded in isolating the *Pfiesteria* toxin—the crucial first step in determining its chemical structure and developing tests for detecting its presence. In 1998, North Carolina State University opened a new laboratory dedicated to research on this dinoflagellate.

According to a 1997 interview by *People* magazine, the neurological effects of this toxin on humans became clear to Dr. Burkholder in 1993, when she rubbed her eyes with a gloved hand that she had previously dipped in an aquarium containing *Pfiesteria*. She immediately felt unsteady, and soon developed stomach cramps, breathing difficulty, and a temporary problem with memory and recognition. A number of fishermen and others exposed to *Pfiesteria* have also reported similar effects, but there appear to be no confirmed reports of long-term injury.

CONSEQUENCES

Although there can be little question that the *Pfiesteria* toxin and its effects are real, inevitably some people have jumped on the bandwagon or succumbed to the power of suggestion. There are home test kits and support groups and testimonials. Some fishermen and other workers have made questionable claims of personal injuries related to *Pfiesteria*, and some doctors have reported miraculous cures. One such doctor—who specializes in the treatment of patients exposed to *Pfiesteria* and other biotoxins—received a warning letter in 2004 from the U.S. Food and Drug Administration for allegedly giving unapproved veterinary drugs to human subjects. As of 2010, this doctor's novel diagnostic and treatment methods for *Pfiesteria* exposure have not gained wide acceptance, but the jury is still out.

WHAT WENT WRONG?

As a general rule, scientists get scared when a new factor accelerates a global environmental crisis, such as the ongoing collapse of fish populations. By contrast, the general public gets scared when the media report a dangerous new poison that may cause personality change and memory loss. These effects strike at the heart of personal identity and may seem more frightening than death. But with so many new health scares appearing every year, how is it possible to know which ones to take seriously?

At the time this book was written, the human health hazards associated with *Pfiesteria* were still controversial, but the consensus appeared to be that the media overreacted to early research reports. By contrast, public response was moderate and dignified, for the most part. A 1998 review by doctors at the University of Maryland concluded that the recent outbreak of human symptoms related to *Pfiesteria* did not meet the criteria for mass psychogenic illness. Once it became apparent that the effects of this new menace were physical, temporary, and largely avoidable, this health scare fizzled.

REFERENCES AND RECOMMENDED READING

Burkholder, J. "Ongoing Controversy over *Pfiesteria*." *Science*, Vol. 304, 2004, pp. 46–47.

Burkholder, J., et al. "New 'Phantom' Dinoflagellate is the Causative Agent of Major Estuarine Fish Kills." *Nature*, Vol. 358, 1992, pp. 407–410.

Burkholder, J., et al. "Demonstration of Toxicity to Fish and to Mammalian Cells by *Pfiesteria* Species: Comparison of Assay Methods and Strains." *Proceedings of the National Academy of Sciences U.S.A.*, Vol. 102, 2005, pp. 3471–3476.

Collier, D. N., and W. A. Burke. "*Pfiesteria* Complex Organisms and Human Illness." *Southern Medical Journal*, Vol. 95, 2002, pp. 720–726.

Diaby, S. "Economic Impact of the Neuse River Closure on Commercial Fishing." North Carolina Division of Marine Fisheries, 1996.

Drgon, T., et al. "Characterization of Ichthyocidal Activity of *Pfiesteria piscicida*: Dependence on the Dinospore Cell Density." *Applied and Environmental Microbiology*, Vol. 71, 2005, pp. 519–529.

Friedman, M. A., and B. E. Levin. "Neurobehavioral Effects of Harmful Algal Bloom (HAB) Toxins: A Critical Review." *Journal of the International Neuropsychological Association*, Vol. 11, 2005, pp. 331–338.

Glasgow, H. B., et al. "Insidious Effects of a Toxic Estuarine Dinoflagellate on Fish Survival and Human Health." *Journal of Toxicology and Environmental Health*, Vol. 46, 1995, pp. 501–522.

Gordon, A. S., et al. "Characterization of *Pfiesteria* Ichthyocidal Activity." *Applied and Environmental Microbiology*, Vol. 71, 2005, p. 6463.

Greenberg, D. R., et al. "A Critical Review of the *Pfiesteria* Hysteria Hypothesis." *Maryland Medical Journal*, Vol. 47, 1998, pp. 133–136.

Hudnell, H. K. "Chronic Biotoxin-Associated Illness: Multiple-System Symptoms, a Vision Deficit, and Effective Treatment."*Neurotoxicology and Teratology*, Vol. 27, 2005, pp. 733–743.

Kaiser, J. "The Science of *Pfiesteria*: Elusive, Subtle, and Toxic." *Science*, Vol. 298, 2002, pp. 346–349.

Magnien, R. E. "State Monitoring Activities Related to *Pfiesteria*-Like Organisms." *Environmental Health Perspectives*, Vol.109 (Suppl. 5), 2001, pp. 711–714.

Morris, J. G., et al. "Occupational Exposure to *Pfiesteria* Species in Estuarine Waters is Not a Risk Factor for Illness." *Environmental Health Perspectives*, Vol. 114, 2006, pp. 1038–1043.

Samet, J., et al. "*Pfiesteria*: Review of the Science and Identification of Research Gaps." *Environmental Health Perspectives*, Vol. 109 (Suppl. 5), 2001, pp. 639–659.

Schmechel, D. E., and D. C. Koltai. "Potential Human Health Effects Associated with Laboratory Exposures to *Pfiesteria piscicida*." *Environmental Health Perspectives*, Vol. 109 (Suppl. 5), 2001, pp. 775–779.

"Scientists Successfully Isolate Fish-Killing Organism *Pfiesteria* Toxin in Lab Tests." Press Release, North Carolina State University, 1 September 1997.

Shoemaker, R. C., and W. Lawson. "*Pfiesteria* in Estuarine Waters: The Question of Health Risks." *Environmental Health Perspectives*, Vol. 115, 2007, pp. A126–A127.

Swinker, M. "Neuropsychologic Testing Versus Visual Contrast Sensitivity in Diagnosing PEAS." *Environmental Health Perspectives*, Vol. 111, 2003, pp. A13–A14.

Tillett, T. "Remember *Pfiesteria*? Occupational Exposure Unlikely to Cause Cognitive Effects." *Environmental Health Perspectives*, Vol. 114, 2006, p. A429.

Weinhold, B. "Diving Deeper into the *Pfiesteria* Mystery." *Environmental Health Perspectives*, Vol. 110, 2002, p. A666.

32

Shoo Fly

The time may come when a fly will be as much of a disgrace in a room as a bedbug is now.
—Attributed to Dr. Samuel J. Crumbine (1908)

SUMMARY

Flies can transmit many infectious diseases and are generally perceived as dirty and annoying. The ancient Greeks had a minor god whose sole responsibility was to drive flies away from animal sacrifices. During the first half of the twentieth century, public health authorities in the United States encouraged people to kill as many flies as possible. The result was a temporary reduction in the number of flies in key locations, such as kitchens and dairies, where flies were most likely to come in contact with food. During the same time period, the incidence of typhoid, tuberculosis, polio, and other diseases also declined, although the connection (if any) was controversial. After these diseases largely disappeared from developed countries, the fear of flies appeared to fizzle—but did it, really? In 2002, German scientists proposed that biting flies might be capable of transmitting HIV, the virus that causes AIDS. Ever since the discovery of HIV in 1982, people have worried that mosquitoes or other vectors might be able to spread this modern plague. The recent discovery, although unconfirmed, may have reawakened an ancient fear of contagion.

SOURCE

Starting in about 1906, public health agencies in the United States and Europe launched a massive campaign to reduce the abundance of flies, particularly in places where these insects might land on food or garbage and facilitate the spread of disease. It was not humanity's first or last war on flies, but it launched a health scare that survives to the present day. The appealing slogan "Swat that fly!" lasted well into the Cold War era and inspired many a school science project. School children designed fly traps, and chemical manufacturers deployed an arsenal of pesticides.

When certain targeted diseases showed a dramatic decline during the same era, people felt like stakeholders, although most of these public health victories probably had other explanations. Two major diseases blamed on flies, typhoid and polio, succumbed to water treatment and vaccination programs, respectively. Others, such as tuberculosis, promptly returned in ever more deadly forms. Flies probably were never a major factor in transmission of any of these diseases, but they are annoying enough to serve as convenient scapegoats.

SCIENCE

Flies (other than the flightless ones) are two-winged insects in the order Diptera. The common housefly, *Musca domestica*, is the one that urban dwellers most often swat. This fly and its close relatives do not bite, but studies have shown that a single housefly can carry as many as six million bacteria and other microorganisms on its feet. Depending on where the fly acquired them, these germs may be harmless, or they may include the agents of diseases such as cholera, typhoid, amebic dysentery, E. coli, poliomyelitis, infectious hepatitis, campylobacteriosis, toxoplasmosis, trachoma, and even stomach ulcers (associated with the bacterium *Helicobacter pylori*). The fact that pathogens can stick to a fly's feet does not prove that these insects are major disease vectors, but few people want to risk finding out. Many other organisms also hitchhike on a fly's feet and legs, including harmless insects called pseudoscorpions and the eggs of some parasitic worms.

A second group of annoying dipterans, collectively known as garbage flies, have shiny metallic colors and tend to aggregate around decaying meat, dog feces, and exposed food at barbecues. These flies do not bite either, but whatever materials stick to their feet or mouthparts may travel back and forth among their preferred hangouts. Garbage flies are sometimes called blow flies, because they lay their eggs in dead animals, which tend to swell up as they decay. The swelling results from internal gases, but somebody apparently thought the flies came along and inflated the corpse like a balloon. An even sillier explanation of the name "blow fly" is the once-popular belief that these insects could blow their eggs into a corpse from a great distance, like an airplane on a strafing run.

Stable flies (*Stomoxys calcitrans*) are similar to houseflies, but with two major differences: they are more common near stables or farms where horses or other livestock are present, and they feed on blood, which they obtain by biting. Stable flies are known to transmit some viral diseases between horses, and they also bite humans. In 2002, German investigators cited laboratory evidence that stable flies might have transmitted SIV (the simian form of HIV) to humans who butchered chimpanzees for meat. Wire services and popular magazines immediately picked up this story because of its public health implications. If it happened once, far away and long ago, could it happen again? As of 2010, there appears to be no proof one way or the other.

Deerflies are another group of unpopular biting flies that are known to spread disease, including a nasty bacterial infection called tularemia or rabbit fever. Although anything linked to rabbits might seem benign, tularemia is a serious disease that has been studied for decades as a potential biological weapon. According to some reports, deerflies may also be capable of transmitting bartonellosis (cat-scratch fever) and even cutaneous anthrax. These flies are about the same size as houseflies, but have green or gold eyes and distinctive dark brown patterns on their wings. Deerflies occur mainly in damp forests and are seldom a problem for most urban dwellers.

HISTORY

We fully expected to begin this section with a discussion of the Biblical "Lord of the Flies," the popular translation of the name Beelzebub—in other words, the Devil. Ancient people knew that dead animals or food left in the sun quickly brought flies, and Baal or Beel was a sun god. (As it turns out, however, the name Beelzebub probably has nothing to do with flies.)

The ancient Greeks did not think highly of flies either; according to classical mythology, the hero Heracles either banished the flies from Mount Olympus by his own efforts, or persuaded Zeus to do it for him. In yet another version of the story, a minor deity called Myiagros or Myagron was responsible for getting rid of flies, mice, and other pests that might interfere with sacrifices to the more senior gods.

Since window screens and organophosphate pesticides were not invented until much later in history, it isn't clear how ancient people rid themselves of flies, but burning certain plants might do the trick. As recently as 1910, some public health officials still recommended a natural insecticide called pyrethrum, which was made from chrysanthemum flowers: "To destroy a large number of flies in a room close it tightly and burn pyrethrum which will give off a dense white smoke fatal to flies but harmless to man."[1] Pyrethrum is less effective than modern pesticides, but also less dangerous to humans and pets. As a result, it has regained some of its lost popularity and is widely used today, sometimes in combination with other chemicals to increase its stability.

In the early twentieth century, Dr. Samuel J. Crumbine of the Kansas State Board of Health spearheaded the U.S. public health campaign to control fly populations. The original slogan was actually "Swat the fly," later changed to the more specific directive "Swat that fly." It was not Dr. Crumbine's only achievement; a lifelong advocate of health education, he began his career as a pharmacist in the Wild West of the 1880s. Other combatants in the war on flies included Frank Rose, a school superintendent and inventor of the fly swatter, and all the unnamed merchants who offered prizes to children who collected the largest number of dead flies.

By the summer of 1908, every American city had deployed fly traps in strategic locations, and some infectious diseases were on the decline. Improved water treatment and sanitation probably accounted for most of the improvement, but the fly campaign helped, if only by raising public awareness of the importance of keeping food clean. At the time, doctors believed that flies were a major factor in the spread of polio, but Yale researchers rejected that hypothesis after a series of field experiments in the 1940s. Fortunately, the polio vaccine came along in 1955 (Chapter 19).

In June 2009, U.S. President Barack Obama reportedly got in trouble with the organization People for the Ethical Treatment of Animals (PETA) for swatting a fly that landed on his arm during an interview. When that event made world news, it was clear that the war on flies had come full circle.

CONSEQUENCES

When people are desperate, they take chances. The early consequences of the fly scare included the invention of some terrible weapons of mass destruction, such as the famous

Shell No Pest Strip, which the USDA approved for indoor use in 1963 over the objections of its own scientists. The No Pest Strip's active ingredient was called DDVP (Dichlorvos or Dimethyl 2,2-dichlorovinyl phosphate), and it *really* worked. Hang one of these babies in an insect-filled room, then go out for a while—or stay there and serve dinner, what the heck. But cover the plates, because within an hour or two it would virtually rain flies and mosquitoes. Even the ones on the ceiling would let go.

After a few years, somebody figured out that this powerful weapon was not particularly good for people, either. There was evidence that it could cause bone marrow damage, aplastic anemia, and neurological problems, and the indoor use of DDVP in the United States was quietly restricted in 1979.

WHAT WENT WRONG?

There are some wars that will never be won. Despite thousands of years of clever fly traps and deadly poisons, flies continue to be a major nuisance wherever exposed garbage accumulates. As landfills run out of space and cities run out of money, this problem can only get worse. Fortunately, in the last half-century, the most serious diseases formerly spread by flies have been largely defeated in developed countries, and the public enjoys the temporary luxury of worrying about pesticides rather than pests.

But old diseases can return, just as new ones can emerge; and thanks to the recent chemical war, many fly populations have now acquired resistance to the most effective pesticides. In his poem "De Culice," the Roman poet Virgil (70–19 B.C.) described how a buzzing gnat saved a sleeping man's life by waking him just as a venomous snake was about to strike. Perhaps Virgil was advising future generations to sleep lightly.

NOTE

1. "Swat the Fly, Each Carries a Million Germs" (*Correctionville News*, 19 May 1910).

REFERENCES AND RECOMMENDED READING

Alam, M. J., and L. Zurek. "Association of *Escherichia coli* O157:H7 with Houseflies on a Cattle Farm." *Applied and Environmental Microbiology*, Vol. 70, 2004, pp. 7578–7580.

Allen, S. J. "Flies and *Helicobacter pylori* Infection." *Archives of Disease in Childhood*, Vol. 89, 2004, pp. 1037–1038.

Blanchard, R. "The War Against Flies in France." *British Medical Journal*, Vol. 2, 1915, p. 612.

Cirillo, V. J. " 'Winged Sponges': Houseflies as Carriers of Typhoid Fever in 19th- and Early 20th-Century Military Camps." *Perspectives in Biology and Medicine*, Vol. 49, 2006, pp. 52–63.

Eigen, M., et al. "Transferability of HIV by Arthropods Supports the Hypothesis about Transmission of the Virus from Apes to Man." *Naturwissenschaften*, Vol. 89, 2002, pp. 185–186.

Ekdahl, K., et al. "Could Flies Explain the Elusive Epidemiology of Campylobacteriosis?" *BMC Infectious Diseases*, Vol. 5, 2005, p. 11.

"Flies and Polio." *Time*, 5 January 1942.

"Fly Control Yields Fewer Trachoma Cases." *Science News*, 29 May 1999.

French, R. E. "Fly Catchers," p. 127 in Tate, K., and J. Tate (Eds.). 2001. *Good Old Days: Country Wisdom*. Berne, IN: House of White Birches.

Goulding, M. "When Bugs Attack." *Men's Health*, Vol. 23, 2008, p. 54.

Graczyk, T. K., et al. "Mechanical Transmission of Human Protozoan Parasites by Insects." *Clinical Microbiology Reviews*, Vol. 18, 2005, pp. 128–132.

Greiner, A. "Pushing the Frontier of Public Health." *KU Med*, Vol. 49, 1999, p. 25.

"How Polio Spreads." *Time*, 28 May 1945.

Kerr, C. "Bloodsucking Fly Blamed for Transmitting HIV." *Lancet Infectious Diseases*, Vol. 2, 2002, p. 265.

Kobayashi, M., et al. "Houseflies: Not Simple Mechanical Vectors of Enterohemorrhagic *Escherichia coli* O157:H7." *American Journal of Tropical Medicine and Hygiene*, Vol. 61, 1999, pp. 625–629.

Lee, R. A. 2007. *From Snake Oil to Medicine: Pioneering Public Health*. Westport: Praeger.

Levine, O. S., and M. M. Levine. "Houseflies (*Musca domestica*) as Mechanical Vectors of Shigellosis." *Reviews of Infectious Diseases*, Vol. 13, 1991, pp. 688–696.

Lundeen, T. "Flies Spread Salmonella to Poultry." *Foodstuffs*, 7 April 2008.

Malik, A., et al. "House Fly (*Musca domestica*): A Review of Control Strategies for a Challenging Pest." *Journal of Environmental Science and Health B*, Vol. 42, 2007, pp. 453–469.

Martinez, M. J., et al. "Failure to Incriminate Domestic Flies (Diptera: Muscidae) as Mechanical Vectors of *Taenia* Eggs (Cyclophillidea: Taeniidae)." *Journal of Medical Entomology*, Vol. 37, 2000, pp. 489–491.

Mlot, C. "Can Houseflies Spread the Ulcer Bacterium?" *Science News*, 7 June 1997.

Nazni, W. A., et al. "Bacteria Fauna from the House Fly, *Musca domestica* (L.)." *Tropical Biomedicine*, Vol. 22, 2005, pp. 225–231.

"PETA Miffed at President Obama's Fly 'Execution.'" Reuters, 18 June 2009.

Raymo, C. "The Point of Flies." *Boston Globe*, 10 July 1989.

Robertson, R. C. "The Fly Menace in Shanghai." *China Journal*, October 1937.

Rogers, N. 1992. *Dirt and Disease: Polio Before FDR*. New Brunswick, NJ: Rutgers University Press.

Shaffer, J., et al. "Filthy Flies? Experiments to Test Flies as Vectors of Bacterial Disease." *American Biology Teacher*, Vol. 69, 2007, pp. 28–31.

"Stable Flies Linked to HIV." *Popular Mechanics*, 1 June 2002.

"What's that Fly Doing in my Soup?" *Newsweek*, 28 July 1997.

Yap, K. L., et al. "Wings of the Common House Fly (*Musca domestica* L.): Importance in Mechanical Transmission of *Vibrio cholerae*." *Tropical Biomedicine*, Vol. 25, 2008, pp. 1–8.

33

Fear of Frankenfood

The anti-GMO movement is an imperialism of rich tastes imposed on the poor.
—Robert L. Paarlberg, Wellesley College (2008)

SUMMARY

For more than two decades, many environmental activists and healthcare advocates have questioned the safety of foods derived from genetically modified organisms (GMOs). Many consumers, particularly in Europe, have expressed aversion to these "Frankenfoods" on general principles. Potential concerns range from the accidental (or deliberate) creation of dangerous monsters, poisonous foods, or killer plagues, to more moderate threats such as the exposure of consumers to allergens transferred from one species to another. To date, genetically engineered crops have not lived up to all promises or expectations, and their existence has created certain legal problems. For example, if patented genes in pollen grains escape from a farmer's field and find their way into a neighbor's crop, who owes money to whom? The ancient lawgiver Hammurabi never anticipated that dilemma, but we have faith in the modern legal profession to work it out. The present scientific consensus appears to be that genetic engineering of agricultural crops is not only safe—in most cases—but increasingly necessary to contain the cost of feeding an overpopulated world. There is some evidence that the deep-rooted fear of genetic engineering has begun to fizzle, now that most people take its products for granted.

SOURCE

Farmers and animal breeders have always found ways to bring about genetic change in plants and animals. Just look at all the high-yield hybrid grains, gigantic pumpkins, and fanciful dog breeds that our ancestors created over the course of centuries by selective breeding alone. Genetic engineering just took the process to the next level, by artificially inserting genes from one organism into the genome of another.

Genetically modified bacteria have produced human insulin for treatment of diabetes since 1982, but few people objected to that breakthrough, since medicine is not quite the same thing as food. The first farming application of this new technology came in 1985, when the U.S. Environmental Protection Agency (EPA) approved field testing of genetically modified bacteria that were designed to prevent frost damage to strawberry plants. The inventors took bacteria that normally promote ice formation on plant stems and modified them to produce a different protein that could not serve as a seed for ice crystal formation. Public reaction was mixed. Not everyone liked the idea of "mutant bacteria" unleashed on the world, but nothing obvious went wrong, and at least the GMO itself was not a food.

The roots of the Frankenfood scare are deeply embedded in history, but every scare must start with some event. The first genetically modified whole food crop was the famous Flavr Savr tomato, which appeared on the market in 1994 after receiving FDA approval in 1992. The new tomato was designed to have a prolonged shelf life, but the rumor mill promptly claimed that the Flavr Savr not only tasted bad, but was square. In fact, it tasted like a tomato and was round. Agronomists developed "square" tomatoes back in the 1950s by the usual method of selective breeding, not to defy the laws of nature, but simply to pack more tomatoes into a square box with less wasted space. Whatever the reason, the Flavr Savr tomato was not a marketing triumph, and the manufacturer withdrew it from the market in 1996.

Meanwhile, several other genetically modified food crops had become available, and consumers faced the fact that the new technology was here to stay. Scientists and journalists on both sides of the debate made extravagant claims that did not pan out. Proponents of genetic engineering promised higher yields to feed the world's starving millions at lower cost, but a 2009 study by the Union of Concerned Scientists found no such benefits to date. Opponents of genetic engineering, by contrast, promised everything from the apocalyptic collapse of ecosystems to economic ruin for Third World farmers. Again, nothing like this has happened to date, but the controversy continues, and the kids hate it when Mommy and Daddy fight.

SCIENCE

Genetic engineering is just what it sounds like—the direct manipulation of an organism's genes to achieve some desired result. Terms such as recombinant DNA technology, gene splicing, molecular cloning, and DNA amplification refer to specific techniques used in this field. Agrogenetics refers specifically to the use of genetic engineering in agriculture. Biotechnology is a more general term that encompasses genetic engineering as well as industrial uses of bacteria and technologies based on cell and tissue cultures.

Genetically engineered food crops are designed to have desirable qualities such as higher yield, improved nutritional content, or resistance to disease, drought, or herbicides. To the extent that these efforts are successful, farmers will be able to feed more people with less land, while also reducing consumption of water, fertilizer, and agricultural chemicals. These are the same as the goals of traditional agronomy, except that biotechnology enables us to get there faster, and to make genetic leaps that would not happen in the course of selective breeding. When discussing the latest developments in genetic engineering, however, the new media tend to ignore these plodding goals in favor of bizarre stories, such as the cloning of fluorescent red cats in South Korea in 2007.

Any discussion of genetic engineering soon turns to the alleged benefits of organic food over genetically modified food. But just what is organic food? For decades, nobody really knew, because the word "organic" has multiple meanings. When chemists refer to organic molecules, they just mean that the substance contains carbon or a carbon-hydrogen bond.

By that definition, all food is organic, and so is gasoline. In the food industry, however, the word usually refers to products that are grown without artificial fertilizers, pesticides, hormones, or biotechnology. In 2010, the U.S. Department of Agriculture (USDA) narrowed the definition of organic milk and meat to exclude any animals that do not spend at least one-third of the year grazing on pasture. When the USDA requested public comments on this issue in 1998, it reported receiving nearly 300,000 letters. People clearly have strong opinions about food.

Genetically modified organisms now account for a large percentage of most major crops. This does not mean the food is poisonous or unnatural, just that agricultural scientists have tinkered with it. For example, about 90 percent of all soybean plants grown in the United States are resistant to certain chemicals used to kill weeds. At first glance, it might be hard to see why anyone would object to genetic shortcuts in the quest for better food, but there are some valid concerns. Biologists have pointed out that some crop plants that have been genetically modified to resist herbicides might outcross with their wild relatives, producing hybrid weeds that would be nearly impossible to kill. Aesthetic concerns are another problem; crops that have been modified to produce their own built-in pesticides may not seem appetizing. Still other consumers worry about allergens. For example, one strain of soybean reportedly has an added gene from the Brazil nut. People who are allergic to Brazil nuts might get sick by accidentally eating these soybeans.

HISTORY

Let us now examine the strange soil in which the fear of biotechnology has its roots. DNA and the methods for manipulating it are recent discoveries, but the idea of taking liberties with Mother Nature is ancient. With the exception of the ever-popular (but usually infertile) mule, crosses between different species throughout history and literature have generally turned out poorly or not at all. A zoo-bred liger is a sad sight. The menacing Sphinx in Greek mythology was a hopeless jumble of woman, snake, eagle, and lion. The Minotaur and most of the centaurs were also antisocial.

In the 1996 motion picture *The Island of Dr. Moreau*, an evil scientist creates seemingly pointless half-human monsters by means of genetic engineering and implanted silicon chips. But H. G. Wells wrote the novel a century earlier, when neither of those technologies existed. The equivalent evil in his day was "vivisection," or experimental surgery that scientists supposedly performed on living animals for no higher purpose than to inflict pain, satisfy curiosity, and make a mess. People have always distrusted any scientist who presumed to tinker with the fundamental processes of life. That fear was alive and well in 1933, when Walt Disney made a Mickey Mouse cartoon called "The Mad Doctor." Pluto escaped from the laboratory, of course, but the title character's monolog is noteworthy:

> I'm a raring, tearing wizard
> When it comes to cutting up
> I can graft a chicken's gizzard
> On the wishbone of a pup

> And here's the great experiment
> I'm just about to tackle
> To find out if the end result
> Will crow or bark or cackle.[1]

In 1982, the year when genetic engineering first began to attract public notice, a Christian minister of our acquaintance told his congregation: "If those scientists have their way, someday you'll have a tree growing out of your head." All too often, the layman's perception is that scientists engaged in biotechnology have no constructive purpose in mind, only the whimsical creation of chaos and suffering and the assumption of powers best left to the Almighty. In recent years, however, the fear of genetic engineering may have begun to diminish as more people understand its purpose. Meanwhile, in any new industry, mistakes are inevitable. Sometimes we really don't know for certain if the result will crow or bark or cackle.

In August 2010, a Federal judge in San Francisco revoked U.S. approval of genetically modified sugar beets, citing environmental concerns. Although the health scare may have fizzled, regulatory oversight is necessary, as in every industry.

CONSEQUENCES

Under English common law, which many American states adopted early in their history, livestock owners were required to confine their animals to their own property by means of a suitable fence, but farmers were not similarly required to build a fence around their crops. Early American colonists reversed this tradition, requiring the farmer to build the fence. In either case, somebody was held responsible for keeping the pig out of the neighbor's turnip field. Meanwhile, pollen continued to move freely back and forth between fields as it had always done, on the wind or on the bodies of bees, and farmers did not pay one another for the exchange of genes.

Now that some genetic traits are protected under patent law as intellectual property, what are the respective property owners to do? Is the owner of the patented genes entitled to compensation if some unavoidable (and largely undetectable) process transfers them to the neighbor's field? If the farmer whose crop receives the patented genes does not want them, how can she give them back? Entire books have been written on this subject, and anyone who believes that fear of litigation does not belong in a book on health scares may be in for a rude awakening.

According to one of our favorite urban legends, the Kentucky Fried Chicken restaurants changed their name to KFC because the genetically modified chickens they used were so abnormal and weird-looking that it was illegal to call them chickens. (This appears to be false.)

WHAT WENT WRONG?

Despite the early promise of enormous profits to startup biotech firms in the 1970s, the scientific community moved cautiously at first, declaring a moratorium on genetic engineering in 1975 while the National Institutes of Health (NIH) developed guidelines for good practice. Issued in 1976, these guidelines were intended not only to avoid potential environmental and social disaster, but also to reassure the general public on that point. It is not clear how well this public relations effort worked, particularly in Europe, where resistance to genetically modified crops has often been stronger than in the United States.

Messing with people's food and farming traditions is like putting fluoride in drinking water or vaccinating children against disease. There are certain basic rights that few people are willing to relinquish. Every innovation encounters resistance, often for good reasons. Even the earliest canned foods (Chapter 13) caused problems, but the world needed the technology, and food processors got it right eventually. Genetic engineering is here to stay, but its long-term impact is unknown at present.

NOTE

1. Walt Disney Productions, "The Mad Doctor" (United Artists, 1933).

REFERENCES AND RECOMMENDED READING

Azadi, H., and P. Ho. "Genetically Modified and Organic Crops in Developing Countries: A Review of Options for Food Security."*Biotechnology Advances*, Vol. 28, 2010, pp. 160–168.

Chomka, S. "Frankenfood or Brave New World?" *Grocer*, 9 February 2008.

De Beer, J. "The Rights and Responsibilities of Biotech Patent Owners." *University of British Columbia Law Review*, Vol. 40, 2007, pp. 343–374.

Elias, P. " 'Frankenfood' or Fruitful Harvest?" Associated, Press, 7 July 2003.

"Genetic Foods Still Mystery to Americans." Associated Press, 24 March 2005.

Goch, L. "Altered Risks." *Best's Review*, June 2000.

Gurian-Sherman, D. "Failure to Yield: Evaluating the Performance of Genetically Engineered Crops." Union of Concerned Scientists, April 2009.

Haslberger, A. G. "Need for an 'Integrated Safety Assessment' of GMOs, Linking Food Safety and Environmental Considerations."*Journal of Agricultural and Food Chemistry*, Vol. 54, 2006, pp. 3173–3180.

Herring, R. J. "Opposition to Transgenic Technologies: Ideology, Interests and Collective Action Frames." *Nature Reviews, Genetics*, Vol. 9, 2008, pp. 458–463.

Hug, K. "Genetically Modified Organisms: Do the Benefits Outweigh the Risks?" *Medicina* (Kaunas, Lithuania), Vol. 44, 2008, pp. 87–99.

Keatley, K. L. "Controversy over Genetically Modified Organisms: The Governing Laws and Regulations." *Quality Assurance*, Vol. 8, 2000, pp. 33–36.

Ladics, G. S., and M. K. Selgrade. "Identifying Food Proteins with Allergenic Potential: Evolution of Approaches to Safety Assessment and Research to Provide Additional Tools." *Regulatory Toxicology and Pharmacology*, Vol. 54 (Suppl. 3), 2009, pp. S2–S6.

Margolis, M. "Crops With Attitude: Poor Nations are Starting to Shake Off the Old 'Frankenfood' Taboo." *Newsweek*, 14 March 2009.

Neuman, W. " 'Non-GMO' Seal Identifies Foods Mostly Biotech-Free." *New York Times*, 28 August 2009.

O'Neill, M. "Geneticists' Latest Discovery: Public Fear of 'Frankenfood.' " *New York Times*, 28 June 1992.

Paparini, A., and V. Romano-Spica. "Public Health Issues Related with the Consumption of Food Obtained from Genetically Modified Organisms." *Biotechnology Annual Review*, Vol. 10, 2004, pp. 85–122.

Pollack, A. "In Lean Times, Biotech Grains are Less Taboo." *New York Times*, 21 April 2008.

Pollack, A. "Monsanto Sees Big Increase in Crop Yields." *New York Times*, 5 June 2008.

Reis, L. F., et al. "GMOs: Building the Future on the Basis of Past Experience." *Anais da Academia Brasileira de Ciências*, Vol. 78, 2006, pp. 667–686.

Rhodes, B., et al. "Frankenfoods? The Debate Over Genetically Modified Crops." National Center for Case Study Teaching in Science, 2003.

Rifkin, J., and T. Howard. "Consumers Reject 'Frankenfoods' (Genetically Engineered Food Products)." *Chemistry and Industry*, 18 January 1993.

Séralini, G. E., et al. "How Subchronic and Chronic Health Effects can be Neglected for GMOs, Pesticides or Chemicals." *International Journal of Biological Sciences*, Vol. 5, 2009, pp. 438–443.

Sparrow, P. A. "GM Risk Assessment." *Methods in Molecular Biology*, Vol. 478, 2009, pp. 315–330.

Thomas, K., et al. "The Utility of an International Sera Bank for Use in Evaluating the Potential Human Allergenicity of Novel Proteins." *Toxicological Sciences*, Vol. 97, 2007, pp. 27–31.

U.S. Environmental Protection Agency. "EPA Approves First Use in Environment of Genetically Altered Bacteria." Press release, 14 November 1985.

Varzakas, T. H., et al. "The Politics and Science behind GMO Acceptance." *Critical Reviews in Food Science and Nutrition*, Vol. 47, 2007, pp. 335–361.

34

Fear of Spiders

You don't stop being frightened of spiders just because the world's blown up.
—Simon Pegg (2005 interview with George A. Romero)

SUMMARY

Many people believe that brown recluse spiders are abundant throughout North America and that their bite causes severe injury or death. In fact, these spiders apparently live only in the south-central Midwestern states, and their bite seldom causes anything worse than a slow-healing skin ulcer. Other recluse species in California and the Southwest have caused no reported deaths. Black widow spiders (of several species) occur throughout the United States and on every continent except Antarctica. At one time, the news media treated the black widow as a major health threat, but in recent decades it has surrendered that title to the brown recluse. A few people have died from brown recluse or black widow bites, but the usual number of U.S. deaths per year from either cause ranges from zero to three. Even in Australia, home of the fabled Sydney funnel web spider, deaths from spider bites are rare. Health scares related to spiders not only cause unnecessary alarm but also contribute to misdiagnosis of skin lesions that are dangerous in themselves, such as necrotizing fasciitis (Chapter 11) and cutaneous anthrax. Although health scares related to spiders have gradually fizzled as new concerns have displaced them, deadly spider bites and horrific "new" spiders remain media staples.

SOURCE

In 1934, at least three respected periodicals—*Science*, *Scientific American*, and *Popular Mechanics*—published warnings about a new global threat that apparently dwarfed such current events as the Dust Bowl, organized crime, the rise of Nazi Germany, and economic recovery from the Great Depression. The new threat was a population explosion of black widow spiders, which, according to *Popular Mechanics*, had become "a menace to mankind." For the next few years, newspapers responded with the purplest of prose, followed in some cases by retractions. This health scare gradually faded by the 1950s, but it is probably fair to say that most people today know the black widow's name. In 2010, on what must have been the slowest news day on record, the wire services reported that a man in Boston found two black widow spiders in a bag of grapes. Oh, the horror!

Scientists have known about the brown recluse spider of the American Midwest since 1940, and a related South American species (the Chilean recluse) was discovered nearly a century earlier. The Chilean recluse drew unfavorable reviews early on, with some reported deaths of people and livestock, and American newspapers ran a few articles about brown recluse bites as early as the 1950s. Yet the brown recluse did not acquire its full reputation until the 1990s, after *Good Housekeeping* and other magazines publicized a Utah woman's severe injury and subsequent battle with gangrene. Although alarming, this 1986 case was not typical, and it is not clear if the spider venom alone or a secondary infection was responsible. Some spider experts pointed out that the brown recluse does not occur in Utah. But published accounts of other cases involving multiple amputations did the trick, and the brown recluse now hails from every state, at least in urban legend.

SCIENCE

The psychiatric term for fear of spiders is arachnophobia, and the fact that nearly everyone knows this word suggests that it must be a common fear (not to mention the title of a 1990 movie). In a 2000 Zogby poll of American adults, spiders as a group ranked third among the most greatly feared animals, after snakes and rats. Fear has little to do with actual risk; dog bites send thousands of people to hospitals every year, whereas most spider bites are harmless.

Journalists often claim that the brown recluse and black widow are the only venomous spiders in the United States. Strictly speaking, nearly all spiders are venomous, but most have mouthparts too small to inject their venom into humans, or else the venom itself is not powerful enough to harm us. An estimated 200 human deaths per year worldwide result from spider bites, but few of those deaths are in the United States. In 2008, the American Association of Poison Control Centers received reports of more than 12,000 spider bites, none of them fatal. The 2007 numbers were similar, with over 13,000 reported spider bites and no deaths. In 2006, there were over 14,000 spider bites, of which one (from a spider of unknown species) was fatal. To put the matter in perspective: Australia's notorious funnel web spider (*Atrax robustus*), said to be the most deadly of all spiders, caused a total of 13 reported deaths over a 53-year period, or less than one-quarter of a death per year. Spider bites in general are not a major problem.

The brown recluse spider (*Loxosceles reclusa*) is hard to identify without a magnifying lens. For example, it has six tiny eyes in a specific arrangement, but most people would prefer not to get close enough to count them. Every year, many reported brown recluse spiders (and their bites) turn out to be something else, so we will not add to the confusion with a sure-fire identification key. When in doubt, put the spider in a jar and take it to a qualified expert for identification. Despite nationwide reports of spiders that look like the brown recluse, experts insist that this species occurs only in the south-central Midwestern states: Kansas, Missouri, southern Iowa, Illinois, Oklahoma, Arkansas, Kentucky, Tennessee, eastern Texas, Louisiana, Alabama, Mississippi, and northwestern Georgia. Other *Loxosceles* species occur in southwestern Texas and parts of New Mexico, Arizona, and California, but these species are not considered dangerous (see the sidebar, "Along Came a Spider").

Along Came a Spider

About ten years ago, the author of this book became bored during a mammal survey in southern Arizona and turned her attention to spiders:

I was sitting in the shade of an acacia [*she wrote*] when I noticed that a medium-sized light brown spider had landed on the back of my left forearm. It was a hot day, and neither of us felt like moving, so I began to examine my passenger idly through a hand lens. Although spider taxonomy is not my area of expertise, I counted six eyes arranged in three pairs and soon recognized this animal as some sort of violin spider, most likely the Arizona recluse (*Loxosceles arizonica*) or the desert recluse (*L. deserta*). The brown recluse (*L. reclusa*), famed in song and story, does not occur in the Arizona desert. Having recently researched and written a book on biological hazards, I knew that the brown recluse seldom lives up to its tabloid image. But what about its lesser-known desert cousins? So I began to poke the spider with a piece of stem, and after a while it fought back, for I felt a slight stinging sensation. Then I gently relocated the spider to the ground and saw what appeared to be a tiny fluid-filled blister where it had stood. Over the next two weeks, the blister broke and a shallow, painless ulcer formed, eventually reaching a diameter of nearly one centimeter (four tenths of an inch). By the end of the fourth week, the bite had healed without treatment.

A 1999 study of 149 confirmed brown recluse bites showed that only 40 percent caused any tissue necrosis, and 43 percent of those healed within two weeks. Only one person in that study had more extensive necrosis that required hospitalization, and there were no deaths. A 2007 study showed that the antibiotic tetracycline may help prevent necrosis in such cases. Brown recluse bites (or allergic reactions to them) have caused circulatory collapse and gangrene on occasion, but such outcomes are rare and possibly related to bacterial infection of the wound. Various skin diseases, such as cutaneous anthrax, skin cancers, herpes lesions, and necrotizing fasciitis (Chapter 11), sometimes are mistaken for recluse spider bites.

The female black widow spider (*Latrodectus mactans* and several related species) causes the majority of reported spider bite injuries in North America. Black widows occur throughout the warmer parts of North America and Hawaii, with related species in Central and South America, Europe, Asia, and Africa. North American black widows are easy to identify, or they should be; the female has a large, shiny black abdomen with a red pattern shaped like an hourglass. The web looks like a tangled mess, not a symmetric orb, and black widows often build their webs in undisturbed corners of rooms. Some sources claim that the death rate for untreated black widow bites is as high as 5 percent, but that number may refer to bites with symptoms severe enough to bring the victim to a hospital; many other bites go unnoticed or unreported. Symptoms often include muscle cramps, sweating, elevated blood pressure, weakness, and rapid pulse. Breathing difficulty, vomiting, and severe pain may occur in some cases. An effective antivenom is available if needed, but it is a good idea to catch or kill the spider (if possible) and take it to the hospital along with the patient. Otherwise, the wrong antivenom might be used.

HISTORY

Loxosceles has come a long way since 1964, when a letter to the editor of the *San Antonio Light* newspaper lambasted the Johnson administration for authorizing (among other federal grants) the grand sum of $4,482 for a "boondoggle" study of the brown recluse spider. When it was just a spider and not an institution, nobody paid much attention to it, other than residents of endemic areas who were actually at risk and a few dedicated researchers. Now this spider has an extensive cult following, and at least one scientist has devoted his life to educating the public about the brown recluse and clearing its good name.

After the scare of 1934 (see Source), the black widow spider never again attained celebrity status in the United States, although it continues to be responsible for more reported bites than the brown recluse. The element of controversy is missing, because the black widow and its webs are so easy to recognize. Also, instead of skin ulcers, the widow's bite often causes uncomfortable but vague symptoms that might easily be mistaken for a bad case of the flu. Eventually, someone must have noticed that almost no actual deaths resulted from black widow spider bites, and the panic died. Yet the legend lives on; in 1995, the port city of Osaka, Japan reported a short-lived health scare when more than 1,000 black widows arrived as stowaways, possibly in shipments of tropical hardwoods from the world's embattled rainforests.

In 2004, a British newspaper ran the absurd story of a man in Berlin who kept 200 pet spiders. One of them, a black widow named Bettina, bit him fatally. Then all the spiders allegedly ate him, with the assistance of his pet snakes and termites and a gecko named Helmut. Finally, the presumably well-nourished menagerie escaped into the city when the heating element on their "tank" exploded. This story is obvious nonsense for several reasons. For example, how would the man know the spider was named Bettina?

In 2005, a team of Chilean researchers reported progress in development of a new pill to combat erectile dysfunction. Their new drug is derived from the neurotoxin found in black widow spider venom.

CONSEQUENCES

To our knowledge, the only beneficiary of the brown recluse and black widow health scare has been the pest control industry. When some people find a black widow spider living behind the toilet or in the attic, they will pay good money to have someone else get rid of it. Brown recluse spiders are another matter, since few exterminators or clients can identify them reliably in the first place.

This health scare had other, less expected consequences that did not become apparent until the postal anthrax incident of 2001. Journalists reported that one of the victims of cutaneous anthrax, a seven-month-old baby, did not receive appropriate treatment for the first two weeks because doctors assumed the lesion must be a necrotic spider bite. Even doctors tend to see what they expect to see, and nobody expected anthrax.

WHAT WENT WRONG?

Spiders run fast and look scary, yet on an individual basis they are easy to kill. This combination of characteristics makes them highly satisfying targets. Maybe this is why the general public often overestimates the dangers of visible threats, while underestimating the danger of microscopic or invisible ones, such as viruses, chemical hazards, contrary viewpoints, and the slow advance of climate change.

The folk traditions of many cultures have depicted spiders in a positive light, as bringers of wealth, luck, or rain. The modern western view of spiders as a deadly menace may reflect a changing relationship with nature.

REFERENCES AND RECOMMENDED READING

Acerrano, A. "Widows of the World." *Sports Afield*, February–March 2007.

Atkins, J. A., et al. "Probable Cause of Necrotic Spider Bite in the Midwest." *Science*, Vol. 126, 1957, p. 73.

Bennett, R. G., and R. Vetter. "An Approach to Spider Bites. Erroneous Attribution of Dermonecrotic Lesions to Brown Recluse or Hobo Spider Bites in Canada." *Canadian Family Physician*, Vol. 50, 2004, pp. 1098–1101.

"Black Widows Found in Bag of Grapes." United Press International, 16 June 2010.

Brunk, D. "Treatment Varies for Severe *Loxosceles* Spider Bite: Clinical Features of Bites Discussed." *Family Practice News*, 1 May 2004.

Cacy, J., and J. W. Mold. "The Clinical Characteristics of Brown Recluse Spider Bites Treated by Family Physicians." *Journal of Family Practice*, July 1999, pp. 536–542.

Dominguez, T. J. "It's Not a Spider Bite, it's Community-Acquired Methicillin-Resistant *Staphylococcus aureus*." *Journal of the American Board of Family Practice*, Vol. 17, 2004, pp. 220–226.

Irish, A. "A Sick Goat Mystery." *Countryside & Small Stock Journal*, July–August 1996.

Isbister, G. K. "Spider Mythology Across the World." *Western Journal of Medicine*, Vol. 175, 2001, pp. 86–87.

Master, E. J. "Loxoscelism." *New England Journal of Medicine*, 6 August 1998, p. 379.

Miller, T. A. "Latrodectism." *American Family Physician*, January 1992, p. 181 ff.

Murphy, M. "Black Widow Venom for Long-Lasting Erections." *Chemistry and Industry*, 6 June 2005.

Nishioka, S. "Misdiagnosis of Brown Recluse Spider Bite." *Western Journal of Medicine*, Vol. 174, 2001, p. 240.

Paixão-Cavalcante, D., et al. "Tetracycline Protects against Dermonecrosis Induced by *Loxosceles* Spider Venom." *Journal of Investigative Dermatology*, Vol. 127, 2007, pp. 1410–1418.

Reed, L. A. "Crawling with Fear." *Washington Post*, 5 February 2002.

Sams, H. H., et al. "Nineteen Documented Cases of *Loxosceles reclusa* Envenomation." *Journal of the American Academy of Dermatology*, Vol. 44, 2001, pp. 603–608.

Swanson, D. L., and R. S. Vetter. "Bites of Brown Recluse Spiders and Suspected Necrotic Arachnidism." *New England Journal of Medicine*, Vol. 352, 2005, pp. 700–707.

Timms, P. K., and R. B. Gibbons. "Latrodectism—Effects of the Black Widow Spider Bite." *Western Journal of Medicine*, Vol. 144, 1986, pp. 315–317.

Trempe, S. "Along Came a Spider." *Good Housekeeping*, April 1993.

Tuohy, C. "Wacky Claims of the Self-Insured." *Risk & Insurance*, December 2005.

Vetter, R. S. "Myth: Idiopathic Wounds are Often Due to Brown Recluse or Other Spider Bites Throughout the United States." *Western Journal of Medicine*, Vol. 173, 2000, pp. 357–358.

Vetter, R. S. "Arachnids Misidentified as Brown Recluse Spiders by Medical Professionals and Other Authorities in North America."*Toxicon*, Vol. 54, 2009, pp. 545–547.

Vetter, R. S., and S. P. Bush. "Reports of Presumptive Brown Recluse Spider Bites Reinforce Improbable Diagnosis in Regions of North America where the Spider is Not Endemic." *Clinical Infectious Diseases*, Vol. 35, 2002, pp. 442–445.

White, J. "Debunking Spider Bite Myths—Necrotising Arachnidism should be a Diagnosis of Last Resort." *Medical Journal of Australia*, Vol. 179, 2003, pp. 180–181.

"Woman Faces Amputation after Bite from Brown Recluse Spider." Associated Press, 21 August 1992.

Zambrano, A., et al. "Severe Loxoscelism with Lethal Outcome: Report of One Case." *Revista Médica de Chile*, Vol. 133, 2005, pp. 219–223. [In Spanish]

35

Fear of Killer Bees

Alas! Alas! I am dying,
I have been bitten
By a little serpent
Who has however wings,
The country people call them bees.

—Thomas Stanley (translator), *Anacreon* (1651)

SUMMARY

Many people are afraid of Africanized "killer" honeybees, which became established in the United States in 1990. Despite early tabloid accounts of marauding swarms of crazed bees killing everything in sight, documented casualties have been low, and only an expert can tell the difference between the newcomers and the familiar European honeybees that arrived in North America centuries ago with colonists. Killer bees are more aggressive than their European cousins, and make less honey, but they may also have more resistance to parasitic mites. Although the new bees are here to stay, the health scare itself has largely fizzled, probably because the predicted carnage did not materialize. In the 30 years following their release, these Africanized bees killed an estimated 1,000 people in South America, or an average of 33 per year; but that number is not as bad as it sounds, because somewhere between 30 and 100 North American residents died from bee stings in a typical year even before the Africanized bees arrived. Bee stings (by killer or nonkiller bees) remain a significant threat to individuals who are allergic to bee venom—an estimated 1 to 2 percent of the U.S. population.

SOURCE

In the 1970s, the American news media treated the impending arrival of "killer bees" from Africa via South America as a millennial event. It was not hard to convince people to be very afraid, because many Americans were already allergic to the venom of ordinary honeybees, and many others had an exaggerated fear of being stung. This fear was not entirely unjustified, since early reports indicated that hundreds or even thousands of Africanized bees might attack the same person.

Many more people die from bee stings every year than from shark attacks, and bees are much harder to avoid than sharks. Also, people have always projected both positive and negative human characteristics onto bees. They are hardworking, live peacefully in large communities, take good care of their mothers, make a pleasant sound among the flowers, pollinate our crops, and give us honey and other useful products if we treat them well—but they are also known to hold a grudge, and will literally rip out their own guts in defense of the hive. A worthy adversary, indeed.

SCIENCE

All honeybees in North America belong to the species *Apis mellifera*, which is native to Africa, Asia, and Europe. Many native bee species also occur in North America, but centuries of competition with introduced European bees may have reduced their numbers. Biologists do not know for certain where *Apis mellifera* originated, but similar bees were present in Europe and Asia 35 million years ago. People in Egypt and the Middle East have raised honeybees in portable hives for several thousand years, and the practice probably spread from there to the rest of the world. When Europeans began to explore and colonize other continents, they took along their beekeepers and bees, and the European honeybee was well established in colonial North America by about 1622.

Every continent has its own honeybee subspecies and strains, each adapted to local conditions with a unique combination of traits, such as disease resistance, honey production, climate preference, and aggressiveness. When bees arrive in new habitats, some of these traits may confer an advantage, whereas others have the opposite effect. Before 1990, residents of North America were accustomed to rather mellow European honeybees (*Apis mellifera mellifera* and *A. m. ligustica*), originally imported from northern and southern Europe, respectively. Some sources claim that hybrids of these two European subspecies tend to sting more readily than either parent.

The African honeybee (*Apis mellifera scutellata*), and the "Africanized" hybrids that have resulted from its interbreeding with European honeybees, appear to be even more aggressive, less inclined to make large amounts of honey, more inclined to desert the hive when conditions are unfavorable, and more resistant to certain bee mites and other parasites. From the viewpoint of beekeepers, the last characteristic is good, but the others are not. Africanized bees are also reputed to invade European honeybee colonies, substitute their own queen, and take over. African honeybee venom is no more dangerous than that of its European counterpart; the problem is that larger numbers of bees may sting the same person. Thus far, the African honeybees are confined to warmer parts of North America and may be unable to survive cold winters.

Honeybee venom (African or otherwise) contains a mixture of proteins and peptides that can cause pain, swelling, inflammation, damage to cell membranes, low blood pressure, and a rapid heartbeat. At least 1 percent of people also have an allergic reaction, which may be mild or severe. The honeybee's stinger is barbed and tends to remain embedded in the skin, causing further pain and itching. More severe effects may include kidney failure, acute pancreatitis, and even myocardial infarction (heart attack).

The LD_{50} for bee venom—the dose necessary to kill 50 percent of recipients—is about 19 stings per kilogram of body weight, or 8.6 stings per pound. In other words, for an untreated 150-pound (68-kilogram) adult stung by 1,300 bees, the probability of death would be about 50 percent, disregarding other factors such as allergy or age. That's a lot of bees, but it can happen. With fewer stings, the probability of death is lower, but not zero. Of course, a person who is severely allergic to bee venom can die after just one sting.

Bee stings kill hundreds of people every year worldwide, but contrary to popular belief, anaphylaxis (severe allergic reaction to venom) is not the only reason. Many of the victims are elderly and have underlying health problems, such as heart disease and atherosclerosis. Environmental temperature, the number of stings, the amount of venom injected, and the location of the sting are also important factors. According to most sources, there is no evidence that people with a history of previous stings are at greater risk. Beekeepers typically report many stings each year, but few find it necessary to leave the profession for that reason.

HISTORY

In about 1956, biologists in Brazil imported a number of queen honeybees from Tanzania, intending to crossbreed them with local honeybees to produce a strain that made more honey and was better adapted to tropical conditions. In 1957, the African bees escaped into the wild, and the original plan backfired. Not only did honey production in the region drop sharply, but according to a 1965 report, hundreds of Brazilian dogs, pigs, and chickens were stung to death. In 1986, a Costa Rican student reportedly died after an estimated 8,000 killer bees stung him.

The U.S. news media reacted with alarm, and Hollywood gave us such classics as *Killer Bees* (made for TV, 1974), *The Swarm* (1978), *The Bees* (1978), and *Killer Bees* (2002). The usual storyline is that deadly African bees invade American cities and kill thousands of screaming people. Between 1975 and 1978, *Saturday Night Live* (SNL) countered this grim trend with a series of hilarious skits about killer bees, featuring the entire SNL cast in striped bee costumes. Soon, the advertising industry jumped on the bandwagon with commercials in which a hapless victim locked in a phone booth must decide which brand of plastic zipper bag will best contain a swarm of angry killer bees.

In real life, the bee invasion was more subtle, and few people other than beekeepers, entomologists, and first responders would even have noticed it without the help of the media. In 1988, the United States and Mexico reportedly shared the cost of a $6 million project designed to trap and kill the Africanized bees. But no border could stop these immigrants, which continued to spread northward at the rate of 200 to 300 miles per year and finally colonized Texas in 1990. A few stragglers actually reached California and other states as early as 1985, but did not become established there until later. Africanized bees now occupy parts of Texas, New Mexico, Arizona, California, Louisiana, Florida, Arkansas, Utah, and probably other states by the time this book goes to press. One of the more restrained TV documentaries about African killer bees stated the matter as follows: "These monsters are going north. . . . They don't stop until whatever they're attacking is dead."[1] At the other extreme, some journalists have claimed that negative remarks about African bees are racist.

Although the health scare itself has largely fizzled, the underlying cause is alive and well. Africanized bees can inflict serious injuries on occasion. In 2010, for example, a swarm of these bees reportedly killed two horses at a ranch in southern California.

CONSEQUENCES

Few people have ever felt entirely cozy with bees, but both the reality and the mythology of "killer bees" have made the situation worse. Beekeepers reportedly face new problems, not only from aggressive Africanized bees invading their hives but also from neighbors who object to living near honeybee farms. Some beekeepers have relocated to colder climates outside the killer bee range to avoid these issues.

Africanized bees have, however, benefited tropical agriculture in at least one unexpected way: their pollination efforts have increased coffee yields in Panama. A 2002 study showed that insect pollination of coffee shrubs, mainly by Africanized bees, increased overall yield by 58 percent as compared with self-pollinated plants.

Several chapters in this book note the tendency for health scares to generate miracle cures, on the theory that a powerful enemy can become a powerful friend. Some alternative medical practitioners have long recommended bee venom as a cure for hundreds of maladies, including cancer, multiple sclerosis, lupus, arthritis, and Lyme disease. There is little evidence that this approach works, but the claims continue, with a new twist: if ordinary bee venom sounds like a potent remedy, killer bee venom must be dynamite! In 2010, a team of doctors in India even proposed that bee venom might help control the H1N1 swine flu pandemic. It probably would have worked in this case, because by the time the paper was published, the H1N1 pandemic had largely fizzled on its own (Chapter 8).

WHAT WENT WRONG?

The original thing that went wrong, of course, was the accidental release of African honeybees in Brazil in 1957. But if it did not happen that year, it would have happened some other year. Throughout human history, numerous animal and plant species and strains have found their way from one continent to another, either by accident or design. Crossbreeding experiments are essential in agriculture, and some of these experiments work out better than others. Non-native species often cause environmental or social problems; familiar examples include the introduction of European rabbits to Australia, zebra mussels to the Great Lakes, and the Mediterranean fruitfly (Medfly) to California. Once established, such species may prove impossible to eradicate.

When the Africanized honeybees got loose in Brazil, journalists simply did their jobs and reported the invaders' northward progress. If the subject matter was inherently unnerving, so much the better. The impending arrival of various alien plant diseases in North America, such as soybean rust in 2004 and citrus canker in 1999, posed far greater economic threats and were tracked just as carefully, but drew less media attention. Bees are simply scarier, possibly because they form large groups and make an ominous buzzing sound, like a rumor passing through a crowd.

NOTE

1. "Giant Killer Bees" (MonsterQuest, 4 March 2010).

REFERENCES AND RECOMMENDED READING

"About 250,000 Bees Removed from Home." United Press International, 23 July 2009.

Adams, S. "The Buzz." *Forbes Global*, 14 March 2005.

Begley, S. "Invasion of the Killer Bees! Really, They're Coming." *Newsweek*, 6 April 1987.

Borrell, J. "Rising Unease about Killer Bees—but a Surprise Awaits the U.S.-Bound Invaders in Mexico." *Time*, 30 May 1988.

Fisher, A. "A Chip on the Old Bee." *Popular Science*, October 1988.

Gore, R. "Those Fiery Brazilian Bees." *National Geographic*, April 1976.

Graebner, L. "Feeling the Sting of Killer Bees." *Business Journal*, 30 May 1994.

Hall, H. G. "DNA Differences Found between Africanized and European Honeybees." *Proceedings of the National Academy of Sciences*, Vol. 83, 1986, pp. 4874–4877.

Hubbell, S. "Maybe the 'Killer' Bee Should be Called the 'Bravo' Instead." *Smithsonian*, September 1991.

Jacobs, M. "The World's Abuzz with the Coming of Africanized Bees." *The News* (Frederick, MD), 24 August 1982.

"Killer Bees Boost Coffee Yields." *Science News*, 6 July 2002.

"Killer Bees Nasty, but Losing some Sting." United Press International, 12 August 2005.

"Killer Bees, Native Bees can Co-Exist." United Press International, 2 October 2009.

"Killer Bees No Longer a Threat." *Supermarket News*, 12 August 1985.

"Killer Bees Plague Brazil." Reuters, 14 August 1965.

Kim, K. T., and J. Oguro. "Update on the Status of Africanized Honey Bees in the Western States." *Western Journal of Medicine*, Vol. 170, 1999, pp. 220–222.

McNamee, G. "Attack of the Killer Bees." *Tucson Weekly*, 19–25 December 1996.

Pinto, M. A., et al. "Africanization in the United States: Replacement of Feral European Honeybees (*Apis mellifera* L.) by an African Hybrid Swarm." *Genetics*, Vol. 170, 2005, pp. 1653–1665.

Ransome, H. 1937. *The Sacred Bee*. London: George Allen & Unwin.

Schlefer, J. "Stopping Killer Bees with Star Wars." *Technology Review*, May–June 1989.

Sherman, R. A. "What Physicians should Know about Africanized Honeybees." *Western Journal of Medicine*, Vol. 163, 1995, pp. 541–546.

Stover, D. "Bees Cross the Border." *Popular Science*, February 1991.

Tennesen, M. "Going Head-to-Head with Killer Bees." *National Wildlife*, February–March 2001.

Vetter, R. S. "Mass Envenomation by Honey Bees and Wasps." *Western Journal of Medicine*, Vol. 170, 1999, pp. 223–227.

Visscher, P. K., et al. "The Progress of Africanized Bees in the United States (1990–1995): Initial Rapid Invasion has Slowed in the U.S." *California Agriculture*, Vol. 51, 1997, pp. 22–25.

Whitfield, C. W. "Thrice Out of Africa: Ancient and Recent Expansions of the Honey Bee, *Apis mellifera*." *Science*, Vol. 314, 2006, pp. 642–645.

Part Six

Other Chemical and Radiological Exposures

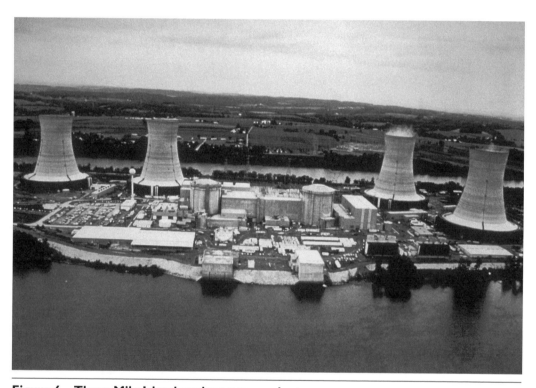

Figure 6   Three Mile Island nuclear power plant.
(*Source:* U.S. Centers for Disease Control and Prevention, Public Health Image Library.)

36

Three Mile Island

Power plants don't blow up like bombs. They blow up like a pressure cooker full of applesauce, only it's radioactive applesauce.

—Attributed to Wisconsin State Senator Douglas J. LaFollette (1973)

SUMMARY

On 28 March 1979, the nuclear power plant at Three Mile Island, near Harrisburg, Pennsylvania, reported a cooling system leak that released radioactive steam from the containment building into the atmosphere and led to an automatic shutdown of the plant. The full scope of the accident did not become apparent until much later, when investigators determined that a partial core meltdown had occurred. Years after the accident, some sources reported increased rates of lung cancer and leukemia in communities downwind from Three Mile Island, but others attributed the apparent increase to newer screening methods. This incident, followed in 1986 by the Chernobyl disaster in Ukraine, severely reduced public enthusiasm for nuclear power. In 2010, however, President Barack Obama awarded $8 billion in loan guarantees to finance the construction of two nuclear reactors in Georgia, the first such projects in 30 years. To the extent that his decision reflects the will of the people, it appears that the Three Mile Island health scare has now officially fizzled.[1]

SOURCE

Americans have worried about nuclear bombs and radioactive fallout ever since Hiroshima. But people can adjust to almost anything, and when the world's first full-scale commercial nuclear power plant (Calder Hill in England) went online in 1956, after a few smaller-scale efforts starting in 1951, we were back on familiar ground: a powerful enemy had become a powerful friend. This innovation was supposed to solve all our energy problems. In the words of Captain Nemo in the 1954 motion picture *20,000 Leagues Under the Sea*, nuclear power would soon provide "enough energy to lift mankind from the depths of hell into heaven."

Thus, by the time of the partial meltdown at Three Mile Island, many people took nuclear power for granted. A 1975 Harris poll showed that 63 percent of Americans wanted to build more nuclear power plants, and only 19 percent actively opposed their construction. The potential for catastrophe was always there, but few Americans really expected this new friend to turn around and bite us—and then in 1979 it did. The main TMI reactor cooling system leaked, radioactive steam escaped into the atmosphere, the plant was evacuated, and the news media went properly berserk and remained so for years. The future had definitely arrived. There is no clear evidence that the radiation leak injured anyone, but it might have been much worse. "Three Mile Island" will most likely remain a metaphor for apocalyptic failure narrowly averted, long after the technology itself is an obsolete footnote.

SCIENCE

Three Mile Island is located in the Susquehanna River, about 15 miles from Harrisburg, Pennsylvania. In 1967, Metropolitan Edison Company chose this location for construction of its nuclear generating station (Figure 6), apparently on the basis of its convenient location and the availability of coolant water. As originally designed, the Three Mile Island station had two pressurized water reactors: TMI-1, which came online in 1974, and TMI-2, which began operation in 1978.

At the time of the 1979 accident, TMI-1 was offline for refueling. Accounts vary, but it appears that the accident began when the pumps that supplied water to the TMI-2 steam generators stopped working because a pressure relief valve was stuck open. The safety system then automatically shut down the steam turbine and generator, but fission in the core continued until the system dropped the control rods into the core to shut it down. Temperatures in the core continued to rise as the products of fission heated the water, and the technicians on duty at the time had inadequate training to deal with the problem. By some accounts, they misinterpreted a water level gauge readout and took inappropriate actions that resulted in core damage.

The first in a long series of wire service reports that morning stated that there was no radiation leak. The next report stated that there was a small leak, but nobody was exposed. The next said that about 20 exposed workers had been treated and released, and that a general state of emergency had been declared, but that nobody was in danger and everybody should relax and stay home—except for pregnant women, who should not come within 5 or 10 miles of the plant, just in case. Another report said the air in neighboring communities should be safe to breathe, but that milk might be unsafe to drink after about a week—apparently because radioactive material might settle on the grass where cows would eat it, but this was not clearly explained. Then there was a hydrogen explosion inside the containment building. With one unfamiliar crisis after another, it was a day that America would not soon forget, particularly since it arrived on the heels of a new action-suspense movie called *The China Syndrome* (see History).

Since no one was certain exactly what would happen next, the U.S. Food and Drug Administration (FDA) acted quickly to protect people in nearby cities who might have been exposed to radiation that would increase their risk of thyroid cancer. Within 72 hours after the accident, FDA had contracted with firms in Missouri, Michigan, and New Jersey to deliver nearly 250,000 doses of potassium iodide to Harrisburg, Pennsylvania.

In other words, contrary to rumor, the government *was* doing something. As it turned out, few people were exposed, and the public health consequences were minimal, but some appropriate preparations were made.

Just what is a meltdown? In everyday usage, this word means an accident in which the core of a nuclear reactor overheats and melts, and radiation escapes into the environment. "Meltdown" has also become a useful figure of speech to describe a personal or economic crisis. In all three contexts, the term lacks precision, and it does not appear in the respective glossaries of the International Atomic Energy Agency and the U.S. Nuclear Regulatory Commission. There is general agreement that the 1986 Chernobyl disaster was a meltdown, and other meltdowns apparently also occurred in the former Soviet Union. The Three Mile Island accident appears to qualify as a large-scale *partial* meltdown. In 1982, engineers inspecting the TMI-2 core found that the top five feet of the fuel assembly had been destroyed. Smaller partial meltdowns have occurred with less fanfare at other U.S. locations, including two military reactors in Idaho in 1955 and 1961, and the Santa Susana Field Laboratory in southern California in 1959.

HISTORY

Public concern about the Three Mile Island reactors (and nuclear power in general) did not start in 1979. Before the station was even built, some people worried about its proximity to Harrisburg and the potential for catastrophic accidents or sabotage. In 1974, the same year TMI-1 came online, environmental journalists around the world—citing a recently released Atomic Energy Commission study known as the Rasmussen Report—warned readers of the nature and consequences of a core meltdown, the difficulty of designing adequate safeguards, the importance of backup cooling systems, and the urgency of funding alternative energy sources such as fusion, solar, geothermal, and wind power. Thirty-six years and an unknown number of partial meltdowns later, these options remain as elusive as ever, and public opinion has once again shifted in favor of nuclear energy.

In 1975, a curious incident at Three Mile Island called attention to its vulnerability to sabotage. Two guards who worked at the power plant allegedly loosened the bolts that secured the gate of a water intake facility, for the sole purpose of embarrassing some rival guards. After losing their jobs, these fun-loving guards approached consumer activist Ralph Nader, who requested a federal investigation and warned of the potential for a core meltdown.[2] The press release went on to describe specific weak spots in plant security, apparently as a service to any would-be saboteur who might otherwise overlook them.

If emergencies were planned in advance, the timing of this one would be exceptionally bad, because the TMI accident happened just 12 days after release of the motion picture *The China Syndrome*—the story of a TV reporter who witnesses a near-meltdown at a nuclear power plant and becomes involved in a subsequent cover-up. Despite the title, a core meltdown cannot bore a hole through the center of the Earth and come out in China (or wherever). But the movie had audiences scared enough to overreact when the real crisis came.

CONSEQUENCES

If the accident at Three Mile Island taught us any lessons, it is unclear what they were. Certain dangers are inherent in nuclear reactor operations, but people need energy, and the alternatives are limited. For the next century or two, we might be stuck with this technology. Harris polls showed that, between 1975 and 1979, public support for new nuclear power plants dropped from 63 percent to about 50 percent, but never went much lower than that. For many, the danger inherent in nuclear power is better than dependence on foreign oil.

But nuclear power is neither renewable nor clean, despite some advocates' claims to the contrary. Eventually, we will run out of fissionable materials and invent something else. Fast-breeder reactors (FBRs) are one renewable alternative, but this technology has the clear disadvantage of creating plutonium and inviting terrorists to steal it. Nor is FBR technology immune to operational problems. During the 1990s, a series of accidents at fast-breeder reactors in Japan and Germany led to shutdown of those facilities.

The Three Mile Island accident also called attention to a host of largely unrelated health and safety issues, such as indoor radon (Chapter 43), the international arms race, and the controversial effects of irradiated food. On the bright side, Three Mile Island also brought a source of unprecedented humor and wisdom into our lives. Without Blinky the Three-Eyed Mutant Fish, and the entire cast of *The Simpsons*, America would be ill-prepared for the realities of a nuclear world. The 1991 episode in which Homer Simpson nearly caused a core meltdown at the Springfield Nuclear Power Plant, and then averted disaster at the last minute by pushing buttons at random, proved that one person could make a difference after all.

WHAT WENT WRONG?

There is no shortage of opinions about what went wrong at Three Mile Island. The incident generated hundreds of reports and commentaries, most of which attribute the accident to inadequate staff training and contingency planning. Yet most authorities concede (more or less grudgingly) that occasional accidents are unavoidable in this industry. Perhaps paying higher salaries to security guards and technicians, and giving them more training and respect, would motivate them to take the job more seriously than Homer Simpson does.

NOTES

1. This book was in press when a major earthquake and tsunami damaged several nuclear reactors in Japan. It was too soon to evaluate the extent of the damage or the long-term impact on public acceptance of nuclear power.

2. "State's Nuclear Generator Plants Target of Many Questions" (Associated Press, 30 June 1975).

REFERENCES AND RECOMMENDED READING

Allen, J. "Radiation Leak Investigated at Three Mile Island." Reuters, 23 November 2009.

Behr, P. "Three Mile Island Still Haunts U.S. Nuclear Industry." *New York Times*, 27 March 2009.

Church, G. J. "Radiation Sickness." *Time*, 26 October 1981.

DeMott, J. S. "An Industry Still in Disarray." *Time*, 11 April 1983.

Evangelinos, K., et al. "Implementation of Responsible Care in the Chemical Industry: Evidence from Greece." *Journal of Hazardous Materials*, 6 January 2010.

Field, R. W. "Three Mile Island Epidemiologic Radiation Dose Assessment Revisited: 25 Years After the Accident." *Radiation Protection Dosimetry*, Vol. 113, 2005, pp. 214–217.

Gatchel, R. J., et al. "A Psychophysiological Field Study of Stress at Three Mile Island." *Psychophysiology*, Vol. 22, 1985, pp. 175–181.

Greenwald, J. "Deadly Meltdown." *Time*, 12 May 1986.

Jones, R. R. "When Failure is Built In." *Research and Development*, June 1986.

Lefever, E. W. "Green at Any Cost?" *Weekly Standard*, 3 March 2007.

Levin, R. J. "Incidence of Thyroid Cancer in Residents Surrounding the Three Mile Island Nuclear Facility." *Laryngoscope*, Vol. 118, 2008, pp. 618–628.

Miller, K. L. "The Nuclear Reactor Accident at Three Mile Island." *Radiographics*, Vol. 14, 1994, pp. 215–224.

"Neighbors Complain about Nuclear Power Plant." Associated Press, 2 November 1978.

Reed, S. "Ten Years Later, Nuclear Ghosts Still Haunt Three Mile Island." *People Weekly*, 3 April 1989.

Shulman, S. "Legacy of Three Mile Island." *Nature*, Vol. 338, 1989, p 190.

"Stress Lingers after Nuclear Accident." *Science Digest*, March 1984.

Sturgis, S. "Revelations about Three Mile Island Disaster Raise Doubts over Nuclear Plant Safety." *New Solutions*, Vol. 19, 2009, pp. 481–492.

Talbott, E. O., et al. "Long-Term Follow-Up of the Residents of the Three Mile Island Accident Area: 1979–1998." *Environmental Health Perspectives*, Vol. 111, 2003, pp. 341–348.

"Three Mile Island: Fallout of Fear." *Time*, 11 April 1983.

Tilyou, S. "Three Mile Island—Ten Years Later. No Health Consequences Seen, but Studies Continue to Assess Potential Effects."*Journal of Nuclear Medicine*, Vol. 30, 1989, pp. 427–430.

Von Hippel, F. "Looking Back on the Rasmussen Report." *Bulletin of the Atomic Scientists*, February 1977.

Wald, M. L. "Normal Cancer Rate Found Near Three Mile Island." *New York Times*, 1 November 2002.

Wing, S. "Objectivity and Ethics in Environmental Health Science." *Environmental Health Perspectives*, Vol. 111, 2003, pp. 1809–1818.

Wood, M. S., et al. "A Medical Library's Response to Three Mile Island." *Bulletin of the Medical Library Association*, Vol. 68, 1980, pp. 242–244.

"Workers Evacuate Nuclear Plant." UPI, 28 March 1979.

37

The Alar Scare of 1989

And then she went to a secret lonely chamber, where no one was likely to come, and there she made a poisonous apple. It was beautiful to look upon . . . but whoever ate even a little bit of it must die.

—Jacob and Wilhelm Grimm, *Snow-White* (1812)

SUMMARY

In 1989, the apple industry in the United States suffered from a major cancer scare that resulted from controversial studies of Alar, a plant growth regulator (not a pesticide). Many supermarkets stopped selling apples, and many parents were afraid to allow their children to eat fruit. Public concern had begun a few years earlier, when the Environmental Protection Agency (EPA) issued a series of ambiguous statements about Alar, but concern escalated into full-fledged panic when the CBS news program *60 Minutes* presented a 1989 report prepared by an environmental advocacy group. Although there can be no justification for exposing consumers to known or suspected carcinogens, it appears that the *60 Minutes* warning was overblown. Apple growers stopped using Alar, and the scare eventually fizzled as a result of conflicting data and loss of interest. As of 2010, Alar and related chemicals are still used in the United States, but only on nonfood crops, such as ornamental flowers. Some other countries still use it on fruits, and available data indicate that the risk is probably minimal. The worst outcome of this health scare may be its contribution to consumers' fear of raw produce in general.

SOURCE

In 1985, the U.S. Environmental Protection Agency (EPA) completed a five-year study of a plant growth regulator called Alar (daminozide) and classified it as a probable human carcinogen. Instead of banning the chemical outright, however, EPA set restrictions on its use and asked the manufacturer for more data. Although the news media covered the Alar controversy both before and after 1985, the real health scare did not start until a February 1989 episode of the CBS news magazine *60 Minutes* presented a terrifying indictment of this chemical, featuring such subtle images as an apple decorated with a skull and crossbones.

A few weeks earlier, EPA and the Natural Resources Defense Council (NRDC) had released their respective reports on daminozide. Although the EPA's estimate of risk was substantially lower than that of NRDC, both reports reached the same conclusion: apple growers must stop using Alar, and they did. The manufacturer voluntarily withdrew the product in 1989, but the incident was a public relations mess. The EPA had only scientists to defend its delayed action, whereas NRDC had actress Meryl Streep, who condemned Alar on TV talk shows and even testified before Congress. *60 Minutes* chose to base its program on the findings of NRDC, and in so doing scared the daylights out of many Americans.

Had we poisoned our children? Would everybody who ate apples be dead within a year? Some worried consumers reportedly asked EPA if it was safe to pour apple juice down a drain. They were afraid it might melt the pipes, contaminate the water table, or kill the bacteria in their septic tanks.

SCIENCE

The chemical daminozide (CAS 1596-84-5) is the active ingredient in plant growth regulators sold under various trade names, including Alar, Kylar, and our personal favorite, B-NINE (presumably a pun on the word "benign"). At the time of this 1989 health scare, the main role of daminozide in agriculture was to strengthen the stems of apples and keep them on the trees until harvest, to ensure that they were red, ripe, and firm when they reached the consumer. Only a small percentage of apple growers actually used this chemical, mostly on the apple variety called Red Delicious. The same product was also registered for use with several other crops, such as cherries and peaches, but it was used primarily on red apples.

Some sources claim that the purpose of Alar was to enhance the crunch and color of apples, but that is not precisely true. It does not dye the apple artificially red, or make it artificially crunchy, but simply improves the timing and efficiency of the harvest and the quality of the end product. The U.S. apple crop is huge—an estimated 241 million bushels in 2009, up from 210 million bushels in 1988—and it is not feasible for human pickers to hand-select each individual apple at the peak of perfection, as the owner of a backyard tree might do. It is highly advantageous to both the grower and consumer if the entire apple crop ripens at the same time.

Since daminozide is sprayed on plants and is completely water-soluble, it was assumed at one time that the chemical would be absent by the time the fruit reached the consumer. As it turned out, traces of the chemical penetrated the fruit and could not be washed off. Laboratory testing showed the presence of residues, not only on raw fruit, but also in products such as applesauce and apple juice. Also, daminozide in water breaks down to form a chemical called UDMH (unsymmetrical dimethylhydrazine). In laboratory testing, both chemicals appear to induce tumor formation in mice. As with many such studies, it is not clear if these chemicals affect humans and mice in the same way, or if the residual amounts that actually reach the consumer are high enough to be harmful. With some consumer products, such as cigarettes, it is possible to compare groups of users versus nonusers. But so many people eat apples, or foods and beverages made from apples, that the epidemiological approach was not feasible.

When in doubt, the prudent action is to stop using the product, and so it was with Alar.

EPA and its supporters claimed that NRDC distorted the facts and used bad science; NRDC and its supporters claimed that EPA had concealed the facts and put young children at risk. EPA had the edge in science, although NRDC clearly won the public relations battle. But with children's lives possibly at stake, many consumers wanted the two groups to stop posturing and simply agree on an answer. Do daminozide and UDMH really pose a significant health risk, or not? The question is unanswerable, since the available data are based on laboratory studies of rodents, without supporting epidemiological studies of humans. The chemical is no longer used on food crops, so this particular debate is over, at least in the United States. But efforts to increase the food supply will generate new controversies, and the next Alar lies in wait.

HISTORY

The U.S. Food and Drug Administration (FDA) approved the growth regulator Alar for use on apples in 1968, after two years of laboratory testing indicated that the chemical was safe and that it satisfied the requirements of the Delaney Clause. In the early 1970s, however, published studies of daminozide and its breakdown product UDMH showed that these chemicals caused tumors in mice. In 1977, an EPA scientist called attention to these studies and proposed a special review of Alar.

The EPA began its investigation in 1980, but put it on hold after a meeting with the manufacturer. Finally, in 1984, EPA reopened the investigation and concluded it in 1985 with the finding that Alar and UDMH were probable human carcinogens. A product is normally acceptable by EPA standards only if it can be shown to cause no more than one additional cancer per million exposed people. The available data showed, instead, that these chemicals might cause as many as nine cases per million, which the agency conceded was unacceptable. NRDC, using the same data but different assumptions, concluded that the increased cancer risk to young children would be as high as 1 in 4,200, which clearly was appalling, if true.

In February 1989, CBS News aired its now-famous *60 Minutes* episode "A is for Apples," a melodramatic exposé of Alar based on the NRDC report entitled "Intolerable Risk: Pesticides in our Children's Food." Here is a representative quotation from that broadcast: "The most potent cancer-causing agent in our food supply is a substance sprayed on apples to keep them on the trees longer and make them look better." The clear implication was that the apple industry and the government had knowingly exposed Americans to danger for trivial-sounding reasons, until NRDC came along and revealed the true facts about this chemical.

In May 1989, CBS ran a follow-up *60 Minutes* episode entitled "What About Apples?" in which the interviewer challenged the integrity and motives of two scientists who had disputed the accuracy of the earlier program. Any ties to the chemical industry or agriculture might have been construed as a conflict of interest, but all scientists get their funding somewhere, and the appearance of bias was hard to avoid. NRDC representatives were also interviewed on the same program, but somehow the subject of their funding did not come up. Was the intended purpose of the two programs to protect consumers, or to shock audiences? Perhaps a little of both.

CONSEQUENCES

The Alar scare was a huge financial blow to the apple industry, and some growers reportedly lost their farms to foreclosure. Within two years, however, consumer demand for apples returned to normal. The government helped reduce the surplus by buying $15 million worth of unsold apples, but economists estimated overall losses at $130 million. Once the scare ended, it was not entirely clear what had happened. To this day, some journalists describe the incident as a colossal hoax perpetrated by the environmental left, whereas others depict it as a great victory for consumer advocacy and the organic food movement. Still others scoffed at the incident, claiming that neither side knew what it was doing.

One clear consequence of this health scare (and others) was the passage of agricultural disparagement laws or "veggie libel laws" in some states. In other words, anybody who makes a negative public statement about an agricultural product may be liable for damages, depending on the circumstances. Apple growers in Washington sued CBS News for its 1989 *60 Minutes* broadcast, but lost. Similarly, the cattle industry filed a lawsuit against Oprah Winfrey in 1997 for saying that the mad cow disease scare discouraged her from eating beef, but that industry also lost. In such cases, the burden is on the plaintiff to prove that such a statement shows reckless disregard of the truth.

WHAT WENT WRONG?

Many people seem to assume that scientists are mere pawns of the military-industrial complex, Big Food, or the ivory tower, whereas environmental activists and celebrities act from higher motives. One reason for this bias may be that scientists are often put in the position of having to deny outside influences, and the very act of denial may seem to imply guilt. Many scientific journals require authors to disclose any conflict of interest, such as funding by a special interest group, or ownership of stock in a company that might benefit from the study. Advocacy groups, by contrast, need not disclose such motives in privately published studies, and are free to editorialize to their heart's content. Activists and celebrities as a group are also more attractive and charismatic than scientists, and thus more believable.

As for the science itself, it is always difficult to extrapolate from studies of laboratory animals, which are exposed to much higher dosages of chemicals and may metabolize them differently. It is necessary to protect consumers, but it is also necessary to feed them. This may become increasingly difficult as the human population grows larger and one agrichemical after another fails to meet safety standards.

REFERENCES AND RECOMMENDED READING

Blum, D. "Who Killed Fido? We All Did." *New York Times*, 28 March 2007.
Brookes, W. T. "The Wasteful Pursuit of Zero Risk." *Forbes*, 30 April 1990.

Cochran, D. E. "State Agricultural Disparagement Statutes: Suing Chicken Little." Harvard University Law School, 2001.

Edelson, E. "The Man who Upset the Apple Cart." *Popular Mechanics*, February 1990.

Egan, T. "Apple Growers Bruised and Bitter after Alar Scare." *New York Times*, 9 July 1991.

Faber, H. "Apple Growers Hurt by Loss of Alar." *New York Times*, 17 September 1989.

Finkel, A. M. "Alar: The Aftermath." *Science*, Vol. 255, 1992, pp. 664–665.

Finkel, A. M. "Toward Less Misleading Comparisons of Uncertain Risks: The Example of Aflatoxin and Alar." *Environmental Health Perspectives*, Vol. 103, 1995, pp. 376–385.

"Government will Buy Apples Left Over from Alar Scare." Associated Press, 8 July 1989.

Groth, E. "Alar in Apples." *Science*, Vol. 244, 1989, p. 755.

Hansen, S. F., et al. "Categorizing Mistaken False Positives in Regulation of Human and Environmental Health." *Risk Analysis*, Vol. 27, 2007, pp. 255–269.

Huber, P. "Publish or Perish." *Forbes*, 11 June 1990.

Jasanoff, S. "Does Public Understanding Influence Public Policy?" *Chemistry and Industry*, 5 August 1991.

Jenkins, N. "Fruit-Chemical Ban Weighed." *New York Times*, 30 August 1985.

Jukes, T. H. "Alar in Apples." *Science*, Vol. 244, 1989, p. 515.

Marshall, E. "Ethics in Science: Science Advisers Need Advice." *Science*, Vol. 245, 1989, pp. 20–22.

Marshall, E. "A is for Apple, Alar, and . . . Alarmist?" *Science*, Vol. 254, 1991, pp. 20–22.

Mott, L. "Alar: The Aftermath." *Science*, Vol. 255, 1992, p. 665.

Mott, L. "Alar Again: Science the Media, and the Public's Right to Know." *International Journal of Occupational and Environmental Health*, Vol. 6, 2000, pp. 68–70.

Mueller, W. "Who's Afraid of Food." *American Demographics*, September 1990.

Negin, E. "The Alar 'Scare' was Real, and So is that 'Veggie Hate-Crime' Movement." *Columbia Journalism Review*, November-December 1996.

"NRDC Pesticide Study was Flawed, EPA Says." *Chemical Marketing Reporter*, 13 March 1989.

Roberts, L. "Alar: The Numbers Game." *Science*, Vol. 243, 1989, p. 1430.

Rodgers, K. E. "Multiple Meanings of Alar After the Scare: Implications for Closure." *Science, Technology, and Human Values*, Vol. 21, 1996, pp. 177–197.

Saxton, L. "Post-Alar Effects on Apples Surface." *Supermarket News*, 26 August 1991.

Shabecoff, P. "Apple Scare of '89 Didn't Kill Market." *New York Times*, 13 November 1990.

Silverstein, K. "Veggie Libel, Wilted Press." *The Nation*, 20 April 1998.

Whelan, E. M. "Stop Banning Products at the Drop of a Rat." *Insight on the News*, 12 December 1994.

Williams, W. "Polishing the Apple's Image." *New York Times*, 25 May 1986.

38

Fear and Worship of Silver

I sing of him, Silver the unique.

—Ancient Hittite text, *The Song of Silver* (circa 1300 B.C.)

SUMMARY

Colloidal silver—fine particles of silver suspended in gel or water—is one of many magic elixirs that alternative health practitioners recommend as alternatives to modern pharmaceutical products. In the early twentieth century, doctors used patent medicines containing silver (or mercury or lead) to treat many diseases, because they had nothing better. Antibiotics, antiviral drugs, and cancer chemotherapy did not yet exist, and the germ theory of disease was barely understood, but the beauty of silver convinced many people that it must have magic properties. Once scientists learned that silver can be toxic, government bans took effect, and some journalists started calling silver "the new asbestos" or "the new mercury." Even some legitimate uses of silver compounds became suspect, such as the traditional eye drops for newborn babies and topical creams used on burn patients. Popular opinion now seems divided between those who regard nanosilver as a menace that is likely to turn their skin blue or damage the environment, and those who hope to improve their health by infusing their GI tracts with colloidal silver solution (from one end or the other). In a sense, the principal health scare presented in this chapter is really the fear of government encroachment on personal liberty.

SOURCE

The fear of silver—and the closely related fear of government regulation of silver—started in earnest near the end of the twentieth century, when the U.S. Food and Drug Administration (FDA) conducted a review of colloidal silver products and banned their sale as drugs. After the FDA rule became effective in 1999, it was illegal to sell colloidal silver for medicinal purposes without first going through the FDA's lengthy application and approval process, which requires proof that a drug is both safe and effective. Since there is little evidence that colloidal silver products are either, most vendors simply repackaged these products as nutritional supplements, although silver is not a recognized human nutrient. The FDA regulates drugs, but not supplements, so colloidal silver stayed on the market. Public opinion was divided as usual, with some people believing the FDA and fearing that they had poisoned themselves, while others muttered about conspiracy.

But the government was not finished with silver. Starting in the late twentieth century, some environmental scientists warned that nanosilver particles used in antibacterial coatings and other products might cause unintended harm by killing beneficial microbes found in water and soil. In 2006, faced with mounting evidence of this threat, the U.S. Environmental Protection Agency (EPA) moved to regulate the sale of such nanosilver products. From 2006 onward, any company that wanted to sell these products must first provide scientific evidence that no environmental risk would result. The nanotechnology industry did not welcome this new hurdle, but in some cases it was possible to avoid it simply by rewording marketing claims.

SCIENCE

Silver metal, nanosilver, colloidal silver, silver salts, and reactive silver are not the same thing, although some sources use these terms interchangeably. All are forms of the chemical element silver, abbreviated Ag (for *argentum*, the Latin word for silver).

- *Silver metal* is the familiar solid material used in jewelry, utensils, and coins. It may be pure or alloyed with copper or other metals to increase its hardness or other properties.
- *Nanosilver* means silver metal in the form of tiny particles, usually between 1 and 100 nanometers (nm) in diameter. A nanometer is one billionth of a meter.
- *Colloidal silver* is the same thing as nanosilver, but suspended in a liquid or gel base that keeps the particles from settling. Ironically, some of these suspensions contain an emulsifier called lecithin, which health food advocates condemn as poison when food processors use it for similar purposes (Chapter 28).
- *Silver salts* are chemical compounds of silver, such as silver nitrate ($AgNO_3$). These salt molecules dissolve in water or other solvents.
- *Reactive silver* refers to any form of silver that can react with other chemicals. For example, silver metal reacts with traces of sulfur in air to produce a dark layer of tarnish (silver sulfide, Ag_2S).

In some forms, and in a few specific circumstances, silver really can kill germs. Long before most people had heard of bacteria, someone figured out that dropping a silver dollar into a container of milk or fruit juice might prevent spoilage. Sometimes it worked, and sometimes the milk or juice spoiled anyway. Safer and more effective methods are now available, such as refrigeration and pasteurization.

Silver also has legitimate medical uses. For example, silver sulfadiazine ($C_{10}H_9$ AgN_4O_2S) ointment was once widely used to prevent bacterial infections in burn patients, but it has fallen out of favor in recent years. The same ointment also works on some resistant forms of acne, but doctors seldom use it for this purpose either, because if used to excess it can turn the patient's skin permanently blue. Also, note the "sulfa" in the name silver sulfadiazine. Although this compound contains about 30 percent silver by weight, it is also a derivative of sulfonamide, one of the early miracle drugs used to control infection in the 1930s before antibiotics were widely available.

Topical silver sulfadiazine is not the only form of silver that can make people blue. To the extent that it exists at all, the popular fear of silver poisoning results mainly from a few highly publicized cases in which cosmetic damage resulted from ingestion of colloidal silver. Several years ago, the media reported that Libertarian politician Stan Jones had turned blue after ingesting large amounts of colloidal silver for unknown reasons. Doctors have known about argyria for centuries, because it formerly affected workers in certain industries who were exposed to silver in the days before protective clothing. The media have dubbed this condition the "disease of the living dead," because its victims have a dark blue-gray color not unlike that of Hollywood zombies.

Until recently, the other well-known example of medicinal silver was silver nitrate ($AgNO_3$), the caustic solution placed in the eyes of newborn babies to kill bacteria and prevent infections such as gonorrhea. For more than a century, most people were delighted to allow doctors to prevent their children from becoming blind; but then some advocacy groups objected to this statutory requirement, on the grounds that it interfered with bonding and seemed to accuse the mother of having a sexually transmitted disease. By 2006, all 50 U.S. states had stopped requiring silver nitrate drops, but most required antibiotics or other drugs that can serve the same purpose with less irritation. Some states also offered religious exemptions.

HISTORY

It has been common knowledge for centuries that silver bullets can kill vampires, and it must have worked, because we rarely see vampires about nowadays. Silver, like gold, also represents wealth and power. Rich children are said to be born with silver spoons in their mouths, and "crossing the palm with silver" enables fortunetellers and authors to predict the future. There is an ancient Persian legend about a silver statue that always laughed when someone told a lie; if that statue has Internet access today, it must be convulsing on the floor by now.

The following item from a 1903 newspaper illustrates the popular perception of silver in that era. Similar advertisements still appear on Internet Web sites more than a century later; the main differences are that (1) the older ads used better grammar and spelling, (2) the newer ads focus on modern maladies, such as Lyme disease and chronic fatigue syndrome, and (3) the newer ads generally exploit the reader's desire for something ancient and Asian, rather than modern and European.

THE WORST DISEASE Can be Eradicated by Newly Discovered Silver Treatment, According to Claims of Paris Physicians. Paris, Feb. 23.—Drs. Matter and Solomon, attached to the Paris hospital, claim they have discovered a new silver treatment which will eradicate the most serious disease if applied in the first stages, and if not applied till later, assures a speedy recovery. The treatment consists of a special preparation of colloidal silver mixed with vaseline. This preparation is rubbed into the skin thus entering the circulation. It has already been successfully tried in cases of typhoid, cerebrospinal meningitis, tubercular pneumonia and other diseases.[1]

As early as 1914, doctors at Columbia University and other major research institutions conducted more objective trials of colloidal silver in the treatment of cancer and other diseases, and reported disappointing results.

Yet fear of unseen evil sometimes brings out the alchemist in all of us. The 2001 postal anthrax incident reportedly caused a major spike in sales of colloidal silver, which many people continue to regard as a panacea for all diseases, particularly those of bacterial origin. To paraphrase the words of one health food dealer, the antibiotic ciprofloxacin cures anthrax only about half the time, and it can give you a headache, but silver cures everything. (The first part of that statement is true, but the last part unfortunately is not.)

In 2008, the EPA imposed a $208,000 fine on a California company for selling computer keyboards that were coated with nanosilver. Since the manufacturers claimed that the product killed germs, they had violated the Federal Insecticide, Fungicide and Rodenticide Act (FIFRA) by not registering the product and proving its effectiveness. It is unclear if this action will prevent other companies from marketing nanosilver-coated products, or if it will simply restrict advertising claims.

CONSEQUENCES

The 1999 FDA restriction on marketing of colloidal silver for medicinal purposes had at least one predictable consequence: a sudden increase in demand for these products. It is natural and healthy for free people to resist authority, up to a point. This conflict has also given us a new conspiracy theory, which holds that colloidal silver is safe and effective for treating practically everything, but Big Drug doesn't want us to know that, because they are unable to patent it and get rich from it.

The other possibility—that colloidal silver really is not safe, and really does not work—seems to have less audience appeal. It might seem that anyone who wants to swallow this stuff should be at liberty to do so, but parents who dose their children with silver or other potentially harmful alternative medicines may be crossing the line. Also, many people turn to alternative medicine as a last resort, because they are gravely ill and cannot afford health insurance or conventional treatment. Colloidal silver may not cure anything, but it costs far less than a quadruple bypass.

The consequences of recent EPA action on industrial nanosilver may not become apparent for some time, until further studies can determine how much of this material we are actually releasing into the environment every year and how it is likely to affect ecosystems. Even nanosilver that is ingested for medical purposes ultimately ends up in the environment, but this source is minor compared with nanosilver leached from industrial waste and landfills.

Perhaps the saddest consequence of the silver war came in 2009, when several Web sites urged people to use colloidal silver instead of Tamiflu to fight the allegedly deadly H1N1 influenza pandemic (Chapter 8). As it turned out, chicken soup and a box of tissues sufficed in most cases.

WHAT WENT WRONG?

Surveys show that many Americans dislike and distrust modern medicine, and that many more are unable to afford it. Even for people with health insurance, medical bills have become the leading cause of bankruptcy. Under these circumstances, more people are likely to embrace alternative medicine and defend the right to choose.

In addition, anything as beautiful and powerful as silver tends to polarize public opinion. One camp fears that the government will take away their God-given colloidal silver, while the other fears that nanosilver in the form of toxic waste will destroy the Earth's resources. Available data suggest that both fears overshoot the mark, but for now, the anti-regulatory group appears to have the edge. If our government could somehow devote as much time and effort to increasing people's freedom as to restricting it, some health scares might be averted.

NOTE

1. *Lima Times-Democrat* (23 February 1903).

REFERENCES AND RECOMMENDED READING

Anderson, E. L., et al. "Argyria as a Result of Somatic Delusions." *American Journal of Psychiatry*, Vol. 165, 2008, pp. 649–650.

"Argentum Argumentum: The Next Asbestos? America Worries about Silver Additives." *Global Agenda*, 1 December 2006.

Chen, X., and H. J. Schluesener. "Nanosilver: A Nanoproduct in Medical Application." *Toxicology Letters*, Vol. 176, 2008, pp. 1–12.

Clark, C. "Forever Blue." *People Weekly*, 28 January 2008.

Cutting, K., et al. "The Safety and Efficacy of Dressings with Silver—Addressing Clinical Concerns." *International Wound Journal*, Vol. 4, 2007, pp. 177–184.

Drake, P. L., and K. J. Hazelwood. "Exposure-Related Health Effects of Silver and Silver Compounds: A Review." *Annals of Occupational Hygiene*, Vol. 49, 2005, pp. 575–585.

"Drug Turned Candidate Blue." *New York Times*, 3 October 2002.

Edwards-Jones, V. "The Benefits of Silver in Hygiene, Personal Care and Healthcare." *Letters in Applied Microbiology*, Vol. 49, 2009, pp. 147–152.

"EPA to Regulate Some Nanosilver Products." *Washington Post*, 23 November 2006.

"FDA Bans Colloidal Silver Products, Cites Lack of Data." *FDA Consumer*, November 1999.

Fung, M. C., and D. L. Bowen. "Silver Products for Medical Indications: Risk-Benefit Analysis." *Journal of Toxicology, Clinical Toxicology*, Vol. 34, 1996, pp. 119–126.

Hill, J. W. 2009. *Colloidal Silver: Medical Uses, Toxicology and Manufacture*. Rainier, WA: Clear Springs Press.

Hori, K., et al. "Believe it or Not—Silver Still Poisons!" *Veterinary and Human Toxicology*, Vol. 44, 2002, pp. 291–292.

Lansdown, A. B. "Silver in Health Care: Antimicrobial Effects and Safety in Use." *Current Problems in Dermatology*, Vol. 33, 2006, pp. 17–34.

Lansdown, A. B. "Critical Observations on the Neurotoxicity of Silver." *Critical Reviews in Toxicology*, Vol. 37, 2007, pp. 237–250.

Luoma, S. N. "Silver Nanotechnologies and the Environment: Old Problems or New Challenges?" Woodrow Wilson International Center for Scholars, Project on Emerging Nanotechnologies, September 2008.

Macintire, D., et al. "Silver Poisoning Associated with an Antismoking Lozenge." *British Medical Journal*, Vol. 2, 1978, pp. 1749–1750.

Marquez, M. "An Anthrax Antidote: Pork-Belly Laugh." *Orlando Sentinel*, 31 October 2001.

Okan, D., et al. "So What If You Are Blue? Oral Colloidal Silver and Argyria Are Out, Safe Dressings Are In." *Advances in Skin & Wound Care*, Vol. 20, 2007, pp. 326–330.

Pala, G., et al. "Ocular Argyrosis in a Silver Craftsman." *Journal of Occupational Health*, Vol. 50, 2008, pp. 521–524.

Prescott, R. J., and S. Wells. "Systemic Argyria." *Journal of Clinical Pathology*, Vol. 47, 1994, pp. 556–557.

Rohdenburg, G. L. "Colloidal Silver with Lecithin, in the Treatment of Malignant Tumors." *Journal of Medical Research*, Vol. 31, 1915, pp. 331–338.

Sullivan, R. "A Case of the Blues." *New Yorker*, 11 November 2002.

"Tarnishing Nanosilver." *Appliance Design*, November 2008.

Wadhera, A., and M. Fung. "Systemic Argyria Associated with Ingestion of Colloidal Silver." *Dermatology Online Journal*, Vol. 11, 2005, p. 12.

39

The Cranberry Scare of 1959

They that can give up essential liberty to obtain a little temporary safety deserve neither liberty nor safety.

—Benjamin Franklin, *Historical Review of Pennsylvania* (1759)

SUMMARY

About three weeks before Thanksgiving Day in 1959, the U.S. Food and Drug Administration (FDA) issued an unprecedented public warning about chemical contamination of cranberries grown in Washington and Oregon. The chemical in question, a weed killer called aminotriazole, caused thyroid cancer when fed to laboratory animals in large doses. Only small traces of aminotriazole were present on a small percentage of cranberries by the time they reached markets, but that was enough to pull the plug. It was the first major test of the 1958 Delaney Amendment to the U.S. Federal Food, Drug, and Cosmetic Act, which prohibited FDA approval of any food additive or contaminant that caused cancer in laboratory animals. In 1959, product recalls and health scares had not yet become routine, and the public took this warning quite seriously. For a time, all cranberries were suspect. The cranberry industry lost an estimated $100 million and spent the next few years trying to repair its image. But for most consumers, this health scare fizzled quickly. Cranberries soon regained and exceeded their former popularity, finally becoming Überfruit, renowned for their nutritional content.

SOURCE

This health scare began abruptly on Monday, 9 November 1959, when the U.S. Secretary of Health, Education, and Welfare announced that the FDA had found chemical contamination on cranberries grown in Washington and Oregon in 1958 and 1959. Radio and television stations and newspapers all picked up the story, and urged Americans to avoid eating cranberries until somebody could figure out how to identify the safe batches. The contaminant was a weed killer called aminotriazole, which appeared to increase the risk of thyroid cancer when fed in high doses to laboratory rats. The cranberry industry protested, and the FDA issued a series of clarifications, but the damage was largely done.

This health scare also ended more abruptly than most, thanks to consumer loyalty, fair media reporting, and a swift, effective response by the cranberry industry. On 1 May 1960,

President Eisenhower issued an executive order that partly reimbursed cranberry growers for their losses. Consumers soon lost their fear of cranberries, and demand returned to normal, but wholesale distributors reportedly took a bit longer.

SCIENCE

Farmers, railroad workers, and road crews have used aminotriazole (also called amitrole, Amizol, Cytrol, and Weedazole) since the 1950s to control unwanted weeds and grasses in fields and along roads. In 1958, the U.S. Department of Agriculture (USDA) approved this weed killer for use on fields after harvests, but its role in thyroid cancer and the tests for detecting residues were not established until 1959. The chemical apparently interferes with the formation of thyroid hormones by blocking the ability of some precursor compounds to bind iodine.

Laboratory rats and mice exposed to high doses of aminotriazole developed thyroid and liver cancer, although hamsters and some other animals were not affected. Studies showed that workers who sprayed this chemical outdoors and absorbed large amounts of it were also at increased risk for various forms of cancer. Since aminotriazole breaks down rapidly in the environment, however, residues on any exposed food crops were usually minimal, and consumers were exposed at very low levels. A 2001 report by the International Agency for Research on Cancer (IARC) concluded that aminotriazole is unlikely to cause cancer in humans unless it is present at levels high enough to reduce circulating levels of thyroid hormones. In other words, the trace amounts present on the cranberries in 1959 probably never posed a threat, but nobody knew that at the time, and the Delaney Clause required government intervention.

Ironically, the chemist who discovered aminotriazole—and determined that it caused cancer in rats—was among the most outspoken critics of the 1959 cranberry scare. Dr. Boyd Schaffer, a toxicologist at American Cyanamid Co., told reporters that a human would need to eat 15,000 pounds of cranberries every day for many years before absorbing a dose of the weed killer sufficient to cause cancer. In other words, if it is reasonable to extrapolate from the rat experiments to humans, and if the extremely small trace amounts of chemical found on some cranberries were typical of all, then the cranberries posed no threat to consumers, and the scare was unnecessary.

Aminotriazole is also one of many environmental chemicals that advocacy groups have identified as possible causes for autism. In 2007, this hypothesis gained some credibility when an academic researcher proposed that fetal exposure to antithyroid agents—which include not only aminotriazole and other herbicides and industrial chemicals but also some common vegetables, such as turnips—might be responsible for changes in brain development. As of 2010, there is no clear evidence of such a connection, but additional studies are in progress.

HISTORY

The first government announcement of the cranberry crisis was simple and to the point, but Americans at the time were unaccustomed to frequent food recalls and warnings, and public reaction was mixed:

The Food and Drug Administration today urged that no further sales be made of cranberries and cranberry products produced in Washington and Oregon in 1958 and 1959 because of their possible contamination by a chemical weed killer, aminotriazole, which causes cancer in the thyroids of rats when it is contained in their diet, until the cranberry industry has submitted a workable plan to separate the contaminated berries from those that are not contaminated.[1]

The U.S. government did not actually ban the sale of cranberries in 1959, but simply advised consumers to avoid them. Some shipments of cranberries were also inspected and seized by regulatory agencies. In response, some warehouses reportedly dumped tons of cranberries without waiting to find out if they were contaminated or not. Many families planning their Thanksgiving dinners quickly crossed cranberries off the shopping list; others called members of Congress to ask if canned cranberry sauce they had already purchased might be safe to eat, or if they should bury it in the yard. Still others thought the whole thing must be a mistake or possibly a prank, something along the lines of the 1938 Orson Welles *War of the Worlds* broadcast, which many people remembered. Some journalists began referring to cranberries as "cancer berries."

Meanwhile, the cranberry industry saw the iceberg ahead, and acted quickly to deflect public wrath and minimize the damage. An agricultural cooperative of cranberry growers (which had recently changed its name to Ocean Spray Cranberries, Inc.) requested the opportunity to make its case, and reportedly sent the following telegram to the Secretary of Health, Education, and Welfare:

We demand that you take immediate steps to rectify the incalculable damages caused by your ill-formed and ill-advised press statements yesterday. You are killing a thoroughbred in order to destroy a flea. You must know that there is not a shred of evidence that a single human being has been adversely affected by eating allegedly contaminated cranberries.[2]

The government backed off somewhat on its original position, and cranberry package labels were devised to reassure the consumer that the contents met FDA safety standards. About two weeks after the original announcement, consumers were told that the scare was over and that it was fine to serve cranberries on Thanksgiving. Unfortunately, many people were unable to change gears quite that fast, and the industry suffered major losses.

On a lighter note, the incident inspired a song called "Cranberry Blues," which was on the radio a few times in 1959. (We cannot quote the lyrics here without paying the copyright holder.) Then presidential candidates Richard M. Nixon and John F. Kennedy proclaimed their confidence in the cranberry industry. Mr. Nixon reportedly ate five servings of cranberry sauce, while Mr. Kennedy drank a large quantity of cranberry juice. And on the day after Thanksgiving 1959, in another attempt to put the matter in perspective, a newspaper reporter interviewed a spot removal instructor from the National Institute of Dry Cleaning, who advised readers that "This Thanksgiving you're more likely to stain your clothes by spilling cranberries than you are to get cancer by eating them."[3] There is something faulty about this comparison, but we present it as a time capsule from a simpler era.

In 1996, Congress amended the Delaney Clause so that it no longer required proof that exposure to a chemical carried zero risk of cancer. Instead, the safety of the chemical must be proven with "reasonable certainty," a vague enough requirement to satisfy almost everyone.

CONSEQUENCES

The cranberry scare of 1959 was the first of many nails in the coffin of the Delaney Clause, but the cranberry industry itself survived without long-term harm. Even before the scare, the industry had advised its members not to use aminotriazole or other unapproved weed killers on their crops, so the incident served as an expensive reminder. Yet no residual suspicion clung to cranberries, because consumers blamed the chemical industry and the government, not the growers or the fruit itself.

As it later turned out, less than 1 percent of the cranberry crop was contaminated, and only with trace amounts of the weed killer. The next half-century would see cranberries evolve from a Thanksgiving specialty into Überfruit, a year-round snack food and salad garnish, an effective remedy for urinary tract infections, and an awesome source of antioxidants and bioflavonoids and things that most people in 1959 could not even spell.

WHAT WENT WRONG?

The cranberry scare of 1959 served to illustrate the problems with "zero risk" laws, such as the Delaney Amendment. In principle, it sounds like a good idea to keep carcinogens (cancer-causing agents) out of the food supply. In practice, the amendment was unenforceable. There are very few chemicals that reliably "cause" cancer, but there are hundreds of thousands of chemicals that might increase the risk of cancer at least slightly, if the exposure level is high enough. We evaluate that risk in terms of the number of additional cancers that are likely to result per million people exposed to a given chemical or other carcinogen. But it would be virtually impossible to get that number down to zero, and any attempt to do so could only result in one crisis after another. Getting a tan, drinking orange juice, having sex, working the night shift, and a host of other popular activities and substances all increase the risk of cancer.

NOTES

1. B. Constable, "Cranberry Scare of 1959" (Eisenhower Library, March 1994).
2. E. T. O'Donnell, "The Great Cranberry Scare of 1959" (*Irish Echo*, 25 November 2005).
3. "Cranberries Warning Given by Cleaners" (Associated Press, 27 November 1959).

REFERENCES AND RECOMMENDED READING

"Airing Asked of Cranberry Scare Report." United Press International, 12 November 1959.
Blank, C. H. "The Delaney Clause: Technical Naïveté and Scientific Advocacy in the Formulation of Public Health Policies." *California Law Review*, Vol. 62, 1974, pp. 1084–1120.

Blum, D. "Who Killed Fido? We All Did." *New York Times*, 28 March 2007.

Brucker-Davis, F. "Effects of Environmental Synthetic Chemicals on Thyroid Function." *Thyroid*, Vol. 8, 1998, pp. 827–856.

Capen, C. C. "Mechanisms of Chemical Injury of Thyroid Gland." *Progress in Clinical and Biological Research*, Vol. 387, 1994, pp. 173–191.

"Changes His Mind About Cranberries." United Press International, 12 November 1959.

Clark, T. "The Thanksgiving Without Cranberry Sauce: Contamination by Weed Killer Almost Destroyed Market in 1959." *Yankee*, Vol. 44, 1980, p. 308.

Comarow, A. "Less-than-Scary Health Scares." *U.S. News and World Report*, Vol. 129, 2000, p. 70.

Constable, B. "Cranberry Scare of 1959: Guide to Historical Holdings in the Eisenhower Library." Abilene, KS: Dwight D. Eisenhower Presidential Library and Museum, March 1994.

"Cranberry Tests Speeded; Nixon Eats 5 Servings." United Press International, 13 November 1959.

Cross, C. E. "Recent Activity in the Massachusetts Cranberry Business." *Economic Botany*, Vol. 17, 1963, pp. 331–332.

Flieger, K. "The Delaney Dilemma." *FDA Consumer*, September 1988.

Goodrich, W. W. "Cranberries, Chickens and Charcoal." *Food Drug Cosmetic Law Journal*, Vol. 15, 1960, p. 87 ff.

"Here's How Public Health is Protected from Poisons." Associated Press, 20 November 1959.

Landi, H. "Straight from the Bog to the Bottle." *Beverage World*, 15 December 2005.

Material Safety Data Sheet: Amitrole. International Programme on Chemical Safety, April 1994.

Merrill, R. A. "Food Safety Regulation: Reforming the Delaney Clause." *Annual Review of Public Health*, Vol. 18, 1997, pp. 313–340.

O'Donnell, E. T. "Hibernian Chronicle: The Great Cranberry Scare of 1959." *Irish Echo*, 25 November 2005.

Pape, S. M. "New Pesticide Law Reforms Delaney." *Prepared Foods*, September 1996.

Román, G. C. "Autism: Transient In Utero Hypothyroxinemia Related to Maternal Flavonoid Ingestion During Pregnancy and to Other Environmental Antithyroid Agents." *Journal of the Neurological Sciences*, Vol. 262, 2007, pp. 15–26.

Santodonato, J., et al. "Monograph on the Potential Carcinogenic Risk to Humans: Amitrole." Syracuse, NY: Center for Chemical Hazard Assessment, Report No. SRC-TR-84-737, 1985.

Scholliers, P. "Defining Food Risks and Food Anxieties Throughout History." *Appetite*, Vol. 51, 2008, pp. 3–6.

Sharp, D. S., et al. "Delayed Health Hazards of Pesticide Exposure." *Annual Review of Public Health*, Vol. 7, 1986, pp. 441–471.

Timmons, F. L. "A History of Weed Control in the United States and Canada." *Weed Science*, Vol. 18, 1970, pp. 294–307.

Weisburger, J. H. "The 37 Year History of the Delaney Clause." *Experimental and Toxicologic Pathology*, Vol. 48, 1996, pp. 183–188.

Zimbelman, R. G. "Scientific Basis for Interpretation of Delaney Clause." *Journal of Animal Science*, Vol. 48, 1979, pp. 986–992.

40

Fear of Aluminum Containers

We took from the goddess' hand the cups she gave us, and drained them greedily . . . My body bent forward and down, until my face looked straight at the ground.

—Ovid, *Metamorphoses* (A.D. 8)

SUMMARY

Many people have heard that food prepared in aluminum cookware may cause Alzheimer's disease (AD) and other health problems. Similar concerns have focused on foods and beverages stored in aluminum cans, and water that contains aluminum salts as a result of treatment to remove suspended material. Some antacid drugs, buffered aspirin, antiperspirants, and vaccines also contain aluminum. In fact, the element is so widely distributed that it would be nearly impossible to avoid exposure. The health scare began in the 1970s, when doctors found high levels of aluminum in the brains of AD patients. As of 2010, the relationship (if any) between aluminum exposure and AD remains unknown. Over the years, the aluminum scare has alternately fizzled and reemerged in new forms. It is unclear if drugs that remove or block aluminum might help prevent AD, because the disease might cause or accelerate aluminum buildup in the brain rather than vice versa. Although some journalists have dismissed aluminum as just another unproven health scare, suspicion continues to focus on this metal.

SOURCE

In the 1920s and 1930s, a series of bogus medical reports claimed that it was dangerous to eat food stored or prepared in aluminum containers. One likely source of this rumor was the stainless steel industry, and the most famous alleged casualty was the actor Rudolph Valentino, who died in 1926 from complications after abdominal surgery—not from aluminum poisoning, as some journalists claimed. It is not clear how aluminum became part of the Valentino legend, but the story persists to the present day. Another popular theory was that a jealous lover fed him arsenic.[1] Some journalists and snake-oil salesmen of that era claimed that aluminum caused cancer, polio, and osteoporosis.

The first highly publicized warnings of a possible connection between aluminum and Alzheimer's disease were published in the late 1970s, although a few related reports appeared in the medical literature as early as the mid-1960s. Researchers who examined the brains of deceased Alzheimer's patients found that certain proteins contained high levels of aluminum. This finding alone does not prove that aluminum causes the disease, any more than the accumulation of copper in the body causes Wilson's disease. In Wilson's, the disease causes the copper buildup, not vice versa; similarly, a brain already damaged by AD may allow more aluminum to enter.

Yet other unnerving discoveries followed during the next two decades. For example, a 1985 study showed that some dialysis patients developed a form of dementia that resulted from the buildup of aluminum in their tissues. Healthy kidneys can eliminate most aluminum from the body, but dialysis does the job less efficiently. This finding was not conclusive either, because the dementia in those patients was not the same as AD. Another scare resulted when a 1994 article showed that exposure to aluminum could cause protein tangles similar to those seen in AD, but the people in that study did not have AD either. As of 2010, the scare appears to be dormant.

SCIENCE

Aluminum (Al) is a chemical element that makes up more than 8 percent of the Earth's crust by weight. It is not only the most abundant metal, but the third most abundant element after oxygen and silicon. Most aluminum exists in the form of compounds with one of these elements, such as aluminum oxide (Al_2O_3). People extract aluminum metal from ores such as bauxite and use it to make a variety of familiar products, including many food and beverage containers, kitchen utensils, and building materials.

Less obvious forms of aluminum include compounds used in antiperspirants, antacids, buffered aspirin, vaccines, and many industrial products, such as paints. Many valuable gemstones, such as rubies and sapphires, are aluminum-based minerals. Aluminum ammonium sulfate, also called ammonium alum, is widely used in water flocculation (treatment to remove suspended materials), in stone form as a "natural" deodorant, and as an additive to improve the color and texture of some foods. Green tea and soy milk reportedly contain more aluminum than most other beverages.

If aluminum intake may be somehow related to the onset or progress or Alzheimer's disease, then it is important to determine how much aluminum people normally ingest in a lifetime, and how much of this is avoidable. Dietary intake of aluminum is usually between 3 and 30 milligrams per day, of which we absorb less than 1 percent. By one estimate, a person who uses uncoated aluminum pans and containers for all cooking and food storage would ingest about 3.5 mg of aluminum per day from that source alone. But people who take certain aluminum-based antacid drugs may get as much as 50 to 1,000 milligrams of aluminum per day, and at present there is no evidence that such drugs are an AD risk factor. Most of this ingested aluminum ends up in the urine and feces.

Alzheimer's disease is a form of senile dementia that affects an estimated 25 million people. By 2050, it may affect as many as one in every 85 people worldwide. This prospect is alarming, because of both the human suffering involved and the enormous cost of care. As of the early twenty-first century, AD costs the United States economy an estimated $100 billion per year. It is not clear if AD is actually increasing, due to some unknown environmental factor or pathogen, or if the apparent increase is the result of better diagnosis and longer life expectancy.

AD symptoms include confusion, mood swings, and memory loss. Usually it appears after age 65, but about 5 percent of patients develop the disease earlier in life, probably due to genetic factors. Other forms of dementia may appear similar, but in AD, plaques (abnormal patches) of a protein called beta amyloid are deposited in the brain. The disease also involves loss of nerve cells in the brain and the formation of characteristic tangled protein structures. Again, the exact relationship of these changes to the disease has eluded researchers.

Some reported interventions that may help remove aluminum from the body, or reduce the actual probability of developing Alzheimer's disease, include drinking beer—no, we are not kidding—taking vitamin C and other antioxidants, going for a walk every day, and keeping the mind active. Although most of these measures have some intuitive appeal, it is hard to see how mental activity, for example, could reduce aluminum in the brain. Again, cause and effect may be reversed here. Medical treatments that remove amyloid plaques do not seem to reduce AD symptoms or slow its progress; on the contrary, in 2009, researchers reported encouraging preliminary results using a drug that actually *increased* beta amyloid. As of 2010, the secrets of AD remain elusive.

HISTORY

People have known since ancient times that elderly people often showed signs of memory loss and emotional disturbance. The majority of people who lived to extreme old age could look forward to this fate. Thus, the word *senile* came to mean either old or dotty (frequently both).

As early as 1897, scientists knew that exposure to high levels of aluminum (or any of several other metals) could cause damage to the central nervous system in laboratory animals. In 1901, a German doctor named Alois Alzheimer (1864–1915) described a human patient who had what would later be recognized as the early-onset form of Alzheimer's disease. In 1906, after that patient died, Dr. Alzheimer examined sections of her brain and found the amyloid plaques and neurofibrillary tangles (abnormal proteins inside nerve fibers) that soon became the hallmark of this "new" disease, later named for its discoverer. Researchers and advocates have proposed so many possible causes for AD that it would take a separate book to review them all.

Until about 1977, anyone who developed symptoms of dementia between the ages of 45 and 65 was likely to receive a diagnosis of Alzheimer's disease or presenile dementia. The definition changed somewhat after a medical conference that year, and the diagnosis became independent of age. Suddenly, millions of people over age 65 had Alzheimer's disease too. This change in terminology may account for part of the apparent AD epidemic, but by any other name, the disease remains just as dreadful. Small wonder that potential risk factors, such as aluminum, have inspired health scares.

CONSEQUENCES

According to some sources, sales of cast aluminum cookware declined precipitously after reports of a possible link to Alzheimer's disease. As a result, sales of cast iron and stainless steel cookware increased. Yet other products that contain aluminum, such as green tea and some antiperspirants, remained popular.

Although the AD question remains unresolved, many health advocates now urge reasonable steps to reduce aluminum consumption, just in case. Aluminum may be an essential micronutrient, but it is present in so many foods that it would be virtually impossible to develop a deficiency. Harmless precautions to limit aluminum intake might include switching to stainless steel cookware, installing a water filter, drinking something other than green tea or soy milk, and checking the labels of products such as antiperspirants and antacids to avoid brands that contain aluminum. A 2009 study showed that boiling water in aluminum cookware greatly reduced subsequent aluminum leaching into food.

The AD-aluminum controversy has also contributed to some parents' distrust of vaccines, because some vaccines use aluminum salts as adjuvants to increase the immune response. As of 2010, these adjuvants are present in the diphtheria-tetanus-pertussis and hepatitis A and B vaccines, but not in the polio, MMR, or influenza vaccines. People who are concerned about this ingredient should ask their doctors about it, but at present there is no evidence that it is harmful. Pharmaceutical companies would like to invent vaccines that are 100 percent effective, have no possible side effects, and contain nothing that anyone might find objectionable, but these goals have proven elusive thus far.

There is such a thing as too much precaution. If people acted in accordance with every published study of Alzheimer's disease risk factors, they would drink large quantities of beer, avoid using antiperspirants, go back to college, walk everywhere instead of driving—and die young, since age is the most important AD risk factor of all. In other words, the planet would undergo a 1960s revival.

WHAT WENT WRONG?

Alzheimer's disease is greatly feared, for excellent reasons. As a result, the news media leap on any report of anything that might possibly cause it, such as prions (or the absence of prions), free radicals, pesticides, solvents, head injuries, genetic mutations, electromagnetic fields, or exposure to various metals, including iron, copper, zinc, or aluminum. According to one study—described in Chapter 41 and based solely on experiments with mice—using a cell phone may actually reduce the risk of AD. Until doctors identify the real cause of AD, or proven methods for treating or preventing it, multiple health scares and lifestyle recommendations may be inevitable.

NOTE

1. "Did Arsenic Cause Film Star Death?" *Sioux City Journal*, 24 August 1926.

REFERENCES AND RECOMMENDED READING

Begley, S. "Are We Taking the Wrong Approach to Curing Alzheimer's?" *Newsweek*, 16 July 2009.
Bharathi, P., et al. "Molecular Toxicity of Aluminium in Relation to Neurodegeneration." *Indian Journal of Medical Research*, Vol. 128, 2008, pp. 545–556.
Blumenthal, D. "Is that Newfangled Cookware Safe?" *FDA Consumer*, October 1990.
Comarow, A. "Less-than-Scary Health Scares." *U.S. News and World Report*, Vol. 129, 2000, p. 70.

Crapper, D. R., et al. "Brain Aluminum Distribution in Alzheimer's Disease and Experimental Neurofibrillary Degeneration."*Science*, Vol. 180, 1973, pp. 511–513.

Edwards, D. D. "Aluminum: A High Price for a Surrogate?" *Science News*, 18 April 1987.

Exley, C., and M. M. Esiri. "Severe Cerebral Congophilic Angiopathic Coincident with Increased Brain Aluminium in a Resident of Camelford, Cornwall, UK." *Journal of Neurology, Neurosurgery, and Psychiatry*, Vol. 77, 2006, pp. 877–879.

"Expert Claims Senility Not 'Natural' to Aging." Associated Press, 15 January 1979.

Ferreira, P. C., et al. "Aluminum as a Risk Factor for Alzheimer's Disease." *Revista Latino-Americana de Enfermagem*, Vol. 16, 2008, pp. 151–157.

Frisardi, V., et al. "Aluminum in the Diet and Alzheimer's Disease: From Current Epidemiology to Possible Disease-Modifying Treatment." *Journal of Alzheimer's Disease*, 7 January 2010.

Hachinski, V. "Aluminum Exposure and Risk of Alzheimer's Disease." *Archives of Neurology*, Vol. 55, 1998, p. 742.

Karbouj, R., et al. "A Simple Pre-Treatment of Aluminium Cookware to Minimize Aluminium Transfer to Food." *Food and Chemical Toxicology*, Vol. 47, 2009, pp. 571–577.

Kramer, S. M. "Fact or Fiction: Antiperspirants Do More than Block Sweat." *Scientific American*, 9 August 2007.

Kukull, W. A., et al. "Solvent Exposure as a Risk Factor for Alzheimer's Disease: A Case-Control Study." *American Journal of Epidemiology*, Vol. 141, 1995, pp. 1059–1071.

McLachlan, D. R., et al. "Would Decreased Aluminum Ingestion Reduce the Incidence of Alzheimer's Disease?" *Canadian Medical Association Journal*, Vol. 145, 1991, pp. 793–805.

Miu, A. C., and O. Benga. "Aluminum and Alzheimer's Disease: A New Look." *Journal of Alzheimer's Disease*, Vol. 10, 2006, pp. 179–201.

Munoz, D. G., and H. Feldman. "Causes of Alzheimer's Disease." *Canadian Medical Association Journal*, Vol. 11, 2000, pp. 65–72.

Patz, A. "Can You Spot Which Baby Hasn't Been Vaccinated?" *Baby Talk*, September 2009.

Peña, A., et al. "Influence of Moderate Beer Consumption on Aluminium Toxico-Kinetics: Acute Study." *Nutrición Hospitalaria*, Vol. 22, 2007, pp. 371–376. [Spanish].

Perl, D. P. "Relationship of Aluminum to Alzheimer's Disease." *Environmental Health Perspectives*, Vol. 63, 1985, pp. 149–153.

Perl, D. P. "Exposure to Aluminium and the Subsequent Development of a Disorder with Features of Alzheimer's Disease." *Journal of Neurology, Neurosurgery, and Psychiatry*, Vol. 77, 2006, p. 811.

Petrovsky, N., and J. C. Aguilar. "Vaccine Adjuvants: Current State and Future Trends." *Immunology and Cell Biology*, Vol. 82, 2004, pp. 488–496.

Rondeau, V., et al. "Analysis of the Effect of Aluminum in Drinking Water and Transferrin C2 Allele on Alzheimer's Disease."*European Journal of Neurology*, Vol. 13, 2006, pp. 1022–1025.

Ross, M. "Many Questions But No Clear Answers on Link Between Aluminum, Alzheimer's Disease." *Canadian Medical Association Journal*, Vol. 150, 1994, pp. 68–69.

U.S. Department of Health and Human Services, Agency for Toxic Substances and Disease Registry. "Toxicological Profile for Aluminum." September 2008.

41

Fear of Cell Phones

Around the world thoughts shall fly
In the twinkling of an eye.
> —Attributed to Mother Shipton (1488–1561), but more likely an 1862 forgery

SUMMARY

Many people have heard that long-term use of cellular phones may cause brain tumors or other health problems, such as male sterility or skin infections. Many others, including some cell phone manufacturers, dismiss such fears as urban legend. In fact, a few studies have appeared to confirm the risks of cell phone use, and long-term health effects (if any) may not be apparent yet. Also, self-reported data on cell phone use is often unreliable. Since no clear, consistent proof of risk has materialized, and cell phones have become a convenience that would be hard to abandon, no major authority has yet discouraged their use—except in specific circumstances, such as driving, when talking or texting on the cell phone becomes dangerous for other reasons. As of 2010, it is not clear if this health scare has completely fizzled or not. Regardless of how people feel about the safety of cell phones, their popularity has reached an all-time high. By 2000, nearly half of all American adults had a cell phone, and by 2009 that was up to 85 percent.

SOURCE

Concern about the possible health effects of electromagnetic fields (EMFs) did not start with cell phones, but with an unrelated health scare related to high-voltage power line exposure (Chapter 42). As more people started using hand-held cellular phones in the early 1990s, epidemiologists took a closer look at this technology and its possible relationship to brain tumors or other health problems. The scare arrived in April 1992, when a Florida woman sued the cell phone manufacturer NEC America, claiming that a hand-held cell phone was responsible for her brain cancer. She died a month later, but her husband pursued the case and went public. In January 1993, he appeared as a guest on the *Larry King Live* television program, and the interview started a near-panic among America's cell phone users, who numbered only about 15 million at the time.

The Cellular Telecommunications Industry Association (CTIA) countered this adverse publicity by funding health studies and by launching an effective public relations campaign of its own. One of the first studies appeared to show that acoustic neuroma (a benign tumor of the auditory nerve) was more common in people who used cell phones than in the general population. In 1995, the Florida case was dismissed, reportedly because there was no proof of a connection. Several similar cases followed, but most (if not all) were dismissed. During the next 15 years, cell phones became a national obsession. The associated health scare never quite went away, but has alternately fizzled and defizzled with each new study.

SCIENCE

If cell phones really can cause tumors in the user's brain or inner ear, the problem is most likely the location of the antenna, not the phone itself. In 1993, when this health scare started, some mobile phones were mounted in cars, whereas others were the portable variety that we take for granted today, with a built-in antenna. When the portable device communicates with a cell tower, the antenna transmits radio-frequency energy close to the user's head. The concern is that people who talk on their cell phones for long periods of time every day are essentially microwaving their brains and ears. It is possible to minimize this exposure by using a Bluetooth headset or other hands-free device, but not everyone finds them convenient. The same problem did not occur with the now-obsolete mobile car phones, which had an outside antenna that was not near the user's head.

Some key studies and interviews to date have yielded the following results:

- A 2004 study concluded that cell phone users were twice as likely as others to develop acoustic neuroma (a benign, slow-growing inner ear tumor).
- Another 2004 study found that cell phone users were *not* more likely than others to develop acoustic neuroma.
- A 2008 study concluded that cell phone users might be at increased risk for salivary gland tumors.
- Another 2008 report noted that cell phone use can cause skin irritation.
- Another 2008 report claimed that men who keep a cell phone in their pockets or on their belts (while using an earpiece) may have reduced sperm quality.
- A 2010 study showed that prolonged cell phone use may be a risk factor for tinnitus (noises in the ear).
- In 2008, three neurosurgeons told Larry King that they avoid holding their own cell phones next to their heads.
- A 2009 study concluded that cell phone users have a 2 percent greater chance of developing a malignant or benign tumor, as compared with non-phone users.
- Another 2009 study, this one involving 60,000 people who developed brain tumors between 1974 and 2003, found that cell phone use was *not* a risk factor. The frequency of brain tumors in the population stayed the same after the introduction of cell phones.
- In 2009, the World Health Organization (WHO) reported that extensive mobile phone use for 10 years or longer might be associated with increased tumor risk.

Consumers often ask why scientists cannot make up their minds. Are cell phones harmful, or not? One problem is that interviewers collecting data must rely on the subject's memory and honesty. It is not possible to confine people to a laboratory for years and experiment on them under controlled conditions. For example, if the interviewer asks an acoustic neuroma patient about her past cell phone habits, she may overestimate usage, hoping to find an explanation for the tumor. As another example, suppose a teenager spends five hours per day talking to acquaintances on his cell phone instead of socializing with them in person. He might not want to admit that, so he tells the interviewer that he uses the phone for maybe a few minutes per day. Also, suppose he lives in a state where it is illegal to drive while talking on a cell phone without a hands-free device. He might claim that he always uses such a device in his car, even if he doesn't. Some studies have checked the accuracy of self-reported data, and the results are not encouraging.

Studies of laboratory animals have other design limitations, such as the fact that rats and mice have very small brains and never use cell phones. Some studies have exposed them to similar electromagnetic radiation, but the results can be hard to interpret. For example, a 2010 study appeared to show that cell phone exposure *cured* some laboratory mice that had been genetically altered to develop Alzheimer's disease. To our knowledge, no one has yet claimed that cell phones can cure human AD patients.

HISTORY

Unlike some health scares, cell phones do not have roots in antiquity. They are similar in concept to smoke signals or mental telepathy, without the disadvantages of either. The communicators on the original *Star Trek* television series resembled modern flip phones, yet they served as convenient plot devices, not as a substitute for social interaction. Also, communicators functioned in subspace, a fictional construct where signals can travel faster than light and probably do not interact with living tissue.

Whenever someone invents a new technology, someone else will suspect that it is potentially harmful, and often it is. Cars, airplanes, and household electric wiring have killed many people. If subspace communicators existed, somebody would be studying their health effects. The question is not whether a thing is dangerous, but whether we want it badly enough to accept the risk.

When cell phones became widely available in about 1990, consumer reaction was mixed. Hardly anyone, other than a few engineers, anticipated that this technology might prove harmful. To everybody else, a cell phone sounded like a good thing to have in case of a flat tire or other emergency. But why, we asked, would anybody want to talk on the phone while walking through a mall or driving a car? Today, an estimated 85 percent of American adults use a cell phone every day. A typical mall is filled with blank-faced people conversing with invisible friends, while small shrines mark the graves of drivers (and airline pilots) who found texting more urgent than the task at hand.

CONSEQUENCES

The 1993 health scare that resulted from the Florida court case reportedly drove down the price of some related stocks, but the effect was temporary, and it said more about the power of Larry King than about cell phones. But as studies alternately condemn and exonerate these phones, many parents remain in a quandary. Is a child safer with or without one? The advent of cheap, prepaid cell phones solved this problem in many cases by relieving parents of the decision.

As of 2010, it appears that the risk of developing a brain tumor as a result of long-term cell phone use is small, but possibly real. With billions of cell phone users worldwide, even a very small added percentage of risk would translate into a great many suffering people. Acoustic neuromas are seldom fatal, but they can cause pain and hearing loss.

When any technology comes under fire, it may become the focus for a host of seemingly unrelated fears. Some advocates have now blamed cell phones for both autism and fibromyalgia—two conditions that appear frequently throughout this book, because nobody knows what really causes them, and people blame them on virtually everything. A less expected claim, also unconfirmed, is that cell phone radiation may be responsible for the recent reduction of North American honeybee populations.

WHAT WENT WRONG?

As noted earlier, people often tend to overestimate the risk inherent in creepy things they can see and sense, like black widow spider bites, killer bee stings, and French cheese that smells like feet, while underestimating the risk from invisible forces associated with pleasant lifestyle choices, such as skipping a vaccination, smoking cigarettes, or using a cell phone. The latter health scare has largely fizzled in the face of overwhelming demand, but the scientific findings are ambiguous at best. No matter how much the world needs cell phones, it needs a clear answer even more.

Specifically, researchers need to find the causal connection (if any) between radio-frequency radiation and tumors. Numbers are not enough; coincidence is not causality. We know that ionizing radiation such as X-rays can damage nucleic acids and cause cancer, but cell phones emit nonionizing radiation that does not appear energetic enough to have a similar effect. It is generally best to solve a mystery such as this before allowing it to fizzle.

REFERENCES AND RECOMMENDED READING

Adams, G. "Maine to Consider Cell Phone Cancer Warning." Associated Press, 20 December 2009.

Arendash, G. W., et al. "Electromagnetic Field Treatment Protects Against and Reverses Cognitive Impairment in Alzheimer's Disease Mice." *Journal of Alzheimer's Disease*, 11 September 2009.

Beckford, M., and R. Winnett. "Long-Term Use of Mobile Phones 'May Be Linked to Cancer.'" *The Daily Telegraph*, 24 October 2009.

Bondy, M. L., et al. "Brain Tumor Epidemiology: Consensus from the Brain Tumor Epidemiology Consortium." *Cancer*, Vol. 113, 2008, pp. 1953–1968.

Cardis, E. "Brain Tumour Risk in Relation to Mobile Telephone Use." *International Journal of Epidemiology*, 17 May 2010.

Christensen, H. C., et al. "Cellular Phone Use and Risk of Acoustic Neuroma." *American Journal of Epidemiology*, Vol. 159, 2004, pp. 277–283.

Deltour, I., et al. "Time Trends in Brain Tumor Incidence Rates in Denmark, Finland, Norway, and Sweden, 1974–2003." *Journal of the National Cancer Institute*, Vol. 101, 2009, pp. 1721–1724.

"Doctors Downplay Cellular Phone Risk." Associated Press, 3 February 1993.

Dolan, M., and J. Rowley. "The Precautionary Principle in the Context of Mobile Phone and Base Station Radiofrequency Exposures." *Environmental Health Perspectives*, Vol. 117, 2009, pp. 1329–1332.

Dreyfuss, J. H. "Mixed Results on Link between Cellular Telephones and Cancer." *CA: A Cancer Journal for Clinicians*, 16 December 2009.

Field, K. "I Think I Feel an EMF Headache Coming On." *Design News*, 1 December 2009.

Hardell, L., et al. "Tumour Risk Associated with Use of Cellular Telephones or Cordless Desktop Telephones." *World Journal of Surgical Oncology*, Vol. 11, 2006, p. 74.

Interlandi, J. "How Safe are Cell Phones?" *Newsweek*, 19 December 2007.

Inyang, I., et al. "How Well do Adolescents Recall Use of Mobile Telephones? Results of a Validation Study." *BMC Medical Research Methodology*, Vol. 9, 2009, p. 36.

Jones, J. "Can Rumors Cause Cancer?" *Journal of the National Cancer Institute*, Vol. 92, 2000, pp. 1469–1471.

Kohli, D. R., et al. "Cell Phones and Tumor: Still No Man's Land." *Indian Journal of Cancer*, Vol. 46, 2009, pp. 5–12.

Kundi, M. "The Controversy about a Possible Relationship between Mobile Phone Use and Cancer." *Environmental Health Perspectives*, Vol. 117, 2009, pp. 316–324.

Kundi, M., et al. "Electromagnetic Fields and the Precautionary Principle." *Environmental Health Perspectives*, Vol. 117, 2009, pp. A484–A485.

Lönn, S., et al. "Long-Term Mobile Phone Use and Brain Tumor Risk." *American Journal of Epidemiology*, Vol. 16, 2005, pp. 526–535.

Madhukara, J., et al. "Cell Phone Dermatitis." *Indian Journal of Dermatology, Venereology and Leprology*, Vol. 74, 2008, pp. 500–501.

Myung, S.-K., et al. "Mobile Phone Use and Risk of Tumors: A Meta-Analysis." *Journal of Clinical Oncology*, Vol. 27, 2009, pp. 5565–5572.

Osterhout, J. E. "Exposure to Radiation from Cell Phones Could Help Protect against Alzheimer's Memory Loss." *New York Daily News*, 7 January 2010.

Parker-Pope, T. "Experts Revive Debate over Cellphones and Cancer." *New York Times*, 3 June 2008.

Raymond, J. "Is That a Phone in your Pocket?" *Newsweek*, 18 September 2008.

Schüz, J., et al. "Cellular Telephone Use and Cancer Risk: Update of a Nationwide Danish Cohort." *Journal of the National Cancer Institute*, Vol. 98, 2006, pp. 1707–1713.

Stang, A., et al. "Mobile Phone Use and Risk of Uveal Melanoma: Results of the Risk Factors for Uveal Melanoma Case-Control Study." *Journal of the National Cancer Institute*, Vol. 101, 2009, pp. 120–123.

Wood, A. W. "How Dangerous Are Mobile Phones, Transmission Masts, and Electricity Pylons?" *Archives of Disease in Childhood*, Vol. 91, 2006, pp. 361–366.

42

Fear of Power Lines

The awful shadow of some unseen Power
Floats though unseen among us.
                    —Percy Bysshe Shelley, *Hymn to Intellectual Beauty* (1816)

SUMMARY

In the 1980s and 1990s, many people believed that exposure to electromagnetic fields associated with high-voltage power lines could cause childhood leukemia and other forms of cancer. Some studies appeared to show a relationship between clusters of leukemia cases and proximity to sources of extremely low frequency (ELF) electromagnetic fields, but other studies refuted these findings. The subject became highly controversial, thanks to several inflammatory articles published in 1989. Later studies expanded these concerns to include not only power lines but common household appliances, electric blankets, computer screens, and other products. As of 2010, this health scare remains unresolved, and it has fizzled only in the sense that the media and the public seem to have largely lost interest in it. Related concerns about radio frequency (RF) exposure from cell phones (Chapter 41) have largely displaced this issue, possibly because of the element of choice. It is possible to break the habit of placing a cell phone antenna against one's head, but proximity to power lines and the design of indoor wiring are issues beyond most people's control.

SOURCE

Long before Mary Shelley wrote the science-fiction classic *Frankenstein* (reportedly to while away the gloomy summer that followed a volcanic eruption), scientists and philosophers pondered the effects of electricity on biological systems. Many ancient deities could hurl lightning bolts, for symmetry seemed to demand that a force powerful enough to take life must also be capable of restoring it. Doctors have used magnetic fields to treat cancer and other diseases for centuries, with mixed results. In 1979, however, an epidemiological study of childhood cancer in Colorado put the matter in a new light. The investigators found what appeared to be an excess number of cancers in children who lived in houses with certain electrical wiring configurations—specifically, those with high current flow, which produced magnetic fields associated with the household plumbing that served as ground.

That report further noted that adults whose occupations might expose them to AC magnetic fields also appeared to be at risk for cancer, but for most readers, the scary part was the possible threat to children. The reasons for these associations were unknown, and would remain so for the next thirty years or longer, but a new health scare was born. The EMF scare attained the level of near-hysteria in 1989, thanks to a series of three dramatic but misleading articles published in the *New Yorker* magazine.

SCIENCE

High-voltage transmission lines (collectively known as "the grid") transfer electricity from power plants to substations, and distribution lines connect the substations to meters at homes and businesses. The current passing through these power lines generates electromagnetic fields (EMF), and we measure the strength or density of such a field in units called gauss (G) or milligauss (mG, one thousandth of a gauss). In most countries, the AC power supply frequency is either 50 or 60 hertz (Hz), within a range that many sources define as extremely low frequency (ELF) and others call super low frequency (SLF). By contrast, the electromagnetic radiation produced by a cell phone antenna (Chapter 41) is in a much higher frequency range, usually above 800 *million* Hz (800 mHz). Higher frequency means shorter wavelength and higher energy per photon. That is why many investigators find cell phones a more likely hazard than magnetic fields from power lines, but a great deal remains to be learned about the interaction of electromagnetic waves with living systems.

The purpose of a cellular phone is to emit a radio-frequency signal, and the user whose head gets in the way runs the (very low) risk of collateral damage. AC power lines, by contrast, are designed to conduct electricity from point A to point B, just as toasters are designed to make toast. The electromagnetic fields that these devices create in the process are unwanted side effects. Household wiring configurations and appliances can be redesigned to produce a weaker field, and some utilities and manufacturers have made such changes in response to consumer demand.

Not all these upgrades were equally successful. For example, in 1992, a leading manufacturer of electric blankets and heating pads announced that its new models had greatly reduced electromagnetic radiation, and urged all consumers to upgrade to these safer products. In 1993, the author bought one of the new "safe" heating pads, and used a standard gauss meter—of a type that was de rigueur in the environmental consulting industry at the time—to compare its magnetic flux density to that of an older pad of the same brand purchased about 10 years earlier. The EMF readings for the old and new heating pads were the same.

Many epidemiological studies have focused on possible health effects of EMF associated with power lines or various household products, but the results, although sometimes troubling, have been inconsistent or have suffered from design problems. For example, at least one large study showed that pregnant women who used electric blankets were more likely than others to have children who later developed leukemia or brain tumors. This problem, if real, is easily solved—pregnant women can stop using electric blankets. But is the connection real? Investigators in such studies must rely on subjects' memories, and the parents of sick children often feel guilty and try to remember what they did wrong. Determining exposure level is particularly complicated in the case of EMF exposure, because people move around during the day and throughout their lifetimes. Unlike cigarettes or dental fillings, which go with us, electromagnetic fields are often stationary and always invisible.

As of 2010, no one really knows how these weak magnetic fields could damage genetic material and cause cancer, although there is no shortage of possible explanations. One of the most promising is that EMF may not directly damage DNA, but instead interfere with the ongoing process of DNA repair in children with a specific gene mutation. In that case, EMF would not be harmful for everyone. Another explanation is that EMF may somehow produce free radicals that are capable of damaging DNA. A third suggestion is that the electric fields around power lines may attract aerosol pollutants, and that those aerosols, not the field itself, may explain any excess morbidity.

HISTORY

Like many a meme, the recasting of mankind's big friend electricity as the source of invisible danger began in the 1960s, although not everyone noticed at the time. In 1966, two Russian scientists reported that workers at a high-voltage power switchboard developed headaches, fatigue, loss of sex drive, and other symptoms that might indicate a neurological problem (or simply Cold War tensions). Western scientists sneered at first, but soon found similar problems related to nonionizing electromagnetic radiation (NIEMR) exposure at a Naval communications facility.

People have been suspicious of high-voltage power lines for a long time, as witness the decades-old "Taos Hum" phenomenon, in which people report a persistent humming sound and blame it on whatever they like least. UFO researchers have reported that alleged alien spacecraft appear to hover near power lines, either because the pilots need to recharge their batteries, or because arcing may produce flashes of light that look like UFOs. Nearly everyone has walked under a high-voltage line and heard or felt something strange. When preliminary reports indicated that power lines might be making children sick, these pent-up fears seemed to explode.

As noted earlier, the public phase of this health scare started in 1979 with a specific publication and intensified in 1989 with three more. In an early draft of a 1990 report, some Environmental Protection Agency (EPA) scientists even recommended classifying EMF as a Class B carcinogen, but this recommendation was deleted from the final draft amid charges of conspiracy. In fact, the agency had to proceed with caution, because the legal implications would have been huge. In practical terms, how could human civilization continue in its present form without the grid?

For the next 10 years, public and scientific opinion oscillated. Although the main issue was (and is) proximity to high-voltage power lines as a possible risk factor for childhood leukemia, the controversy soon expanded to include the possible role of household wiring configurations and appliances in several forms of cancer, plus Alzheimer's disease, autism, infertility, and fibromyalgia—and, of course, a host of general complaints including headaches, fatigue, stress, high blood pressure, and insomnia. Such competing claims may have confused the issue and made it harder for legitimate researchers to take it seriously.

CONSEQUENCES

Starting in about 1990, the EMF controversy created a demand for environmental consultants who could measure exposures in homes, schools, and offices and make educated guesses about the level of risk. Any college graduate with a science major could complete a self-administered training course, buy a small gauss meter, and hang out a shingle. Consumer demand for this service has declined over the last two decades, thanks to competing issues, such as radon and toxic mold.

EMF protection products also enjoyed their heyday, although most of these products could not possibly work. The same copper bracelets and pendants that vendors had long advertised as sure-fire cures for arthritis or demonic possession were suddenly marketed for their alleged ability to redirect magnetic fields away from the head or solar plexus or something. A few people even lined their homes or bedrooms with protective copper mesh cages.

The EMF issue was alive and well in 2010, when public utilities in California announced the installation of "smart" residential electric meters, only to encounter resistance from customers who believed the meters might pose a health risk. That same year, at least one Web site advertised silver-lined belly shields to protect pregnant women and their fetuses from the alleged effects of electromagnetic radiation.

Thanks to the power of the dark side, the EMF health scare also created the matching phenomenon of "magnetic field deficiency syndrome," which meant not having *enough* EMF exposure, or the wrong kind, or from the wrong sources. The Earth itself generates a powerful magnetic field, within which all life evolved, but apparently that field is not good enough for everyone. Again, magnetic bracelets and pendants and meditation crystals came to the rescue. The magnet therapy industry alone now reports worldwide sales in excess of $1 billion per year, depending on the source and the definition of magnet therapy. That billion does not include legitimate (mostly experimental) medical uses of magnets and EMF, such as treatment of bone fractures and tendonitis.

WHAT WENT WRONG?

A wonderful 1954 book entitled *How to Lie with Statistics* (still in print) explains many of the techniques that some EMF investigators would later adopt, whether intentionally or not. One 1989 EMF article, for example, claims that a certain office had seven pregnant women all working at video display terminals, and four of them had children with birth defects. Four out of seven—my God, that's 57 percent! But the problem with this reasoning is that it ignores all the offices where pregnant women who used computer screens or other EMF sources had perfectly normal babies. Also, the example lumps together all birth defects, including those that could not be linked to EMF exposure. Some birth defects are hereditary, and others may result from unrelated exposures, such as certain viruses and drugs.

Another problem is the precautionary principle. Any scientist or layperson who thinks EMF (or anything else) might be harming children is morally obligated to report his or her findings, but all too often, the general public and the news media interpret preliminary findings as absolute. Eventually, most people got tired of this issue and moved on to the next, but the EMF puzzle is far from solved.

REFERENCES AND RECOMMENDED READING

Baker, D. "PG&E Considers SmartMeter Compromise." *San Francisco Chronicle*, 20 November 2010.

Bernard, N., et al. "Assessing the Potential Leukemogenic Effects of 50 Hz Magnetic Fields and their Harmonics Using an Animal Leukemia Model." *Journal of Radiation Research*, Vol. 49, 2008, pp. 565–577.

Brain, J. D., et al. "Childhood Leukemia: Electric and Magnetic Fields as Possible Risk Factors." *Environmental Health Perspectives*, Vol. 111, 2003, pp. 962–970.

Brodeur, P. The Hazards of Electromagnetic Fields. I—Power Lines. *New Yorker*, 12 June 1989.

Brodeur, P. The Hazards of Electromagnetic Fields. II—Something is Happening. *New Yorker*, 19 June 1989.

Brodeur, P. The Hazards of Electromagnetic Fields. III—Video Display Terminals. *New Yorker*, 26 June 1989.

Campion, E. W. "Power Lines, Cancer, and Fear." *New England Journal of Medicine*, Vol. 337, 1997, pp. 44–46.

Draper, G. "Childhood Cancer in Relation to Distance from High Voltage Power Lines in England and Wales: A Case-Control Study." *British Medical Journal*, 4 June 2005.

Feychting, M., et al. "EMF and Health." *Annual Review of Public Health*, Volume 26, 2005, pp. 165–189.

Field, K. "I Think I Feel an EMF Headache Coming On." *Design News*, 1 December 2009.

Jackson, J. D. "Are the Stray 60-Hz Electromagnetic Fields Associated with the Distribution and Use of Electric Power a Significant Cause of Cancer?" *Proceedings of the National Academy of Sciences U.S.A.*, Vol. 89, 1992, pp. 3508–3510.

Kay, J. "Transmission Lines, Appliances Dangerous to your Health?" *San Francisco Examiner*, 9 December 1987.

London, S. J., et al. "Exposure to Residential Electric and Magnetic Fields and Risk of Childhood Leukemia." *American Journal of Epidemiology*, Vol. 134, 1991, pp. 923–937.

Macklis, R. M. "Magnetic Healing, Quackery, and the Debate about the Health Effects of Electromagnetic Fields." *Annals of Internal Medicine*, Vol. 118, 1993, pp. 376–383.

Myers, A., et al. "Childhood Cancer and Overhead Powerlines: A Case-Control Study." *British Journal of Cancer*, Vol. 62, 1990, pp. 1008–1014.

Schüz, J., et al. "Nighttime Exposure to Electromagnetic Fields and Childhood Leukemia: An Extended Pooled Analysis." *American Journal of Epidemiology*, Vol. 166, 2007, pp. 263–269.

Sharick, C. "Do Belly Blankets Protect Baby from Radiation?" *Time*, 3 September 2010.

U.S. Environmental Protection Agency. "Evaluation of the Potential Carcinogenicity of Electromagnetic Fields." EPA/600/6-90/005B (External Review Draft), October 1990.

Verkasalo, P. K., et al. "Risk of Cancer in Finnish Children Living Close to Power Lines." *British Medical Journal*, Vol. 307, 1993, pp. 895–899.

Vince, G. "Large Study Links Power Lines to Childhood Cancer." *New Scientist*, 3 June 2005.

Wertheimer, N., and E. Leeper. "Electrical Wiring Configurations and Childhood Cancer." *American Journal of Epidemiology*, Vol. 19, 1979, pp. 273–284.

Woolston, C. "On Different Wavelengths over EMFs." *Los Angeles Times*, 15 February 2010.

World Health Organization. "Electromagnetic Fields and Public Health Cautionary Policies." WHO Backgrounder, March 2000.

43

Fear of Radon

Radon is an odd pollutant. None of us is responsible for it and all of us are exposed to it.
—Dr. Anthony V. Nero, Jr. (1986)

SUMMARY

A radioactive gas called radon (the chemical element Rn) occurs naturally in soil, rocks, and groundwater. Inhalation of radon at sufficiently high levels can increase the risk of lung cancer, and about 10 percent of all lung cancers may result from radon exposure. This gas can reach harmful levels in confined spaces, such as mine tunnels and poorly ventilated basements and attics of well-insulated modern houses. Older, more porous structures allow more radon to escape into the atmosphere. Some granite countertops, clay bricks, and even cat litter can emit radon, but it usually reaches high indoor levels only in areas where soil has a high uranium content. Most houses can be retrofitted to reduce exposure. Fear of radon qualifies as a health scare only to the extent that people have capitalized on it by discouraging new construction or by selling dubious products and services, such as "radon spas" that are said to cure a great variety of ailments. This health scare has largely fizzled in the media in recent years, but radon remains a source of legitimate concern, despite some exaggerated early reports.

SOURCE

Unlike some health scares in this book, radon is not a modern invention or an industrial byproduct, but a naturally occurring gas that is older than the Earth. Chemists discovered radon in 1900, but the general public gave it little thought until the 1920s, when doctors started using radon treatment for some forms of cancer, just as more modern forms of radiotherapy are used today. By the 1950s, doctors had determined that radon gas was responsible for the high rate of lung cancer in uranium miners. The first hint of a health scare began in 1976, when Swedish researchers found high radon levels in some houses.

The journal *Nature* reported the Swedish radon problem in 1979, the same year when the poster child for all manmade disasters—the nuclear accident at Three Mile Island (Chapter 36)—brought the unrelated issue of radon into the national spotlight.

In the aftermath of that accident, researchers began monitoring nearby homes for radiation, and southern Pennsylvania just happens to be a region with fairly high radon levels because of the type of soil. By the mid-1980s, it became apparent that many American houses had a radon problem, particularly in the Northeast and Midwest. Radon was suddenly big news, and the U.S. Environmental Protection Agency (EPA) recommended testing of every American house. Since an estimated 1 in 15 homes (about 7%) have elevated radon levels, this goal proved impractical. In 2005, the EPA modified its recommendation to focus on geographic areas with the highest risk.

This health scare took an unexpected turn in 1995, when a trade journal reported that some granite countertops—a minor fad at the time—emitted radon at levels that were marginally unsafe by EPA standards. This finding drew yelps from the granite industry, which saw it as a ploy by the competing formica industry and manufacturers of radon detectors. The problem finally came to a head in 2008, by which time many people who had installed granite countertops in their kitchens reportedly ripped them out again. A study by the Marble Institute of America largely exonerated granite, and there was a brief media feeding frenzy before the issue faded to its normal background level.

SCIENCE

When a uranium or thorium atom in a grain of mineral soil undergoes radioactive decay, it releases an alpha particle (two neutrons and two protons) from its nucleus and gives rise to radium. When the radium atom decays, it releases another alpha particle and produces radon gas. The location of the radon atom determines what happens next. If it is deep inside the mineral grain, it stays there and causes no harm. Otherwise, it may move into the pore space between the grains of soil or fractures in the rocks, and from there into the atmosphere, or the basement of any overlying house.

Radon has a half-life of only a few days, after which it decays to a sequence of short-lived isotopes ("radon daughters") and finally to lead, releasing three more alpha particles and other forms of radiation in the process. If those steps take place in the lining of someone's lung, DNA damage and cancer may result. As usual, the potential for harm depends on dose. Radon causes about 10 percent of all lung cancers and is the second most frequent cause of that disease, after cigarette smoke.

Not all indoor radon comes from the soil under the house. Minor sources include granite countertops (see Source), common building materials such as concrete blocks, cat litter made from bentonite clay, and even rock collections that contain radioactive minerals. Critics object that we are bombarded with radiation from multiple sources every day, and that the small increase attributable to radon makes no difference. Even fruits and vegetables that contain potassium can emit some measurable radiation.

However, the relationship between radiation exposure and cancer appears to be complex, and it is probably best to avoid needless radon exposure. Examples of bad ideas might include living in the basements of houses in high-radon areas, installing granite countertops without first having the material tested, and allowing children to keep radioactive mineral collections in their bedrooms. The radon level in cat litter apparently is insignificant, but pregnant women should avoid handling this material for other reasons, including the risk of an infectious disease called toxoplasmosis.

As of 2010, a joint Web site of the Lawrence Berkeley National Laboratory and Columbia University has an interactive online map that enables consumers to make a preliminary assessment of their radon risk, and provides instructions for testing and remediation if needed: www.stat.columbia.edu/~radon.

HISTORY

Although the actual discovery and description of radon had to await the invention of modern chemistry, people have recognized its effects since at least 1530, when the Swiss alchemist and physician Philippus Aureolus Paracelsus (1493–1541) and others described a lung disease that affected miners who spent long periods of time working underground. At that time, doctors had no idea what caused the disease, only that ventilation of mine shafts helped prevent it.

If one person deserves credit for the discovery of high radon levels in some American homes, it is probably Stanley J. Watras, a former construction engineer at the Limerick Nuclear Power Plant in eastern Pennsylvania, about 60 miles from Three Mile Island. When Mr. Watras arrived at work one day in 1984 and unexpectedly set off the radiation alarms, other employees searched his home in nearby Boyertown and found radon leaking into the cellar. It seems ironic that a man who worked in a nuclear power plant was safe at work, but exposed to dangerous radiation in his own home.

Radioactivity is often measured in units called picocuries (pCi), and the highest indoor radon level that the EPA considers reasonably safe or acceptable for human occupancy is 4 pCi per liter of air (pCi/L). By contrast, the Watras house contained about 4,400 pCi/L in the cellar, 3,200 pCi/L in the living room, and 1,800 pCi/L in the bedroom. The family reportedly moved out for several months while exhaust fans and other remediation measures were installed.

CONSEQUENCES

Like many health scares, this one was good for toxic tort attorneys and entrepreneurs, legitimate and otherwise. Radiation monitoring companies and building contractors profited from the sale of products and services that would enable consumers to determine if their homes contained harmful radon levels. In some parts of the United States, radon testing has become a routine part of most real estate transactions. Inexpensive radon test kits and guidelines are available from a number of Web sites.

The radon health scare apparently did not diminish the appeal of "radon spas," where people pay for the privilege of immersing themselves in water from underground springs with high radon content. This therapy is supposed to harness the life-giving and life-taking properties of ionizing radiation to cure arthritis and other diseases. It is unclear why these people do not simply buy houses in high-radon areas and live in the basement. The owners of such houses sometimes find it hard to sell them, and this solution would appear to help everyone.

Our favorite moment of the radon scare came when it temporarily merged with the brown recluse spider scare in the early 1990s. Suppose these spiders (Chapter 34) live in a cellar that also has a high level of radon. Will they become giant venomous radioactive mutants? We have found nothing in the literature to confirm this.

WHAT WENT WRONG?

After the discovery that radon caused lung cancer in uranium miners, why did it take nearly three decades for scientists to figure out that the same gas could also accumulate in houses and put the occupants at risk? For the same reason that it took so long to figure out that there was something wrong with cigarettes, asbestos insulation, and lead-based paint. The world is full of unanticipated problems, and it often takes a long time to find each one—and even longer to convince consumers. Many people do not want their homes tested for radon, because the results might reduce property values and wipe out their life savings. The demand for a former "radon house" may be limited, even after mitigation has brought the exposure level down to normal.

Some journalists in the mid-1980s noted that the EPA may have overreacted to this latest crisis, so that the public soon became tired of hearing about radon. Although it is one of the most serious health threats discussed in this book, radon is invisible and odorless, and thus easily dismissed as the latest media scare.

REFERENCES AND RECOMMENDED READING

Barnaby, W. "Very High Radiation Levels Found in Swedish Houses." *Nature*, Vol. 281, 1979, p. 6.
Berreby, D. "The Radon Raiders: Turning Perils into Profits." *New York Times*, 25 July 1987.
Copes, R., and J. Scott. "Radon Exposure: Can We Make a Difference?" *Canadian Medical Association Journal*, Vol. 179, 2007, pp. 1229–1231.
Cowley, G., and C. Kalb. "The Deadliest Cancer." *Newsweek*, 22 August 2005.
Dales, R., et al. "Quality of Indoor Residential Air and Health." *Canadian Medical Association Journal*, Vol. 179, 2008, pp. 147–152.
Darby, S., et al. "Radon: A Likely Carcinogen at All Concentrations." *Annals of Oncology*, Vol. 12, 2001, pp. 1341–1351.
Darby, S., et al. "Radon in Homes and Risk of Lung Cancer: Collaborative Analysis of Individual Data from 13 European Case-Control Studies." *British Medical Journal*, 21 December 2004.
Edelstein, M. R., and W. J. Makofske. 1998. *Radon's Deadly Daughters: Science, Environmental Policy, and the Politics of Risk*. Lanham, MD: Rowman and Littlefield.
Fairfield, H. "In a New Map, Radon Looks Less Likely for Many." *New York Times*, 11 January 2005.
Gray, A., et al. "Lung Cancer Deaths from Indoor Radon and the Cost Effectiveness and Potential of Policies to Reduce Them." *British Medical Journal*, 6 January 2009.
Murphy, J. "The Colorless, Odorless Killer." *Time*, 22 July 1985.
Murphy, K. "What's Lurking in Your Countertop?" *New York Times*, 24 July 2008.
Nero, A. V. "The Indoor Radon Story." *Technology Review*, January 1986.
Pavia, M., et al. "Meta-Analysis of Residential Exposure to Radon Gas and Lung Cancer." *Bulletin of the World Health Organization*, Vol. 81, 2003, pp. 732–738.
Puskin, J. S., and D. J. Pawel. "Attributable Lung Cancer Risk from Radon in Homes May Be Low." *British Medical Journal*, Vol. 330, 2005, p. 1151.
Radford, E. P. "Potential Health Effects of Indoor Radon Exposure." *Environmental Health Perspectives*, Vol. 62, 1985, pp. 281–287.

"Radon Revisited: The Early Warnings May have been Overblown, but Research Since has Shown that Lung Cancer Risk from the Gas is Real." *Harvard Health Letters*, Vol. 32, 2007, pp. 4–5.

Roach, M., and K. A. Weaver. "Indoor Radon—What Is to be Done?" *Western Medical Journal*, Vol. 156, 1992, p. 86.

Scheberle, D. "Radon and Asbestos: A Study of Agenda Setting and Causal Stories." *Policy Studies Journal*, Vol. 22, 1994, pp. 74–86.

U.K. Childhood Cancer Study Investigators. "The United Kingdom Childhood Cancer Study of Exposure to Domestic Sources of Ionising Radiation: 1. Radon Gas." *British Journal of Cancer*, Vol. 86, 2002, pp. 1721–1726.

U.S. Environmental Protection Agency. "A Citizen's Guide to Radon: The Guide to Protecting Yourself and your Family from Radon." EPA 402/K-09/001, January 2009.

"Uranium Miners' Cancer." *Time*, 26 December 1960.

Watts, G. "Radon Blues." *British Medical Journal*, Vol. 330, 2005, pp. 226–227.

Witschi, H. "A Short History of Lung Cancer." *Toxicological Sciences*, Vol. 64, 2001, pp. 4–6.

Zdrojewicz, Z., and J. J. Strzelczyk. "Radon Treatment Controversy." *Dose Response*, Vol. 4, 2006, pp. 106–118.

Part Seven

Actions and Reactions

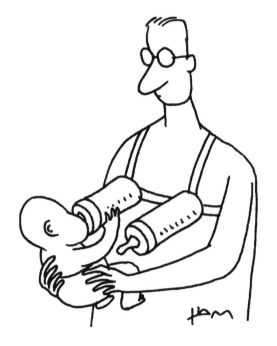

**Figure 7   Breastfeeding has clear
advantages, but there is little evidence that bottlefeeding does any
harm, and it enables the father to
participate.**
(*Source:* **Courtesy of CartoonStock
[artist, Ham Khan].**)

44

Fear of Bottle Feeding

Mothers should breastfeed their children two full years, provided they want to complete the nursing. The family head must support women and clothe them properly. Yet no person is charged with more than he can cope with. No mother should be made to suffer because of her child, nor family head because of his child.

—The Holy Qur'an, Al-Baqarah: 233 (Trans., T. B. Irving)

SUMMARY

Breastfeeding has real benefits for infants and their parents. Breast milk requires no preparation, few babies have allergic or other negative reactions to it, and it is clean and safe (unless the mother is sick, takes drugs, or eats a lot of fish). Although breast milk is deficient in some nutrients by modern dietary standards, vitamin and mineral drops are easily given as a supplement. Antibodies in breast milk also provide temporary protection against some intestinal infections. The majority of American women choose to breastfeed for at least a few months, and some religions even have formal doctrines on the subject. Unfortunately, some breastfeeding advocates have exaggerated its health benefits to the point of lunacy and have even harmed some infants (and mothers) in the process. Some women who are unable to breastfeed, whether for medical or economic reasons, may suffer from unwarranted fears about the effect on their child's development. Those who choose to breastfeed may be equally distressed when their babies grow more slowly than expected, based on growth charts compiled in an era when most infants were raised on formula. Although the fear of bottle-feeding has not entirely fizzled, as of 2010 there are hopeful signs that breast hysteria might be on the wane at last.

SOURCE

Before the invention of the first infant formulas and baby bottles in the mid-nineteenth century, breastfeeding was not a matter of choice. If the mother died, and a wet nurse was not available, the baby also died. With formula, the father or other family members could feed the baby if necessary (Figure 7). Like many medical inventions—such as vaccines and antibiotics—formula feeding saved many lives, and people regarded it as a modern miracle until the original problem faded from memory. By 1972, only about 22 percent of American mothers chose to breastfeed their babies.

Then, in the mid-1970s, things turned around and more women began to breastfeed. At first, this trend resulted mainly from the advice of pediatricians and other healthcare professionals, who in turn were influenced by published studies of breast milk and by the efforts of organizations such as La Leche League. The associated health scare appeared toward the end of that decade, as breastfeeding evolved from a lifestyle choice and nutritional benefit to a dogmatic belief system that extended into many aspects of family life. Upper-middle-class women in particular began to worry that their child would not get into Harvard unless they breastfed her exclusively for at least a year, or maybe six—and bombarded the hapless infant with visual stimuli and classical music and problem-solving toys, and taught her to read words on flash cards before she could sit up. By 1980, about 55 percent of newborns in the United States were breastfed.

SCIENCE

Infant formula is essentially cow or goat milk (or artificial soy milk) that has been diluted with water and sweetened with sugar to approximate the consistency and sweetness of human breast milk. Most infant formulas are also fortified with extra vitamins and minerals. Although there is no scientific evidence that breastfed babies are smarter, healthier, stronger, or in any way "better" than bottle-fed babies, breast milk does have a number of clear advantages that bear repeating:

- Unlike the contents of a bottle that might have sat too long in the sun or sink, breast milk is clean and safe. Exceptions occur when the mother has certain infections, or if she is taking drugs that might harm the baby. Also, women who eat large amounts of fish sometimes deliver potentially harmful amounts of methylmercury (Chapter 21) in their breast milk.
- Some babies are allergic to formula, but very few are allergic to human breast milk. (Contrary to rumor, this can happen, but it is highly unlikely.)
- Human breast milk contains antibodies that protect the baby from certain viruses and bacteria that would otherwise pass through the wall of the intestine. These antibodies cannot enter the infant's blood circulation, however, so they offer only limited protection.
- Some studies show that breastfed babies have reduced long-term risk for asthma, obesity, and some forms of childhood cancer. (Other studies show no such effect.)
- Breastfeeding also benefits the parents, by saving them some money and by making night feedings easier—unless, of course, they forget the baby is in the bed and roll over.

Although breastfeeding clearly has major advantages, nothing is perfect, and fairness requires us to list a few disadvantages as well:

- A 2001 study showed that prolonged breastfeeding is associated with reduced arterial function in adulthood. The reason is unknown.

- Exclusive breastfeeding with inadequate sunlight exposure can cause vitamin D deficiency and rickets. More sunlight or vitamin drops can easily prevent this problem.
- Breastfed infants may also develop deficiencies of iron and vitamins A and K. If the mother is a vegetarian, her milk may also be deficient in vitamin B_{12}. Again, vitamin drops are a simple remedy, unless the mother (or father) somehow interprets the requirement as a personal failing.
- For the first few months, breastfed babies often require feeding every two hours, around the clock. If the mother can afford to stay at home all day, and the father has ear muffs, this is fine. Otherwise, serious financial and interpersonal tensions may develop.

Breastfed babies grow more slowly on average and may end up shorter than bottle-fed babies, but we refuse to call that a "disadvantage." What is so great about being big? Still, there is a paradox here. If breastfeeding made babies grow faster, its advocates would cite that as a clear advantage. So why is the opposite finding not a disadvantage?

In summary, breastfeeding is an excellent choice if it meets the needs of all parties involved. Families should feel free to bottle-feed if prolonged breastfeeding interferes with the mother's role as breadwinner, or with the child's need for socialization or key nutrients. A combination of breast and bottle feeding (with frozen breast milk or formula) can actually make life easier for the baby, by avoiding the trauma of abrupt weaning.

HISTORY

Breastfeeding is not a recent phenomenon. The first mammals were doing it in one form or another when dinosaurs roamed the Earth, and all their descendants followed their example for millions of years—until humans discovered alternatives, such as dairy farming and soybean culture. At that point, breastfeeding became largely a matter of fashion and convenience. Humans no longer rely on Nature's gifts for other aspects of life; most of us grow (or buy) food instead of hunting and gathering, drive cars instead of walking, and use birth control for family planning purposes. Each of these choices has its opponents, and bottle-feeding is no exception.

As noted earlier, breastfeeding enjoyed a renaissance in the 1970s, and most people would agree that the net effect is positive. But this chapter is about health scares, and a trend usually does not produce a scare until somebody stands to benefit. In the case of breastfeeding, the motive for scaremongering appears to be largely ideological rather than financial. Some advocates may profit from the sale of products such as breast-feeding instruction manuals and DVDs, but for the most part, breastfeeding advocacy is more like a religion. Any woman of childbearing age who allows herself to be seen reading infant formula labels at a supermarket will sooner or later be the recipient of a hate stare, often accompanied by a stern lecture about infant bonding and brain development and a woman's role in the universe.

The fact that some female journalists have recently addressed this phenomenon with grace and humor (e.g., in the April 2009 *Atlantic Monthly*) suggests that this health scare may be on the verge of a well-deserved fizzle. Without the pressure of a health scare, more women may even choose to breastfeed, because many adults resent being bullied.

CONSEQUENCES

Several American doctors have actually proposed that all mothers should be *forced* to breastfeed for at least a year. This dystopian vision is too ugly to be a joke, so apparently they are serious. A few advocates insist on exclusive breastfeeding until the child is toilet trained, or even old enough to start school. More moderate voices have pointed out that mandatory prolonged breastfeeding would not only isolate and infantilize the children, but discourage their mothers from pursuing a career—or exercising other rights and responsibilities that most American adults take for granted, such as traveling, training for a marathon, or taking prescription drugs.

Worse, some medical authorities have claimed that a mother and child cannot bond properly unless the mother breastfeeds immediately after giving birth. Where does that leave adoptive mothers, and all fathers? Such claims are on a scientific par with the notion that a man and woman cannot form a pair bond unless the man brings her chocolates or sings outside her window. Regardless of anyone's belief or bias, there is simply no evidence that human relationships depend on the types of stereotypical behavior seen in birds and insects. Love alone will ordinarily suffice.

For a feeding strategy that is just as natural and traditional as breastfeeding, yet seldom utilized in Western cultures, see the sidebar ("Instant Baby Food").

Instant Baby Food

As soon a child is able to ingest solid food, Nature provides an often-overlooked supplemental feeding option that is just as natural as breastfeeding. In some rural communities today, as in most hunter-gatherer societies of the past and probably among early hominids as well, family members chew up ordinary food and spit it into their hands or directly into the child's mouth. This custom is known as half-eating or premastication, and a number of birds and mammals do the same thing. In a more advanced variant, the parent actually swallows the food (usually meat) and partially digests it, then regurgitates it and feeds it to the child.

Premastication is not only totally natural for mothers but also empowers fathers by enabling them to participate fully. The potential drawbacks are essentially the same as those for breastfeeding. Not everyone finds half-eating aesthetically agreeable, it is an awkward thing to do in public, the quid or vomit may be deficient in key nutrients—particularly if the parents live on junk food—and it may transmit disease. Feeding a child on vomit might also draw unfavorable attention from the authorities. But, as we said, nothing is perfect.

(Yes, we are pulling the reader's leg, but only to make an important point. Many behaviors can be natural, traditional, and healthful without necessarily being the best choice for every family.)

WHAT WENT WRONG?

The breastfeeding standoff appears to result from two powerful human drives: the need of parents to give their children the best possible start in life—which cannot always include breastfeeding—and the need of compulsive busybodies to force their personal belief systems on others.

This topic has much in common with the chapters on masturbation, alcohol, and so-called cleansing. The world is full of people who need to control the most intimate details of how others have sex, go to the bathroom, eat, sleep, wash, think, and feed their children. The resulting angry rhetoric about breastfeeding frequently disregards the fact that children need self-esteem and positive role models as much as they need milk. Children who are bottle-fed for any reason are *not* at a disadvantage, and they must not be made to feel that they are.

Another reason for the bottle-feeding scare may be the recent decline of science education. Advocates claim, for example, that breast milk—whether as a result of creation or evolution—must automatically contain everything a baby needs. We cannot speak for the Creator; but if the composition of breast milk is the product of human evolution, it should *not* be perfect baby food, but rather a compromise between the prehistoric survival needs of mother and infant. Early hominids must have encountered food shortages, and if breast milk were super-rich and jam-packed with vitamins and minerals, lactation would soon drain the mother's resources and she would die along with her infant. Thus, it should surprise no one that breast milk is deficient in some nutrients. Fortunately, the evolution of the human brain has also enabled us to manufacture supplements.

REFERENCES AND RECOMMENDED READING

Bhandari, N., et al. "Mainstreaming Nutrition into Maternal and Child Health Programmes: Scaling Up of Exclusive Breastfeeding." *Maternal and Child Nutrition*, Vol. 4, Suppl. 1, 2008, pp. 5–23.

"Breastmilk Can Save 1 Million Lives Yearly." United Press International, 5 August 2004.

Caspi, A., et al. "Moderation of Breastfeeding Effects on the IQ by Genetic Variation in Fatty Acid Metabolism." *Proceedings of the National Academy of Sciences*, Vol. 104, 2007, pp. 18860–18865.

Cattaneo, A. "Breastfeeding by Objectives." *European Journal of Public Health*, Vol. 11, 2001, pp. 397–401.

Cole, T. "Babies, Bottles, Breasts: Is the WHO Growth Standard Relevant?" *Significance*, Vol. 4, 2007, pp. 6–10.

Eckhardt, K. W., and G. E. Hendershot. "Analysis of the Reversal in Breast Feeding Trends in the Early 1970s." *Public Health Reports*, Vol. 99, 1984, pp. 410–415.

Gaur, A. H., et al. "Practice of Feeding Premasticated Food to Infants: A Potential Risk Factor for HIV Transmission." *Pediatrics*, Vol. 124, 2009, pp. 658–666.

Grandjean, P. "Breastfeeding and the Weanling's Dilemma." *American Journal of Public Health*, Vol. 94, 2004, p. 1075.

Grandjean, P., et al. "Human Milk as a Source of Methylmercury Exposure in Infants." *Environmental Health Perspectives*, Vol. 102, 1994, pp. 74–77.

Greer, F. R. "Are Breastfed Infants Vitamin K Deficient?" *Advances in Experimental Medicine and Biology*, Vol. 501, 2001, pp. 391–395.

Greer, F. R. "Do Breastfed Infants Need Supplemental Vitamins?" *Pediatric Clinics of North America*, Vol. 48, 2001, pp. 415–423.

Ip, S. et al. "Breastfeeding and Maternal and Infant Health Outcomes in Developed Countries." Agency for Healthcare Research and Quality, Evidence Report/Technology Assessment No. 153, April 2007.

Knaak, S. J. "The Problem with Breastfeeding Discourse." *Canadian Journal of Public Health*, Vol. 97, 2006, pp. 412–414.

Kovar, M. G., et al. "Review of the Epidemiologic Evidence for an Association between Infant Feeding and Infant Health." *Pediatrics*, Vol. 74, 1984, pp. 615–638.

Kramer, M. S., et al. "Health and Development Outcomes in 6.5-Year-Old Children Breastfed Exclusively for 3 or 6 Months." *American Journal of Clinical Nutrition*, Vol. 90, 2009, pp. 1070–1074.

Leeson, C. P. M., et al. "Duration of Breast Feeding and Arterial Distensibility in Early Adult Life: Population-Based Study." *British Medical Journal*, Vol. 322, 2001, pp. 643–647.

Macrae, F. "So is Breast Not Best?" *Daily Mail*, 21 July 2009.

Mead, M. N. "Contaminants in Human Milk: Weighing the Risks against the Benefits of Breast-feeding." *Environmental Health Perspectives*, Vol. 116, 2008, pp. A427–A434.

Mégraud, F. "Transmission of *Helicobacter pylori*: Faecal-Oral versus Oral-Oral Route." *Alimentary Pharmacology and Therapeutics*, Vol. 9 (Suppl. 2), 1995, pp. 85–91.

Merritt, D. "Mandatory Breastfeeding Questioned." *Birth Gazette*, Vol. 9, 1993, pp. 4–5.

"Question Formula-Feeding by AIDS Moms." *Science Online*, 23 July 2007.

Rabin, R. "Breast-Feed or Else." *New York Times*, 13 June 2006.

Raloff, J. "Pre-Chewed Baby Food Can Spread HIV." *ScienceNews*, 27 July 2009.

Roed, C., et al. "Severe Vitamin B_{12} Deficiency in Infants Breastfed by Vegans." *Ugeskrift for Laeger*, Vol. 171, 2009, pp. 3099–3101. [In Danish]

Rosin, H. "The Case Against Breastfeeding." *Atlantic Monthly*, April 2009.

Skenazy, L. "Mothering as a Spectator Sport." *Newsweek*, 7 May 2009.

Spiesel, S. "Tales from the Nursery." *Slate*, 27 March 2006.

U.K. Royal College of Paediatrics and Child Health. "The UK-WHO Growth Charts: What is the Difference?" Fact sheet, 2009.

Van de Perre, P. "Transfer of Antibody via Mother's Milk." *Vaccine*, Vol. 21, 2003, pp. 3374–3376.

Wright, C. M. "Growth Charts for Babies." *British Medical Journal*, Vol. 330, 2005, pp. 1399–1400.

45

Solitary Pursuits

Let's just do it until we need glasses.

—Extremely Old Joke

SUMMARY

During the eighteenth and nineteenth centuries, many people regarded masturbation as a dangerous practice for a variety of medical, social, and spiritual reasons. The Greek physician Hippocrates (460–375 B.C.) wrote that too much sex was harmful, but masturbation did not emerge as a unique health threat until the early 1700s, when some doctors and clergymen claimed that it caused problems ranging from fatigue, weakness, and a general loss of mental and visual acuity to murder, everlasting damnation, and several infectious diseases. In the nineteenth century, doctors took this idea and ran with it, devising elaborate theories that not only blamed masturbation for mental illness, epilepsy, blindness, and an ever-expanding list of diseases but also warned that its ultimate consequence would be the collapse of society. The Victorian ideal of a proper life was one of self-abnegation and service to others, and from that perspective, the only defensible use of sex was to make babies. Although these medical theories were discredited long ago—notably by the 1948 Kinsey Report—the associated health scare has not entirely fizzled in the modern age, as evidenced by the fact that we had trouble choosing a title for this chapter.

SOURCE

Starting in about 1726—after the publication of an apparently anonymous book called *Onania*—many medical authorities in England and elsewhere started blaming masturbation for blindness, mental illness, epilepsy, pimples, baldness, tuberculosis, and a host of other health problems. A second book with the now-familiar title *Onania*, this one published in France in 1758, expanded on the same theme.

Throughout history, men had undoubtedly noticed that a sudden feeling of lethargy often followed ejaculation and also heralded some diseases, such as influenza. Thus, it made at least a small amount of sense to conclude that any unnecessary sex (whatever that means) was bad for the body. In that era, doctors knew little about the real causes of disease, so instead of admitting defeat, they often resorted to blaming the patient's alleged moral shortcomings. (The same tendency survived well into the twentieth century, when some doctors blamed AIDS on a lifestyle they found morally unacceptable, rather than on a virus they had not yet discovered.)

Many authors have traced the self-service health scare to the Biblical story of Onan, who "spilled it on the ground," after which God killed him (Genesis 38:9–10). Eighteenth-century doctors apparently relied heavily on the Bible and tended to disregard empirical data. A more careful reading shows that Onan was not masturbating anyway, but simply practicing coitus interruptus to avoid getting his brother's widow pregnant. Nevertheless, the misinterpretation stuck, and it gave us the word "onanism" and the titles of those two influential eighteenth-century books.

Nor is this viewpoint uniquely Judeo-Christian, for an oft-quoted Muslim proverb states that "the one who weds his hand is accursed." By contrast, Taoists have maintained that masturbation is acceptable (although not recommended) for men, but potentially dangerous for women. Although this health scare has taken many forms over the centuries, the common denominator appears to be religious tradition, which has often found self-service inconsistent with the need to sustain a high pitch of spiritual fervor—to say nothing of the social imperative to be fruitful and multiply.

SCIENCE

Any habit can be dangerous if taken to extremes. In 2007, for example, doctors reported the case of a man who injured himself by sticking a telephone cable up his urethra. It is not clear what he was trying to accomplish, but if this was an example of masturbation, then yes—it can be harmful. The so-called "vacuum cleaner injury" is another fairly common emergency room scenario. People have even succeeded in electrocuting, dismembering, or hanging themselves, or crashing their cars into trees, while engaged in various autoerotic practices. Harm of a different sort may result when a person focuses on such behavior to the entire exclusion of relationships with other people. Given the limits of common sense, however, masturbation is certainly harmless.

Medical research has shown that this practice actually confers some physical benefits on subscribers. According to a 2003 Australian study, frequent ejaculation (by any method) between the ages of 20 and 50 appears to reduce the risk of later developing prostate cancer. Also, masturbation may serve to maintain a supply of fresh, high-quality sperm cells by periodically flushing the pipes, so to speak. In women, appropriately timed masturbation can help prevent a painful condition called endometriosis, in which a form of tissue that normally lines the uterus escapes through the fallopian tubes and starts growing in other parts of the body. And in people of either sex who are between relationships, alternative outlets may help control the urge to pick up strangers in bars, thus reducing the spread of infectious disease. The syphilis epidemic in Victorian England might have been less severe if men had felt free to spend less time with Venus and Mercury (see Chapter 21) and more with Narcissus.

HISTORY

In the course of researching this section, we found historical material that we would not write on a bathroom wall. Suffice it to say that the body of medical and philosophical opinion on the subject of masturbation is both large and strange.

Several medical authorities in the eighteenth and nineteenth centuries described the pitiful condition of mental patients who sat around all day masturbating. These observations raise several troubling questions. Did these patients have no privacy? Did they have anything else to do? They might have preferred video games, which had not been invented yet. And did many of these patients suffer from organic brain disease that might explain a lack of inhibition? Apparently it took at least a century for doctors to figure out that cause and effect were reversed in this case. The patients also did other things that doctors might just as well have blamed for their condition, such as banging their heads against walls and talking to themselves. But there were no books decrying these practices, probably because they were already unpopular.

The next time the reader eats a bowl of cereal, it might be well to ponder the life of its inventor—John Harvey Kellogg (1852–1943), a medical doctor who also invented peanut butter. In the late nineteenth century, by which time doctors should have known better, Kellogg devised a number of masturbation "cures" that were so sadistic and disturbing that they are not fit for print. He even discouraged sexual relations between husband and wife. Unsurprisingly, Kellogg and his wife had no children of their own, although they raised about 40 children that other people somehow produced.

Many people in that era apparently regarded masturbation—like suicide and refusal of military service—as a supreme act of abandonment of one's responsibility to others. Career women with no children, hermits who lived in caves, and scientists who worked alone in shuttered laboratories were also suspect. If they were not doing what everybody else did, they were potentially dangerous. One influential nineteenth-century doctor actually wrote that it was a healthy sign for boys to masturbate together in groups, rather than doing it alone. School administrators nowadays would probably scratch their heads at that conclusion.

The theory that masturbation causes insanity eventually disappeared, for three main reasons. First, doctors finally figured out that such behavior in hospitalized patients was more likely a symptom than a cause. Second, once doctors started actually listening to their patients instead of reading the Bible, it soon became apparent that most healthy people did it. Most of the doctors themselves probably did it too. Third, doctors could find no cause-and-effect relationship between masturbation and mental illness.

In 1948, Dr. Alfred Kinsey's landmark study *Sexual Behavior in the Human Male* revealed that 92 percent of men admitted masturbating. Like most studies, the Kinsey Report suffered from sampling bias and other problems, but it was highly influential. Thus, the stage was set for the "Me Generation," whose members focused on personal fulfillment rather than on the good of society, while hoping the two would coincide. Instead of "For king, for country," the mantra became "If it feels good, do it."

CONSEQUENCES

No health scare ever really dies. In 1991, police arrested comedian Pee-Wee Herman for allegedly masturbating in an adult theater. In 1994, President Clinton fired Surgeon General Joycelyn Elders for recommending that masturbation should be part of the curriculum in sex education classes. New urban legends have replaced old ones; adolescents now tell one another that masturbation can cause hair to grow on the palms of the hands, certainly a better fate than blindness or insanity.

But at least it is now possible to poke fun at such attitudes without risking excommunication or worse. The 1964 motion picture *Dr. Strangelove* featured an insane Army officer who believed that "loss of essence" through ejaculation was a Communist plot. The 1980 movie *The Blue Lagoon* even included a scene that depicted masturbation as a normal outlet and a charming phase of adolescence.

It might seem that life is already hard enough without worrying about harmless, private matters such as masturbation. We considered including a table of contemporary slang terms and euphemisms for this common practice, to show how much anxiety it inspires to the present day. Less controversial activities, such as walking or breathing, do not seem to require colorful metaphors. Suffice it to say that the table would have included a couple of hundred entries, in the English language alone.

WHAT WENT WRONG?

How could doctors blame so many evils on masturbation? Who stood to benefit from this particular health scare? It might be a copout to blame an entity as vague as the established social order; but political and religious leaders have understood for centuries that redirecting the sexual drive can generate a powerful force for good or evil, or more often for both. In his landmark 1949 novel *1984*, George Orwell gave us the nightmare of a future totalitarian regime that discouraged eroticism in any form:

> There was a direct intimate connexion between chastity and political orthodoxy. For how could the fear, the hatred, and the lunatic credulity which the Party needed in its members be kept at the right pitch, except by bottling down some powerful instinct and using it as a driving force?[1]

NOTE

1. George Orwell, *1984* (Signet Classics, New York, 1977).

REFERENCES AND RECOMMENDED READING

Baker, R. R., and M. A. Bellis. "Human Sperm Competition: Ejaculate Adjustment by Males and the Function of Masturbation." *Animal Behaviour*, Vol. 46, 1993, pp. 861–885.
"Big Whack Attack." *Men's Health*, December 2004.

Braun, S. " 'The Main Cause of His Insanity . . . Self-Pollution.' Attributions to Illness and the Treatment of Insanity in the Siegburg Asylum (1825–1878). The Case of Georg v. G." *Würzburger Medizinhistorische Mitteilungen*, Vol. 25, 2006, pp. 43–61. [German]

"Circle of Jerks." *The Nation*, 2 January 1995.

Darby, R. J. L. "The Masturbation Taboo and the Rise of Routine Male Circumcision: A Review of the Historiography." *Journal of Social History*, Vol. 36, 2003, pp. 737–757.

Esquirol, E. 1838. *Des Maladies Mentales Considérées sous les Rapports Médical, Hygiénique et Médico-Légal*. Paris: J.-B. Bailliere.

Fox, M., and E. L. Barrett. "Vacuum Cleaner Injury of the Penis." *British Medical Journal*, 25 June 1960.

Gilbert, A. N. "Masturbation and Insanity: Henry Maudsley and the Ideology of Sexual Repression." *Albion*, Vol. 12, 1980, pp. 268–282.

"Good for You: Sexual Strategies." *The Economist*, 27 March 1993.

Grumman, R. "How Orgasm Protects Your Health." *Cosmopolitan*, November 2002.

Hall, L. A. "Forbidden by God, Despised by Men: Masturbation, Medical Warnings, Moral Panic, and Manhood in Great Britain, 1850–1950." *Journal of the History of Sexuality*, Vol. 2, 1992, pp. 365–387.

Hare, E. H. "Masturbatory Insanity: The History of an Idea." *Journal of Mental Science*, Vol. 108, 1962, pp. 1–25.

Kellogg, J. H. 1888. *Plain Facts for the Old and Young: Embracing the Natural History and Hygiene of Organic Life*. Burlington, IA: Segner.

Laqueur, T. W. 2003. *Solitary Sex: A Cultural History of Masturbation*. New York: Zone Books.

Nau, J. Y. "Physicians For and Against Masturbation." *Revue Médicale Suisse*, Vol. 5, 2009, p. 1155. [French]

Neuman, R. P. "Masturbation, Madness, and the Modern Concepts of Childhood and Adolescence." *Journal of Social History*, Vol. 8, 1975, pp. 1–27.

Patton, M. S. "Twentieth-Century Attitudes toward Masturbation." *Journal of Religion and Health*, Vol. 25, 1986, pp. 291–302.

Popkin, J. "A Case of Too Much Candor." *U.S. News and World Report*, 19 December 1994.

Rössner, S. "John Harvey Kellogg (1852–1943): 'Masturbation Results in General Debility, Unnatural Pale Eyes and Forehead Acne.' " *Obesity Reviews*, Vol. 7, 2006, pp. 227–228.

Slater, L. "Medical Antiques—The Practice of Phisick." *Medical Ethics*, 19 September 2008.

Spitz, R. A. "Authority and Masturbation: Some Remarks on a Bibliographical Investigation." *Yearbook of Psychoanalysis*, Vol. 9, 1953, pp. 113–145.

Stengers, J., and A. Van Neck. 2001. *Masturbation: The History of a Great Terror*. New York: Palgrave.

"Strong-Arm Tactics." *Men's Health*, October 2003.

Studd, J. "A Comparison of 19th Century and Current Attitudes to Female Sexuality." *Gynecology and Endocrinology*, Vol. 23, 2007, pp. 673–681.

Studd, J., and A. Schwenkhagen. "The Historical Response to Female Sexuality." *Maturitas*, Vol. 63, 2009, pp. 107–111.

Trehan, R. K., et al. "Successful Removal of a Telephone Cable, a Foreign Body Through the Urethra into the Bladder: A Case Report." *Journal of Medical Case Reports*, Vol. 1, 2007, p. 153.

46

Fear of Autointoxication

Purge me with hyssop, and I shall be clean: wash me, and I shall be whiter than snow.
—King James Bible, Psalms 51:7

SUMMARY

The belief that the human body is inherently unclean forms the basis of many alternative health practices and religious purification rituals. This chapter focuses on the centuries-old fear of material that normally passes through the alimentary canal on its own schedule. A multibillion dollar industry serves the consumer's perceived need to hasten the process and remove the fearful residue before it has time to produce so-called autointoxication ("self-poisoning"). Colonic hydrotherapy has no known physical benefits, and it has caused injuries such as perforations and abscesses. The related practice of laxative abuse can cause irritable bowel syndrome, pancreatitis, and even kidney failure. Similar fears focus on contaminants that normally pass out of the body through the skin and urine. Sweat lodges and saunas are intended to remove toxins by increasing perspiration; herbal products that allegedly cleanse the blood are also popular, although healthy kidneys do the same job for free. Finally, "foot detox pads" allegedly draw poisons out of the body through the soles of the feet. Urban legends capitalize on the apparently universal fear of being dirty. This health scare already fizzled once, in about 1920, and it is high time for it to fizzle again.

SOURCE

The roots of this health scare are lost in time, but it may have resulted from the observation that profuse or abnormal-looking body secretions, such as diarrhea, often accompany disease. Modern doctors realize that the disease causes the diarrhea and not vice versa, but maybe it took a while to figure this out. Also, sewage contamination of drinking water has long been associated with deadly epidemics; but in the days before the germ theory of disease, it may have appeared that the sewage itself was responsible, rather than the bacteria and viruses it often contained. Or perhaps the fear of soiling oneself is simply left over from a traumatic period of early childhood.

Modern advertisements bombard consumers with the message that man in his natural state is covered with vile secretions and filled with assorted poisons, some of them homegrown and others derived from environmental or dietary sources. Many of these ads falsely state that 90 percent of all diseases result from improperly cleansed bowels. Some colonic hydrotherapy establishments go so far as to claim that anyone whose stool smells bad is in serious trouble and needs immediate cleansing. (That would appear to include everybody.)

SCIENCE

The alternative healthcare practices discussed in this chapter are usually harmless, and they apparently make some people feel better. But feeling better or worse is a subjective matter, and our job is to present the science, if any.

1. *Colonic Hydrotherapy.* The human gastrointestinal tract normally contains food in various stages of digestion. The colon's job is to absorb some water, salts, and vitamins from feces and resident bacteria before ejecting the residue. In general, it's a fine idea to leave the GI tract alone and let it do its thing, except in unusual circumstances that require medical intervention. Overly aggressive colonic irrigation can interfere with the normal intestinal flora required for good digestion, thus creating the very problem that it seeks to cure. Other adverse outcomes may include perforation of the colon and transmission of infectious diseases such as amebic dysentery.
2. *Laxative Abuse.* Like colonic hydrotherapy, this practice reflects either a feeling of uncleanliness or some perceived need to control exactly when and where bowel movements take place. People with eating disorders who abuse laxatives often report the urge to rid themselves of what they regard as poisonous, rotting filth. The overuse of laxatives can cause a number of well-documented problems, including irritable bowel syndrome, pancreatitis, kidney failure, and, of course, physical or psychological dependence on laxatives.
3. *Cleansing Diets.* The world's great religions have made use of ritual meals and fasting for thousands of years, but in such cases the intended benefits are spiritual, just as eating turkey on Thanksgiving makes a cultural statement. This discussion is limited to special diets that are supposed to have a *physical* cleansing effect on the body. For example, one fad diet in the 1970s required the person to avoid all solid food while drinking up to a gallon of fruit juice or herbal tea per day. All that liquid was supposed to purify the kidneys, and at the end of a week, people reported that their urine was really clean. Then there was the Zen macrobiotic diet, whose practitioners gradually stopped eating all solid food except brown rice. These diets have no known beneficial effects and can eventually lead to deficiency diseases. Some studies have shown that intermittent fasting may improve health, if only by reducing excess weight, but this has nothing to do with "cleansing" per se.
4. *Sweat Lodges and Saunas.* Entering a heated building or tent to induce sweating as a form of purification is an ancient tradition that has existed in Europe for thousands of years. The term "sweat lodge" usually refers to similar Native American traditions, either in their original form or as adopted and modified

by New Age enthusiasts. The ability of a sweat lodge, sauna, or steam room to induce spiritual cleansing is a matter of individual conscience, but doctors have refuted the more specific claim that sweating rids the body of toxins. The function of sweat is to cool the body, not to cleanse it.

5. *Detox Foot Pads.* This is a fairly new gimmick, or at least one that did not achieve global fame until about 2008. Advertisements claim that these products will draw poisons out of the body through the soles of the feet. Indeed, measurable traces of various metals and pesticides sometimes appear on the pad after use—but the source is simply dirt that the adhesive pad pulls off the surface of the skin. Also, the chemical solution on the pad is designed to react with moisture to produce brownish gunk that looks really toxic. This fad is unlikely to last long, and it is incredible that so many people fell for it.

HISTORY

Many ancient cultures went in for purifying ritual baths and the use of enemas and laxative potions. One source estimates that 70 percent of all the medicines described in medieval herbals were purgatives. When people got sick, the doctor immediately cleaned them out, and often bled them for good measure. Depending on the nature of the illness, these interventions often contributed to fatal dehydration.

Some authorities claim that people in ancient times cleansed themselves by standing in a river and inserting a hollow reed. Although we have never seen this in an ancient Egyptian mural, it seems entirely possible. Still, the occasional use of water to move things along is quite different from the compulsive practice of frequent cleansing using patent medicines, high-technology equipment, and the vigorous emptying of wallets. Alternative medical practitioners often claim that people in ancient times knew a lot more about medical science than we know today, but if this is true, it seems strange that life expectancy has increased over the years. An Egyptian medical text called the *Ebers Papyrus* (ca. 1550 B.C.) does, in fact, recommend enemas to cure various ailments—but it also states that tears, urine, and semen pass through the heart, which of course they do not.

John Harvey Kellogg (1852–1943), the same guy who invented corn flakes, peanut butter, and sadistic methods for preventing masturbation (Chapter 45), also recommended replacing the intestinal flora with yogurt administered by enema. It is indeed sobering to contemplate how often individual pathology has transformed human history. How could the fermented milk of a cow possibly be a more "natural" filler for the human colon than the stuff that was already in there?

The popularity of colonic hydrotherapy peaked in about 1900, then declined in 1920–1930 after a series of studies proved it was sheer nonsense. In 1936, the Council on Physical Therapy of the American Medical Association issued a press release that stated, in part:

Colonic irrigation is a method of treatment outrageously exploited not only by the out and out charlatan, but by the ignorant but nearly honest layman . . . These individuals exploit the public by playing on its belief in the great value of "elimination," of "removal of toxins," and of a "clean alimentary tract."[1]

Like some other alternative health practices, however, colonic cleansing has regained much of its lost popularity in recent years. It is hard to say if this trend is a result of declining science education standards, or possibly a reaction to the breakdown of the mainstream healthcare system. People who cannot afford medical treatment, or those who have lost confidence in doctors, may turn to less expensive options that sound appealing. Why this one sounds appealing is anyone's guess.

CONSEQUENCES

The pursuit of inner purity has directly injured a few people and distracted many others from dealing with more serious health issues. For example, colonic hydrotherapy practitioners offer a sure-fire cure for fatigue, headache, memory loss, depression, abdominal pain, lower-back pain, and a dozen other symptoms that might point to a catastrophic illness (or not). But by the time the person discovers that the colonic treatment is useless, it may be too late for other options.

Related urban legends include the often-repeated claim that the human large intestine contains somewhere between 30 and 80 pounds of undigested red meat. This is nonsense, but highly effective nonsense. For one thing, it's gross to think of all that meat in there, and any right-thinking person would want it out. For another, consider the example of a woman who has overindulged for years and now weighs 200 pounds. If this treatment can instantly relieve her of 80 pounds of excess weight, she can be back in her prom dress in no time. And if it fails to work as advertised, well—maybe it takes more than one session.

No health scare would be complete without some courtroom drama. In 2003, the Texas Attorney General filed several lawsuits against colonic hydrotherapy equipment manufacturers and providers after one patient died and four others had serious injuries. Two manufacturers and one clinic reportedly paid civil penalties in 2004, and agreed to work under a doctor's supervision and to stop making false advertising claims. One manufacturer agreed to go out of business. And in 2009, the Lakota Nation filed a lawsuit against a white man who allegedly desecrated a sacred sweat lodge ceremony and caused a woman's death.

If advertisements are any indicator, Americans even worry about the inner purity of their canine companions. In 2010, a dog food manufacturer offered a product that would give a dog "optimum stool quality."

WHAT WENT WRONG?

Maybe the problem is that we are the first species capable of thinking about what goes on inside our bodies. People seem highly susceptible to claims that they are dirty, or in some way socially unacceptable, and alternative practitioners have zeroed in on that vulnerability by identifying a need and offering to fill it—if the reader will pardon the expression.

NOTE

1. I. Galdston, "Colonic Irrigation" (New York Academy of Sciences, 5 March 1936).

REFERENCES AND RECOMMENDED READING

Acosta, R. D., and B. D. Cash. "Clinical Effects of Colonic Cleansing for General Health Promotion: A Systematic Review." *American Journal of Gastroenterology*, Vol. 104, 2009, pp. 2830–2836.

Baron, J. H., and A. Sonnenberg. "The Wax and Wane of Intestinal Autointoxication and Visceroptosis—Historical Trends of Real Versus Apparent New Digestive Diseases." *American Journal of Gastroenterology*, Vol. 97, 2002, pp. 2695–2699.

Beck, M. "Inner Beauty: A Healthy Colon." *Wall Street Journal*, 28 September 2009.

Benjamin, R., et al. "The Case Against Colonic Irrigation." *California Morbidity*, 27 September 1985.

Braden, A. "Colon Hydrotherapy: Will It Benefit You?" *Vibrant Life*, January–February 2007.

Challem, J. "Colonic Therapy: Hydro Irrigation that May Leave You Too Clean for your Own Good." *Natural Health*, December 1996.

Che, C. "Colon Cleansing: Healthful or Just a Load of @$%!" *Clinical Correlations*, 16 July 2009.

Chen, T. S., and P. S. Chen. "Intestinal Autointoxication: A Medical Leitmotif." *Journal of Clinical Gastroenterology*, Vol. 11, 1989, pp. 434–441.

Ernst, E. "Colonic Irrigation and the Theory of Autointoxication: A Triumph of Ignorance over Science." *Journal of Clinical Gastroenterology*, Vol. 24, 1997, pp. 196–198.

Handley, D. V., et al. "Rectal Perforation from Colonic Irrigation Administered by Alternative Practitioners." *Medical Journal of Australia*, Vol. 181, 2004, pp. 575–576.

Harkness, R. "'Detox' Products Debunked." *Prevention*, August 2009.

Kellogg, J. H. 1915. *Colon Hygiene*. Battle Creek, MI: Good Health Publishing Co.

Kellogg, J. H. 1922. *Autointoxication; or, Intestinal Toxemia*. Battle Creek, MI: The Modern Medicine Publishing Co.

Kuriyama, S. "The Forgotten Fear of Excrement." *Journal of Medieval and Early Modern Studies*, Vol. 38, 2008, pp. 413–442.

Laliberte, R. "Mr. Clean." *Men's Health*, April 1995.

Müller-Lissner, S. A., et al. "Myths and Misconceptions about Chronic Constipation." *American Journal of Gastroenterology*, Vol. 100, 2005, pp. 232–242.

Park, A. "Detox, Shmeetox. The Truth about Pollutant-Draining Foot Pads, Colonics and Other Supposedly Healthy Cleansers." *Time*, 16 February 2009.

Ratnaraja, N., and N. Raymond. "Extensive Abscesses Following Colonic Hydrotherapy." *Lancet Infectious Diseases*, Vol. 5, 2005, p. 527.

Schiller, L. R. "The Therapy of Constipation." *Alimentary Pharmacology and Therapeutics*, Vol. 15, 2001, pp. 749–763.

Schneider, K. "How Clean Should Your Colon Be?" American Council on Science and Health, 27 February 2003.

Smith, J. L. "Sir Arbuthnot Lane, Chronic Intestinal Stasis, and Autointoxication." *Annals of Internal Medicine*, Vol. 96, 1982, pp. 365–369.

Sullivan-Fowler, M. "Doubtful Theories, Drastic Therapies: Autointoxication and Faddism in the Late Nineteenth and Early Twentieth Centuries." *Journal of the History of Medicine and Allied Sciences*, Vol. 50, 1995, pp. 364–390.

Tan, M. P., and D. M. Cheong. "Life-Threatening Perineal Gangrene from Rectal Perforation following Colonic Hydrotherapy: A Case Report." *Annals of the Academy of Medicine Singapore*, Vol. 28, 1999, pp. 583–585.

Whorton, J. "Civilisation and the Colon: Constipation as the 'Disease of Diseases.'" *British Medical Journal*, Vol. 321, 2000, pp. 1586–1589.

47

Fear of Not Drinking

If all be true that I do think,
There are five reasons we should drink:
Good wine—a friend—or being dry—
Or lest we should be by and by—
Or any other reason why.

—Henry Aldrich (1647–1710), *Five Reasons for Drinking*

SUMMARY

In the late twentieth century, a number of medical authorities claimed that moderate consumption of alcoholic beverages had major health benefits, especially for people over age 40. Epidemiological studies seemed to support this position. Wine was supposed to help prevent heart disease and stroke, and at least one study showed that beer might reduce the risk of Alzheimer's disease. Some studies suggested that resveratrol, a chemical in red wine, could protect against cancer and other diseases; others pointed to alcohol itself as the miracle ingredient. Next, a few doctors and science journalists claimed that everybody should drink in moderation, and that abstaining from alcohol is actually risky. This belief was widely accepted for years (and had some of us nondrinkers worried), until researchers found methodological problems in some of the earlier studies. Also, religious groups that abstain from alcohol (and tobacco) tend to have *less* heart disease than the general population. Although moderate social drinking may have some health benefits, there is no evidence that people can increase their lifespans by taking up drinking in the absence of other lifestyle changes. The fear of not drinking has largely fizzled, although the quest for new reasons to drink will probably never end.

SOURCE

A large-scale study published in 1976 appeared to show a reduced risk of heart disease in drinkers, but most doctors assumed at first that the benefit resulted from something in the beverages other than alcohol. A 1984 study showed that heavy alcohol consumption appeared to reduce the risk of emphysema in smokers, probably by inhibiting inflammatory cells. Again, the investigators did not advise smokers to increase their alcohol intake; instead, they proposed further study to identify drugs with similar benefits, but without the harmful side effects of alcohol. Not until the early 1990s did the medical establishment begin to recommend therapeutic drinking.

Several studies of the so-called Mediterranean diet (vegetables, fish, and wine) quickly settled on wine as the protective factor. One of the most influential sources of this health scare—that is, the fear of not drinking—was a 1991 *60 Minutes* segment that presented wine as the answer to the "French paradox," the low rate of heart disease in France despite heavy smoking, sedentary lifestyles, and a high-fat diet. Wine advocacy gathered momentum through the 1990s, culminating in several papers that depicted alcohol as a near-miracle drug. And then the long downhill slide began, as investigators discovered problems in earlier studies, such as measurement error and confounding variables. In other words, people did not always respond accurately when asked how much they drank, and moderate wine drinking was associated with other characteristics (such as diet and social habits) that might better explain health outcomes.

SCIENCE

Alcohol supporters and detractors alike agree that *heavy* drinking is a bad idea. It severely damages the liver and other organs, causing diseases such as cirrhosis and liver cancer. Binge drinking can damage the brain and also appears to suppress the immune system. Alcohol abuse in general is a major factor in traffic fatalities and domestic violence. Therefore, this discussion will focus on light to moderate social drinking.

There are no universal definitions of these terms, but for most purposes, one "drink" means one can of beer, one glass of wine, one shot of straight liquor, or one mixed drink. Binge drinking refers to episodic heavy drinking, as when a college student abstains all week and then tosses back 10 or 12 beers on Saturday night. Social drinking is even harder to define, but usually refers to drinking at a shared meal or party, rather than (say) sitting alone in an alley with a bottle of vodka. A 1999 survey of physicians produced the following criteria:

- Light drinking: 1.2 drinks per day
- Moderate drinking: 2.2 drinks per day
- Heavy drinking: 3.5 drinks per day
- Abusive drinking: 5.4 drinks per day

Of course, the physicians in this survey were not recommending fractional drinks; the investigators averaged the results and rounded numbers to the nearest tenth.

Some studies have concluded that the benefits of wine result from a chemical called resveratrol, which is also present in grapes, peanuts, and various other foods. One 2006 report (published in a legitimate medical journal) claimed that resveratrol can prevent heart disease, cancer, Alzheimer's disease, type 2 diabetes, inflammation, and infection! A list this long is usually a red flag for a belief system, and not all doctors agreed with this conclusion. Several investigators have insisted that alcohol itself is the protective factor, and that resveratrol alone is ineffective.

To the extent that wine (or any of its components) reduces the risk of heart disease and ischemic stroke, it may do so by making blood platelets less sticky, and thus less likely to form clots. Another hypothesis is that the apparent health benefit of alcohol results from the presence of so-called confounding or lurking variables that the investigators did not consider. For example, some non-drinkers might abstain due to a preexisting health condition, and light social drinking might reflect a cheerful, relaxed personality that also is conducive to good health.

Several sources have pointed out the excellent cardiac health of Mormons and other religious groups that traditionally avoid both alcohol and tobacco. This observation alone does not prove that alcohol has no benefits, for it is generally accepted that smoking does more harm than drinking can repair. Smoking may double the risk of heart disease, whereas alcohol reduces that risk by less than half, even by the most optimistic estimates. But are people who drink, but do not smoke, healthier than those who do neither? And can a nonsmoking nondrinker improve any objective measure of cardiovascular health (such as HDL cholesterol) by taking up drinking, while holding other factors constant, such as diet and social interactions? We have found no studies to date that clearly answer these questions.

HISTORY

In about 2500 B.C., a wave of technologically advanced immigrants whom we now call the Beaker People, of mixed Spanish and African ancestry, brought the first alcoholic beverage to the British Isles. It was a fermented honey product called mead, and the locals no doubt welcomed their new friends with open arms. The Beaker People also introduced metalworking and sheep raising to a backward society, but no matter; we remember them for their drinking vessels. No trace of their health lore has survived, but alcohol probably made their lives easier or more enjoyable, rather than longer.

During the first half of the twentieth century, several countries banned the manufacture or sale of alcoholic beverages. The possible health benefits of alcohol had not yet been discovered, and the temperance movement was mainly a reaction to domestic violence and other negative effects of abusive drinking. Unfortunately, it is difficult to ban the abuse of a chemical without also banning its legitimate use, and prohibition in most countries was a short-lived experiment.

In 1999, only 66 years after the repeal of Prohibition, the U.S. government came as close as it has ever come to recommending the consumption of alcohol. The wine industry wanted product labels that listed specific health benefits of wine, but the Bureau of Alcohol, Tobacco and Firearms (now part of the Tax and Trade Bureau) stopped short of outright endorsement. Instead, the agency approved wine labels that advised consumers to consult a family doctor or the U.S. Department of Agriculture's *Dietary Guidelines for Americans* for information on the health effects of wine. And as of 2009, those guidelines state:

Alcohol may have beneficial effects when consumed in moderation. The lowest all-cause mortality occurs at an intake of one to two drinks per day. The lowest coronary heart disease mortality also occurs at an intake of one to two drinks per day.[1]

CONSEQUENCES

This health scare had its share of semi-humorous consequences, such as the spectacle of worried nondrinkers across America forcing themselves to swallow a bedtime glass of red wine. (People who like wine cannot imagine how bad it tastes to those who don't.) After the 1991 *60 Minutes* episode on the French paradox, red wine sales in the United States soared by 44 percent. In 2006, after publication of the latest studies touting red wine as the elixir of life, sales again increased by 40 percent. In each case, the increase was temporary; people who liked wine probably already drank it, and those who disliked it soon decided they would prefer a heart attack. There was also a short-lived rush on bottled grape juice in the late 1990s after publication of one of the resveratrol studies. A 2007 paper that associated beer with a reduced risk of Alzheimer's disease may have increased beer sales, but we don't remember.

A less favorable consequence of the fear of not drinking is that heavy or abusive drinkers—who often perceive themselves as moderate social drinkers—now have an excellent excuse not to quit. They must continue boozing to protect their health. This outcome is probably not what any of the pro-alcohol investigators had in mind. Also, since studies have shown that drinking may confer some protection on smokers, an unknown percentage of smokers may have chosen to increase their alcohol intake instead of giving up cigarettes.

Despite all the studies touting the benefits of wine and spirits, in 2009 about 36 percent of Americans still reported drinking no alcohol, either for religious reasons or as a matter of personal choice. Gallup polls show that the percentage of nondrinkers has fluctuated between 30 percent and 45 percent ever since the question was first asked in 1939. Drinking reached its maximum in the mid-1970s, before the wine controversy started, and has declined slightly since then.

WHAT WENT WRONG?

Alcohol, like gun control and breastfeeding, is an emotional topic that discourages rational debate. One camp blames alcohol for all society's ills, from car accidents to birth defects, whereas another firmly believes that moderate drinkers are healthier and better-adjusted than nondrinkers. The public may be more eager to embrace some research findings than others. Dark chocolate is another example of a consumer favorite that enjoyed a recent spike in demand (and price) after medical journals reported that it contains heart-healthy nutrients. Broccoli sales, by contrast, have been relatively flat despite the reported role of cruciferous vegetables in maintaining a healthy colon.

NOTE

1. USDA, *Dietary Guidelines for Americans*, 2005 Edition.

REFERENCES AND RECOMMENDED READING

Caldwell, T. M., et al. "Drinking Histories of Self-Identified Lifetime Abstainers and Occasional Drinkers: Findings from the 1958 British Birth Cohort Study." *Alcohol and Alcoholism*, Vol. 41, 2006, pp. 650–654.

Daley, J. "Overhyped Health Headlines Revealed." *Popular Science*, August 2009.

Díaz, L. E., et al. "Influence of Alcohol Consumption on Immunological Status: A Review." *European Journal of Clinical Medicine*, Vol. 56 (Suppl. 3), 2002, pp. S50–S53.

Djoussé, L., and J. M. Gaziano. "Alcohol Consumption and Heart Failure: A Systematic Review." *Current Atherosclerosis Reports*, Vol. 10, 2008, pp. 117–120.

Foley, D. "Healthy . . . or Harmful?" *Prevention*, October 2006.

Goldberg, I. J., et al. "Wine and Your Heart." *Circulation*, 23 January 2001, pp. 472–475.

Guardia Serecigni, J. "Is Alcohol Really Good for Health?" *Adicciones*, Vol. 20, 2008, pp. 221–235.

Kamholz, S. L. "Wine, Spirits and the Lung: Good, Bad or Indifferent?" *Transactions of the American Clinical and Climatological Association*, Vol. 117, 2006, pp. 129–145.

Klatsky, A. L. "Never, or Hardly Ever? It Could Make a Difference." *American Journal of Epidemiology*, Vol. 168, 2008, pp. 872–875.

Lieber, C. S. "Alcohol and Health: A Drink a Day Won't Keep the Doctor Away." *Cleveland Clinic Journal of Medicine*, Vol. 70, 2003, pp. 945–953 passim.

McVean, M. "Reports Spur Many Americans to Toast their Platelets." Associated Press, 11 March 1992.

Meister, K. 1999. *Moderate Alcohol Consumption and Health*. New York: American Council on Science and Health.

Mukamal, K. J., et al. "Beliefs, Motivations, and Opinions about Moderate Drinking: A Cross-Sectional Survey." *Family Medicine*, Vol. 40, 2008, pp. 188–195.

Nielsen Company. "Sales of Red Wine Surge on Reports of Health Benefits." Press release, 2 April 2007.

Opie, L. H., and S. Lecour. "The Red Wine Hypothesis: From Concepts to Protective Signalling Molecules." *European Heart Journal*, Vol. 28, 2007, pp. 1683–1693.

Pearl, R. 1926. *Alcohol and Longevity*. New York: Alfred A. Knopf.

Peña, A., et al. "Influence of Moderate Beer Consumption on Aluminium Toxico-Kinetics: Acute Study." *Nutrición Hospitalaria*, Vol. 22, 2007, pp. 371–376. [Spanish]

Popkin, B. M., et al. "A New Proposed Guidance System for Beverage Consumption in the United States. *American Journal of Clinical Nutrition*, Vol. 83, 2006, pp. 529–542.

Pratt, P. C. "The Beneficial Effect of Alcohol Consumption on the Prevalence and Extent of Centrilobular Emphysema." *Chest*, Vol. 85, 1984, pp. 372–377.

Saarni, S. I., et al. "Alcohol Consumption, Abstaining, Health Utility, and Quality of Life—A General Population Survey in Finland." *Alcohol and Alcoholism*, Vol. 43, 2008, pp. 376–386.

Turvey, C. L., et al. "Alcohol Use and Health Outcomes in the Oldest Old." *Substance Abuse Treatment, Prevention and Policy*, 29 March 2006.

Twis, L. J., and R. D. Twis. "One-per-Occasion or Less: Are Moderate-Drinking Postmenopausal Women Really Healthier than their Nondrinking and Heavier-Drinking Peers?" *Alcoholism, Clinical and Experimental Research*, Vol. 32, 2008, pp. 1670–1680.

Vidavalur, R., et al. "Significance of Wine and Resveratrol in Cardiovascular Disease: French Paradox Revisited." *Experimental and Clinical Cardiology*, Vol. 11, 2006, pp. 217–225.

Wannamethee, S. G. "Alcohol and Mortality: Diminishing Returns for Benefits of Alcohol." *International Journal of Epidemiology*, Vol. 34, 2005, pp. 205–206.

"Winemakers Bubble Over as Government Approves New Labels." Associated Press, 24 February 1999.

48

Fear of Involuntary Fatness

Your culture will adapt to service us. Resistance is futile.

—Borg saying

SUMMARY

An obesogen is a substance (or sometimes a behavior) that promotes weight gain by increasing fat storage. Despite overwhelming evidence that people become fat as a result of overeating, often combined with lack of exercise, researchers and the media have produced a steady stream of alternative explanations for weight gain. As a result, many people now believe that they cannot lose weight because some factor in their heredity, upbringing, economic circumstances, or environment forces them to overeat and become fat. The search for the perfect obesogen is very much alive, but this chapter examines five specific fat-related health scares that have largely fizzled as of 2010:

- Mental work makes you fat.
- Lack of fresh vegetables makes you fat.
- Diet soda makes you fat.
- Sleeping too much or too little makes you fat.
- Exposure to pesticides makes you fat.

SOURCE

The sources of these five obesity-related health scares are easy to pinpoint, because each one started with a specific publication or series of publications. Somebody did a study, and the news media picked it up and dramatized it. But what is the source of the more general modern obsession with the alleged futility and complexity of weight control? Who first convinced overweight people that they were helpless slaves of circumstance, incapable of simply eating less, and desperately in need of medical intervention?

Dangerous diet pills have been around for more than a century, but the effects of drugs are at least reversible in most cases. When and why did people begin to accept potentially dangerous gastric bypass and stomach-banding surgeries as the weight-loss treatments of choice, and when did medical insurance companies start picking up the tab? Without that desperate mindset, none of these health scares could have happened. The studies that generated them would simply not have been newsworthy.

The "resistance is futile" philosophy of weight control reared its head briefly in the 1950s, when doctors thought most overweight people suffered from an underactive thyroid gland. However, investigators soon figured out that low thyroid hormone levels were usually the result of obesity, rather than the cause. Treatment with beef thyroid extract was not only risky but ultimately ineffective, and the focus soon returned to diet and exercise, with the help of some rather silly fat-jiggling machines.

The U.S. government's 2000 preventive healthcare agenda entitled "Healthy People 2010," and its dismal outcome, may have put one of the final nails in the coffin of rational weight control. In 2000, about 23 percent of Americans were obese, and the goal was to reduce that group to 15 percent by the year 2010, through such familiar interventions as promoting healthy diet and exercise habits. Now 2010 is here, and an estimated 35 percent of Americans are obese. In other words, it didn't work.

SCIENCE

Humans and other animals derive energy from food and store excess energy in the form of several categories of body fat. The amount and distribution of fat vary from one person to another, but the percentage of fat is usually proportional to the body mass index (BMI), calculated as the weight in pounds, multiplied by 703, and divided by the squared height in inches. The following numbers apply to adults only:

- BMI < 18.5   Underweight
- BMI 18.5–24.9   Normal
- BMI 25.0–29.9   Overweight
- BMI 30.0–34.9   Obese
- BMI 35.0–39.9   Severely Obese
- BMI 40.0 or higher   Morbidly Obese

But what do these numbers mean? Do they reflect some sort of value judgment? Although obesity is a risk factor for type 2 diabetes, high blood pressure, heart disease, and certain cancers, obesity itself is not a disease, nor is every obese person automatically at risk. Some individuals can be overweight and healthy at the same time, and a growing social movement in this country seeks respect and the end of "fat jokes." For some people, enjoying food and being heavy are legitimate personal choices. For many others, however, the mere suggestion that obesity results from external factors beyond the individual's control may precipitate a health scare. We selected five examples for their illustrative value:

1. *Mental work makes you fat.* According to a 2008 study, female college students who sat at computers performing stressful mental work tended to eat more than others when offered a buffet. Blood tests further showed that the subjects' glucose and insulin levels fluctuated for unknown reasons. The study was based on exactly 14 people, and it proved nothing, except that stress gives some people the munchies. But the wire services loved it.

2. *Lack of fresh vegetables makes you fat.* Several investigators have proposed variations on this theme over the years to explain why low-income people tend to be overweight. The hypothesis is that they simply cannot afford these relatively expensive and healthful foods. In fact, frozen vegetables are cheap (and often contain more nutrients than fresh produce), and there is no evidence that adding vegetables to the diet causes weight loss, in the absence of other lifestyle changes.

3. *Diet soda makes you fat.* There appears to be a strong association between obesity and the habit of drinking diet soda, but drinking a zero-calorie beverage cannot directly cause weight gain. The soda might somehow increase appetite and food intake, or the association might simply mean that people who are already obese start drinking diet soda in an effort to lose weight.

4. *Sleeping too much (or too little) makes you fat.* This hypothesis makes some sense, because sleeping too much might decrease exercise, and sleeping too little might result in constant snacking to fight daytime fatigue. But even if people suffer from clinical depression or insomnia (both major medical industries in themselves), again the ultimate cause of obesity is excess food intake.

5. *Exposure to pesticides makes you fat.* Scientists have pointed out that increasing numbers of American children are becoming overweight before they are six months old. Since exercise and menu choices cannot be major factors for infants, exposure to environmental chemicals, such as the herbicide atrazine, could be partly responsible for increased fat storage. Breastfed babies (the majority at this age), unlike bottle-fed babies, not only choose the amount of milk they drink, but also ingest whatever contaminants the mother may have absorbed (Chapter 44). This scare is not quite over; but even if some pesticides promote early weight gain, adults (unlike babies) can learn to resist the demands of appetite.

HISTORY

Obesity was not a problem during most of human history. Those few people who found enough food to become overweight had to be doing something right, and being heavy was often a sign of prosperity and high social status. Some cultures that took prosperity for granted felt otherwise; classical Greek comedy often featured a fat clownlike character. It is doubtful that Victorian women really swallowed tapeworm eggs to lose weight, or had their lower ribs surgically removed to make their waists smaller, but they often starved themselves and wore impossibly tight corsets to accentuate their hourglass figures.

In the 1960s, the American ideal of womanhood took a dramatic turn when Marilyn Monroe passed the torch to Twiggy. Now women were expected to look like 12-year-old boys. Over the next few decades, the ideal woman once again sprouted modest curves. But real women (and men) come in all shapes and sizes, and a great deal of suffering resulted from the effort to conform to these successive images, as amphetamines and Fen-phen replaced tapeworm eggs and corsets.

To our knowledge, however, at no time in human history has it been fashionable for people to become so fat that they can barely move or care for themselves. The increasing prevalence of morbid obesity is a new development, and pesticides may indeed have something to do with it. Again, however, resistance is *not* futile. The success of weight loss surgery proves that reduced food intake results in weight loss, pesticides or no. Simply choosing what to swallow would achieve the same result without the risks of surgery.

In a 2010 CBS News opinion poll, 95 percent of Americans said obesity was a serious public health problem—and nearly 90 percent said diet and exercise alone could solve that problem, without the help of junk food taxes or other drastic measures.

CONSEQUENCES

The consequences of these five obesity-related health scares, and many others, may include a growing sense of futility on the part of overweight Americans. In every Gallup poll since 1990, a majority of respondents have expressed the desire to lose weight. According to a 2010 study, obesity in the United States is increasing so rapidly that related costs will account for at least 21 percent of all healthcare spending by 2020. The national obsession with weight control has also contributed to an epidemic of eating disorders, such as anorexia nervosa and bulimia.

Another dangerous trend is the overuse of potentially dangerous surgeries to limit food intake. Many doctors claim that this is the only effective way to lose a large amount of weight and keep it off, but others find the trend appalling. Once reserved as a last resort for the morbidly obese, bariatric surgery is now available to people who want to lose as little as 40 or 50 pounds. During 2008 alone, 220,000 Americans had such procedures, at an average cost of over $50,000 each. Nearly 20 percent of bariatric surgery patients later report major side effects, such as involuntary vomiting or defecation, and significant numbers also have heart attacks and strokes. There must be a better way.

WHAT WENT WRONG?

In a sense, nothing went wrong. Mankind has achieved the age-old dream of freedom from hunger, at least in part of the world. Food tastes good, and with a surplus constantly available, those people who assimilate energy most efficiently have the opportunity to do so. Pesticides, economic hardship, and other factors may have compounded the problem, but the ultimate source of obesity is excess food intake. If this were not so, gastric bypass and banding surgeries could not work. These surgeries do not remove pesticides from the environment, raise the patient from poverty, or rewrite genes. All they do is to reduce the amount of food a person swallows.

As for the periodic obesity-related health scares, they are an inevitable consequence of medical research. Investigators often release preliminary findings that have not been verified, either to justify continued funding or simply to encourage the exchange of ideas. If the finding translates into an appealing sound byte, the wire services pounce on it, accurately or otherwise. Health scares and fads related to the cause or cure of obesity are among the most likely to attract attention, because they affect so many consumers.

REFERENCES AND RECOMMENDED READING

Adámková, V., et al. "Association between Duration of the Sleep and Body Weight." *Physiological Research*, Vol. 58 (Suppl. 1), 2009, pp. S27–S31.

Babey, S. H., et al. "Bubbling Over: Soda Consumption and its Link to Obesity in California." *Policy Brief, UCLA Center for Health Policy Research*, September 2009, pp. 1–8.

Begley, S. "Born to be Big: Early Exposure to Common Chemicals May be Programming Kids to be Fat." *Newsweek*, 21 September 2009.

Bellisle, F., and A. Drewnowski. "Intense Sweeteners, Energy Intake and the Control of Body Weight." *European Journal of Clinical Nutrition*, Vol. 61, 2007, pp. 691–700.

Beydoun, M. A., et al. "The Association of Fast Food, Fruit and Vegetable Prices with Dietary Intakes among U.S. Adults: Is There Modification by Family Income?" *Social Science and Medicine*, Vol. 66, 2008, pp. 2218–2229.

Blake, J. "Researcher Links Food Prices, Obesity." *Seattle Times*, 18 June 2003.

Bursey, R. G. "Letter to Fowler et al., 2008. No Valid Association between Artificial Sweeteners and Weight Gain." *Obesity*, Vol. 17, 2009, p. 628.

Chaput, J.-P., and A. Tremblay. "Acute Effects of Knowledge-Based Work on Feeding Behavior and Energy Intake." *Physiology and Behavior*, Vol. 90, 2007, pp. 66–72.

Chaput, J.-P., et al. "Glycemic Instability and Spontaneous Energy Intake: Association with Knowledge-Based Work." *Psychosomatic Medicine*, Vol. 70, 2008, pp. 797–804.

Chaput, J.-P., et al. "Risk Factors for Adult Overweight and Obesity in the Quebec Family Study: Have We Been Barking Up the Wrong Tree?" *Obesity*, Vol. 17, 2009, pp. 1964–1970.

Christian, T., and I. Rashad. "Trends in U.S. Food Prices, 1950–2007," *Economics and Human Biology*, Vol. 7, 2009, pp. 113–120.

Fowler, S. P., et al. "Fueling the Obesity Epidemic? Artificially Sweetened Beverage Use and Long-Term Weight Gain." *Obesity*, Vol. 16, 2008, pp. 1894–1900.

Hanlon, P., and S. Carlisle. "Do We Face a Third Revolution in Human History? If So, How Will Public Health Respond?" *Journal of Public Health*, Vol. 30, 2008, pp. 355–361.

Hue, O., et al. "Plasma Concentration of Organochlorine Compounds is Associated with Age and Not Obesity." *Chemosphere*, Vol. 67, 2007, pp. 1463–1467.

Landhuis, C. E., et al. "Childhood Sleep Time and Long-Term Risk for Obesity: A 32-Year Prospective Birth Cohort Study." *Pediatrics*, Vol. 122, 2008, pp. 955–960.

Lassiter, T. L., et al. "Exposure of Neonatal Rats to Parathion Elicits Sex-Selective Reprogramming of Metabolism and Alters the Response to a High-Fat Diet in Adulthood." *Environmental Health Perspectives*, Vol. 116, 2008, pp. 1456–1462.

Lim, S., et al. "Chronic Exposure to the Herbicide Atrazine Causes Mitochondrial Dysfunction and Insulin Resistance." *PLoS One*, 13 April 2009.

Mattes, R. D., and B. M. Popkin. "Nonnutritive Sweetener Consumption in Humans: Effects on Appetite and Food Intake and their Putative Mechanisms." *American Journal of Clinical Nutrition*, Vol. 89, 2009, pp. 1–14.

McCabe-Sellers, B., et al. "Challenges in Promoting Fruits and Vegetables for Obesity Prevention." *Experimental Biology*, 20 April 2009.

Patel, S. R., et al. "The Association between Sleep Duration and Obesity in Older Adults." *International Journal of Obesity*, Vol. 32, 2008, pp. 1825–1834.

Smink, A., et al. "Exposure to Hexachlorobenzene during Pregnancy Increases the Risk of Overweight in Children Aged 6 Years." *Acta Paediatrica*, Vol. 97, 2008, pp. 1465–1469.

"Study: Thinking Too Much Leads to Obesity." United Press International, 31 December 2008.

Touchette, E., et al. "Associations between Sleep Duration Patterns and Overweight/ Obesity at Age 6." *Sleep*, Vol. 31, 2008, pp. 1507–1514.

Tremblay, A., and J.-P. Chaput. "About Unsuspected Potential Determinants of Obesity." *Applied Physiology, Nutrition and Metabolism*, Vol. 33, 2008, pp. 791–796.

49

Fear of Sunlight

Can it be that there is a malign influence of the sun at periods which affects certain natures, as at times the moon does others?

—Bram Stoker, *Dracula* (1897)

SUMMARY

For decades, many people have avoided exposing their skin to sunlight because ultraviolet (UV) light is a known risk factor for cancer. Parents smear their children with sunblock and make them wear hats outdoors. Since sunlight converts naturally occurring skin chemicals to vitamin D, overly strict avoidance of sunlight can result in vitamin D deficiencies. The long-term consequences may include loss of bone density in adults and rickets in children. The recent increase in breastfeeding may even have compounded this problem, since breast milk is often deficient in vitamin D (Chapter 44). A low level of this vitamin is also a risk factor for tuberculosis, pneumonia, and other infectious diseases. This dilemma has created twin health scares: fear of sunlight and fear of darkness. Although both reflect valid concerns, the recent popularity of indoor tanning suggests what we might call an asynchronous double fizzle. Tanning establishments claim to provide a solution, in the form of a safe alternative to outdoor sunbathing, but many doctors believe indoor tanning is equally harmful (particularly for teenagers) or even addictive.

SOURCE

The fear of sunlight and its flip side both result from media warnings that started in the 1960s (after the tanning craze of the 1950s) and have continued with variations ever since. Nearly all credible sources now agree that too much sunlight can cause skin cancer, particularly in light-skinned people, and that too little sunlight—in combination with inadequate dietary vitamin D—can also have serious health consequences.

Until recently, the solution appeared to be simple: drink milk that has been fortified with vitamin D, eat salmon or other oily fish that contains a lot of vitamin D, or just take vitamin pills. But many people now prefer "natural" milk, and avoid fish because of mercury contamination (Chapter 21) or high cost. Also, some (not all) forms of vitamin A can interfere with the action of vitamin D. Age, gender, skin color, and other factors also influence vitamin D requirements, and an overdose of vitamin D can cause high blood pressure and kidney failure. The problem here is not too little information, but too much.

SCIENCE

Ultraviolet (UV) light is invisible light with wavelengths in the range between 10 nanometers (nm) and 400 nm. Most of the UV light that reaches the Earth is long-wave UV, called UVA, with wavelengths between 315 and 400 nm. Most of the remainder is UVB (280–315 nm), which some sources call short-wave UV and others call medium-wave UV. The sun and germicidal lamps also produce even shorter-wave ultraviolet light, called UVC (100–280 nm), but the ozone layer normally prevents solar UVC from reaching the Earth. As discussed in Chapter 42, shorter wavelength means higher frequency, higher energy per photon, and often a greater potential for damage.

UVA light penetrates the skin deeply and contributes to the appearance of aging by damaging connective tissue. Unlike UVB, it can also pass through glass windows. UVA light may increase the cancer-causing effect of UVB, but it is less likely to cause sunburn. By contrast, UVB causes sunburn and several forms of skin cancer that often appear many years after exposure. Occasional deep sunburn (particularly in childhood) may result in basal cell carcinoma, a type of skin cancer that doctors can easily remove. Less often, UVB can cause malignant melanoma, which is often fatal, but treatable if caught early. Chronic UVB exposure may cause another form of skin cancer, called squamous cell carcinoma, which is also treatable if caught early.

With enough exposure, UVB can also damage the interior and surface of the eyes, and may even suppress the immune system. UVB exposure appears to be a risk factor for several infectious diseases including malaria, hepatitis B, herpes simplex, cutaneous leishmaniasis, and some bacterial skin infections. (UVB does not directly cause any of these diseases, but it may increase the likelihood that an exposed person will be infected.)

But humans evolved in a world bathed in sunlight, and UVB light is not only our enemy, but also a powerful friend. This is the complicated part. Certain chemical compounds normally found in human skin—and in mushrooms and other organisms—give rise to vitamin D when exposed to UVB light. Humans also get vitamin D from food, particularly certain fish with a high fat content. Other dietary sources include eggs, liver, fortified dairy products, and UV-irradiated mushrooms. A full discussion of the chemical structure and health effects of vitamin D is beyond the scope of this book, but the level of vitamin D in the body influences bone density, immune function, and many other aspects of human health. Children who do not get enough vitamin D often develop a condition called rickets, which causes bone pain, muscle weakness, and sometimes permanent skeletal deformities.

So it is often hard to know which is worse—too much sunlight, or too little. Tanning salons claim to solve this dilemma by providing a safe way for people to absorb just the right amount of ultraviolet radiation, while also becoming tan. The UV lights on tanning beds typically produce about 95 to 98 percent UVA and only 2 to 5 percent UVB. These numbers are misleading, however, because natural sunlight is similar, with about 2 to 3 percent UVB. Tanning beds are a cosmetic convenience for people who want to start their tan before the bikini season, and many find them relaxing, but it is hard to understand how they can be any "safer" than sunlight. This is a point of contention between the healthcare and tanning salon industries. Several recent studies have shown that the use of tanning beds, particularly by teenagers, may be associated with increased risk of later developing malignant melanoma.

HISTORY

Rickets was (and is) largely a disease of civilization, because indoor work and urban smog can reduce exposure to sunlight. Living in near-darkness for much of the year was not a problem for the Inuit and other northern cultures, because their normal diet included high levels of vitamin D. The same could not be said for factory workers in nineteenth-century Europe or America, who seldom dined on fish liver. In 1822, a Polish doctor named Jędrzej Śniadecki (1768–1838) reported that sunlight appeared to cure rickets. In 1827, French physician Pierre-Fidèle Bretonneau (1778–1862) found that cod liver oil, which contains vitamin D, was also effective against rickets. Another century passed before German researchers repeated these findings using artificially produced ultraviolet light. In 1924, American biochemist Harry Steenbock (1886–1967) patented a process of irradiating food to increase its vitamin D content, and rickets became a thing of the past—or so it appeared.

In the eighteenth and nineteenth centuries, light-skinned women in some cultures wore large hats and other protective clothing to avoid sunburn. The link between sunlight and skin cancer was not discovered until the 1930s; before that, pale skin was simply fashionable, perhaps because it implied that the wearer need not resort to hard outdoor work. By the 1940s, however, this fad somehow reversed itself, and light-skinned Americans and Europeans of both sexes went to prodigious lengths to become deeply tanned. That goal has continued into the twenty-first century, with one major plot twist. Many sun-worshippers now prefer tanning salons to actual sunlight, apparently because of the enhanced privacy and sense of control over nature.

CONSEQUENCES

Although most (not all) skin cancers are curable, whereas the skeletal effects of childhood rickets can last a lifetime, the fear of ultraviolet light seems to outweigh the fear of vitamin D deficiency. Once confined to developing nations, rickets has made a comeback in many parts of the world. For example, the people of Saudi Arabia are blessed with economic prosperity and abundant sunshine, yet many Saudi infants reportedly suffer from rickets. The main reason for this trend appears to be exclusive breastfeeding without the use of a vitamin supplement. In Saudi Arabia and some other countries, women are required by law to breastfeed each child for two years, and human breast milk is low in vitamin D.

Thanks to publicity about UV light and skin cancer (and the ozone layer), annual sales of sunblock and sunscreen products now exceed $500 million in the United States alone. Surveys have shown, however, that most consumers either avoid using these products on a regular basis or do not apply them properly. Tanning parlors have also enjoyed an economic boom in recent years, although the two trends would appear to cancel each other. In 2007, the Indoor Tanning Association ran a full-page ad in the *New York Times*, questioning the validity of the link between sun exposure and melanoma, and claiming health benefits such as vitamin D synthesis. At the time this book went to press, the U.S. Health Care Reform Bill included a controversial 10 percent excise tax on the use of tanning beds.

A third industry that has benefited from the sunlight controversy includes the manufacturers and sellers of do-it-yourself home test kits for monitoring vitamin D levels. It is not clear if these test results are either accurate or useful, but they may serve to reassure consumers who feel overwhelmed by competing health scares. In 2009, a prominent diagnostic laboratory announced a major recall of inaccurate vitamin D test results distributed during the previous two years.

Avoidance of natural sunlight may also play a role in seasonal affective disorder (SAD), a controversial form of mental depression that occurs each year in a specific season, usually winter. The prevalence of this disorder in some northern regions may be as high as 10 to 20 percent of the population. Some patients have recovered simply by spending more time outdoors; others may require dawn simulation or other forms of indoor bright light therapy.

WHAT WENT WRONG?

Two opposite health recommendations have collided, and the cosmetic advantages of tanning appear to have trumped both. The idea of sunlight aging the skin is horrifying to westerners, but so is the idea of looking pale at the beach.

Maybe someone should invent an inexpensive (and legitimate) procedure to calculate each individual's optimum sunlight exposure and dietary vitamin D requirement, based on skin pigmentation, latitude, occupation, age, genetics, and a host of other relevant variables. As a cheaper alternative, we recommend eating sardines, which contain vitamin D, but are too low on the food chain to absorb a lot of mercury during their short lives.

REFERENCES AND RECOMMENDED READING

Al-Atawi, M. S., et al. "Epidemiology of Nutritional Rickets in Children." *Saudi Journal of Kidney Diseases and Transplantation*, Vol. 20, 2009, pp. 260–265.

Albert, M. R., and K. G. Ostheimer. "The Evolution of Current Medical and Popular Attitudes toward Ultraviolet Light Exposure: Part 3." *Journal of the American Academy of Dermatology*, Vol. 49, 2003, pp. 1096–1106.

Balasubramanian, S., and R. Ganesh. "Vitamin D Deficiency in Exclusively Breast-Fed Infants." *Indian Journal of Medical Research*, Vol. 127, 2008, pp. 250–255.

Chandra, P., et al. "Tanning Can Be an Alternative Source of Vitamin D in High Risk Populations." *Journal of Nutritional Science and Vitaminology*, Vol. 54, 2008, p. 105.

Chang, Y. M., et al. "Sun Exposure and Melanoma Risk at Different Latitudes: A Pooled Analysis of 5700 Cases and 7216 Controls." *International Journal of Epidemiology*, Vol. 38, 2009, pp. 814–830.

Cranney, A., et al. 2007. *Effectiveness and Safety of Vitamin D in Relation to Bone Health*. Rockville, MD: Agency for Healthcare Research and Quality, Evidence Report/Technology Assessment No. 158.

Fairney, A., et al. "The Effect of Darkness on Vitamin D in Adults." *Postgraduate Medical Journal*, Vol. 55, 1979, pp. 248–250.

Gilchrest, B. A. "Sun Exposure and Vitamin D Sufficiency." *American Journal of Clinical Nutrition*, Vol. 88, 2008, pp. 570S–577S.

Heckman, C. J., et al. "Prevalence and Correlates of Indoor Tanning Among U.S. Adults." *Journal of the American Academy of Dermatology*, Vol. 58, 2008, pp. 769–780.

Holick, M. F. "Sunlight, UV-Radiation, Vitamin D and Skin Cancer: How Much Sunlight Do We Need?" *Advances in Experimental Medicine and Biology*, Vol. 624, 2008, pp. 1–5.

Jacobs, E. T., et al. "Vitamin D Insufficiency in Southern Arizona." *American Journal of Clinical Nutrition*, Vol. 87, 2008, pp. 608–613.

Khattak, I. A., and N. Ullah. "Fundamental Rights of Infants are Guaranteed in Islam—Breastfeeding is Mandatory." *Saudi Medical Journal*, Vol. 28, 2007, pp. 297–299.

Lee, W. T., and J. Jiang. "The Resurgence of the Importance of Vitamin D in Bone Health." *Asia Pacific Journal of Clinical Nutrition*, Vol. 17 (Suppl. 1), 2008, pp. 138–142.

Moan, J., et al. "Addressing the Health Benefits and Risks, Involving Vitamin D or Skin Cancer, of Increased Sun Exposure." *Proceedings of the National Academy of Sciences*, Vol. 105, 2008, pp. 668–673.

Ozzard, A., et al. "Vitamin D Deficiency Treated by Consuming UVB-Irradiated Mushrooms." *British Journal of General Practice*, Vol. 58, 2008, pp. 644–645.

Rajakumar, K. "Vitamin D, Cod-Liver Oil, Sunlight, and Rickets: A Historical Perspective." *Pediatrics*, Vol. 112, 2003, pp. e132–e135.

Saint Louis, C. "Confused by SPF? Take a Number." *New York Times*, 14 May 2009.

Schoenmakers, I., et al. "Abundant Sunshine and Vitamin D Deficiency." *British Journal of Nutrition*, Vol. 99, 2008, pp. 1171–1173.

Stroud, M. L., et al. "Vitamin D—A Review." *Australian Family Physician*, Vol. 37, 2008, pp. 1002–1005.

Tangpricha, V., et al. "Tanning is Associated with Optimal Vitamin D Status (Serum 25-Hydroxyvitamin D Concentration) and Higher Bone Mineral Density." *American Journal of Clinical Nutrition*, Vol. 80, 2004, pp. 1645–1649.

U.S. Food and Drug Administration. "Indoor Tanning: The Risks of Ultraviolet Rays." Consumer Health Information, November 2009.

Wagner, C. L., et al. "Prevention of Rickets and Vitamin D Deficiency in Infants, Children, and Adolescents." *Pediatrics*, Vol. 122, 2008, pp. 1142–1152.

Youl, P. H. "Vitamin D and Sun Protection: The Impact of Mixed Public Health Messages in Australia." *International Journal of Cancer*, Vol. 124, 2009, pp. 1963–1970.

50

Junk Food Addiction: The Twinkie Defense

Researchers have discovered that chocolate produces some of the same reactions in the brain as marijuana. The researchers also discovered other similarities between the two but can't remember what they are.

—Matt Lauer (on NBC's *Today Show*, 1996)

SUMMARY

This chapter is not about food, but about a lifestyle based on a poorly defined class of foods. "Junk food" usually means candy, chips, and snack cakes, plus most of the high-fat, high-salt menu options available at fast-food restaurants. Junk food is not exactly an obesogen (Chapter 48), because it has no clear identity. Nevertheless, many people believe that junk food is physically addictive, like cocaine or heroin. Others claim they must have junk food to save time or money, to make the children stop screaming, or to stay awake while performing sedentary work. There is also a widespread belief that junk food causes hyperactivity in children, pimples in adolescents, depression and criminal behavior in adults, and obesity in everybody. Few of these claims hold up to scrutiny, except for the part about obesity. Foods that are high in fat and sugar, and eaten in large quantities as a remedy for boredom or stress, can really pack on the pounds. This scare officially fizzled sometime before 2010, when 60 percent of Americans in an opinion poll opposed a tax on junk food. Whether they were voting for a way of life or against government regulation, one thing is clear: the scare did not work, and junk food is here to stay.

SOURCE

Many food-related publications claim that a well-known consumer activist coined the term "junk food" in 1972, but in fact it was already in general usage in the 1950s, and appeared in newspaper articles published as early as 1960. For example:

This vacation was going to be perfect . . . And the children were going to eat right. Good solid food—soups, mashed potatoes, meat and gravy. Lots of milk. No junk food. No popcorn for breakfast, no pop, no candy bars, no corn crackies or lemon malted milks.[1]

The source of the media catch phrase "Twinkie Defense" is less controversial, because the news media coined it during the famous 1979 trial of San Francisco City Supervisor Dan White, for the 1978 murder of fellow Supervisor Harvey Milk and Mayor George Moscone. The defense attorney claimed that his client suffered from mood swings, and that one symptom—not the cause—of his depression and diminished capacity was the fact that he had recently started eating junk food. Nobody claimed that eating junk food somehow forced him to commit murder, but that was the meaning that the public later assigned to the so-called Twinkie Defense. In any case, the jury apparently bought the argument. They convicted the defendant of voluntary manslaughter, instead of premeditated murder, and an urban legend was born.

SCIENCE

Junk food, like pornography, is hard to define but easy to recognize. As a general rule, junk foods are high in fat, sugar, or salt, or sometimes all three; and they are sold in a form that is ready to eat with minimal preparation—such as removing the wrapper from a cupcake, or popping a frozen pizza into the microwave oven. Junk foods also tend to be low in fiber and many essential nutrients. Most candies, chips, snack cakes, and cookies qualify as junk food, as do many (not all) entrées available from a fast-food restaurant or grocer's freezer case. But the terms junk food and fast food are not interchangeable, because some fast foods are relatively low in fat, sugar, and salt. Familiar examples of fast non-junk food are Subway's veggie sandwiches and the Jack-in-the-Box chicken fajita pita.

The actual ingredients in food do not necessarily dictate its status as junk or non-junk food either. Something labeled as a high-energy granola bar may have a chemical composition that is oddly similar to that of an ordinary candy bar, yet one is junk food and the other is not. Some yogurt products contain as much sugar and fat as ice cream, and some "energy" drinks contain as much sucrose as a non-diet soda that costs half as much. So junk-food status is partly a matter of packaging and context. Some sources go even further, defining junk food as any food that is highly processed or not "natural." These criteria are also hard to define, because we modify almost all foods in some way before eating them, if only by killing or washing them. And if the criterion is the presence of chemical additives, what about dried fruits? These traditional health foods are often loaded with sulfites and other preservatives.

Having failed to define junk food, what can we say about its merits? There is nothing unnatural, or even uniquely human, about cravings for fat, sugar, and salt. Given a choice between a sea lion and a surfer, any right-thinking shark will choose the sea lion for its higher fat content. Primates often choose the sweetest fruits, and hoofed mammals as well as bats gravitate to salt licks. For wild creatures that cannot count on a year-round food surplus, all these preferences reflect physiological needs.

But does a junk food craving qualify as a physical addiction? Is junk food as hard to abandon as heroin or cocaine? Compulsive overeating in general may qualify as an addiction, but a compulsive overeater deprived of junk food would simply eat something else. Recent studies show that sugar and salt addictions are possible; but sugar and salt are components of many foods, junk and otherwise. We have never heard of people turning to crime or looting their children's college funds to support a banana-flavored Moon Pie habit. Also, the nature of junk food dependence is somehow qualitatively different from what we call a true chemical addiction. The Moon Pie junkie looks for specific branding, and will not settle for a drum of high-fructose corn syrup. For less focused junk-food lovers, the collective contents of snack machines and quickie marts may offer a sense of comfort that qualifies as a psychological addiction. In all these cases, it is entirely possible to stop without a 12-step program.

Finally, what does junk food *do*? Can it make us crazy? Some studies appear to support the notion that children raised on a diet of junk food are more likely than others to be hyperactive or otherwise troubled. The problem with these studies, as some of the investigators admit, is that junk food is hard to define and confounding variables are hard to exclude. How can we separate other aspects of parenting from the practice of serving junk food? Also, to the extent that children choose their own snacks, which came first, the behavioral problem or the jellybeans?

HISTORY

The first snacks were probably things like berries and nuts that were easily picked off a bush and consumed with little or no preparation. A meal, on the days when people were lucky enough to get one, might consist of a lean animal that took hours to cook. Fast-forwarding to the birth of the Planters Peanut Company in 1906, we find a young nation eager for sweet and salty foods to enhance the experience of mass entertainment that did not exist in the Pleistocene. Salted nuts were still nutritious, but then came Cracker Jack and cotton candy and Jujubes. After a day of snacks and meals and sedentary work or school, it was time for the family dinner or social gathering, followed by dessert and cocktails and maybe a taffy pull. Snacks finally merged with regular food, and people ate all day long.

Ever since the invention of junk food—although it was not yet called junk food— some parents have complained that it made their children run wild. On Halloween night, sugar-powered mania toppled many a rural outhouse. Nor were adults immune to the mood-altering properties of junk food. The 1956 book *Spring on an Arctic Island* describes how a group of American naturalists became "tired, nervous, headachy, and dangerously undernourished" after living on nuts, candy, and crackers for two days. Their Inuit guide recognized the problem and solved it by cooking up a dinner of seal liver. Studies confirm that some junk foods may affect mood and behavior, but so can any dietary habit that causes blood glucose levels to fluctuate (see also Chapter 19).

By the late twentieth century, junk food ceased to be a convenient snack and became a way of life for many people who apparently never learned to cook. Taco Bell, in partnership with Big Food, invented the term "Fourthmeal" to legitimize round-the-clock consumption of sugar and grease; the mental health establishment countered with night eating syndrome (NES). In 2008, a California couple became briefly famous in the news media after surviving for a month on a food budget of one dollar per day. For some reason, this couple reported that the cheapest foods available in stores were junk foods, such as candy and chips. In reality, far cheaper alternatives include nutritious non-junk foods, such as beans and rice. But such meals require at least a minimum of knowledge, foresight, and patience. The same foods that are expensive in the form of individual microwaveable portions are cheap when purchased in bulk and cooked using actual heat. The most expensive part of such a meal may be the spices and flavor enhancers required to make it taste like junk food.

In 2007, German physicians reported a profoundly instructive international crisis. An American woman with a psychiatric disorder flew to Germany for unknown reasons, and was hospitalized as a result of a delusion that she was being poisoned. She refused to eat or drink anything for four days, until the German hospital staff won her trust by giving her familiar American junk food.

CONSEQUENCES

Whether or not junk food can cause (or cure) mood swings, attention deficit disorder, or violent behavior, a diet that contains a large proportion of junk food clearly is not in the best interest of public health. Known consequences of excess sugar and fat consumption include obesity, type 2 diabetes, and heart disease. Government agencies and consumer organizations have proposed the same regulatory measures used to control any unwanted commerce: pass a law against it or slap a tax on it.

Public reaction has been decidedly mixed. Although parents want their children to be healthy, too much regulation raises the specter of Big Brother. As noted earlier, a 2010 opinion poll showed that 60 percent of Americans opposed a junk food tax. Other proposed measures, such as removing junk food vending machines from schools, have also been unpopular. Students simply bring "bootleg" junk food and sell it to classmates at a significant markup, while schools lose much-needed revenues.

An alternative approach, called performance-based regulation, is supposed to place the burden on the food manufacturer rather than the consumer. Such regulation requires each manufacturer to find ways to reduce the negative social costs of its products. In other words, the government imposes a tax on public health harm rather than on the products themselves. It is unclear how these businesses would make the required changes without passing the cost along to the consumer.

In 2010, British researchers proposed that fast-food restaurants might add statins (drugs that lower serum cholesterol levels) to fast foods such as burgers and fries. Since these drugs are potentially harmful when used without a doctor's supervision, their indiscriminate use would simply expose consumers to a second health hazard while failing to address the underlying problems of overeating and bad nutrition.

WHAT WENT WRONG?

Employed people in modern industrialized societies spend more time working (and commuting) than ever before in history. The unemployed are under great financial stress, and the underemployed have both problems—long work hours combined with poverty. The prevalence of fatigue and stress makes junk food almost inevitable. After a hard day, it seems natural to want a cupcake, or several.

Perhaps the best way to get rid of junk food is to redefine it. People will not stop wanting convenient, good-tasting snacks and meals, but it is possible to change the composition of such foods. A number of fast food restaurant chains and snack manufacturers have recently reduced salt levels, stopped using trans fats, or otherwise made their products healthier. In the next few years, so-called performance-based regulation may nudge more businesses in that direction.

NOTE

1. Dan Valentine, "Vacation Log" (*Salt Lake Tribune*, 12 June 1960).

REFERENCES AND RECOMMENDED READING

Akbaraly, T. N., et al. "Dietary Pattern and Depressive Symptoms in Middle Age." *British Journal of Psychiatry*, Vol. 195, 2009, pp. 408–413.

Anderson, J. W., and K. Patterson. "Snack Foods: Comparing Nutrition Values of Excellent Choices and 'Junk Foods.'" *Journal of the American College of Nutrition*, Vol. 24, 2005, pp. 155–156.

Avena, N. M., et al. "Evidence for Sugar Addiction: Behavioral and Neurochemical Effects of Intermittent, Excessive Sugar Intake." *Neuroscience and Biobehavioral Review*, Vol. 32, 2008, pp. 20–39.

Brownell, K. D., and K. E. Warner. "The Perils of Ignoring History: Big Tobacco Played Dirty and Millions Died. How Similar is Big Food?" *Milbank Quarterly*, Vol. 87, 2009, pp. 259–294.

Cocores, J. A., and M. S. Gold. "The Salted Food Addiction Hypothesis May Explain Overeating and the Obesity Epidemic." *Medical Hypotheses*, 28 July 2009.

Colantuoni, C., et al. "Evidence that Intermittent, Excessive Sugar Intake Causes Endogenous Opioid Dependence." *Obesity Research*, Vol. 10, 2002, pp. 478–488.

Compton, D. "As-Salt on Science." *New York Post*, 13 January 2010.

Dagher, A. "The Neurobiology of Appetite: Hunger and Addiction." *International Journal of Obesity*, Vol. 33 (Suppl. 2), 2009, pp. S30–S33.

Daley, J. "Overhyped Health Headlines Revealed." *Popular Science*, August 2009.

Fleetwood, B. "From the People Who Brought You the Twinkie Defense: The Rise of the Expert Witness Industry." *Washington Monthly*, June 1987.

Gracey, M. "Junk Food or 'Junk Eating'?" *Nestle Nutrition Workshop Series, Paediatric Program*, Vol. 56, 2005, pp. 143–150.

"Homicidal? Could be Your Diet . . ." *Food Management*, June 2007.

Leo, J. "The It's-Not-My-Fault Syndrome." *U.S. News and World Report*, 18 June 1990.

Naughton, K. "Bring on the Junk Food." *Newsweek*, 10 July 2000.

Ordoñez, J. "Taking the Junk out of Junk Food." *Newsweek*, 8 October 2007.

Pirisi, A. "A Real Sugar High?" *Psychology Today*, January–February 2003.

Rosa, M. A., et al. "Development of a Questionnaire to Evaluate Sugar Abuse and Dependence." *Cadernos de Saúde Pública*, Vol. 24, 2008, pp. 1869–1876. [Portuguese]

Savodnik, I. "Psychiatry's Sick Compulsion: Turning Weaknesses into Defenses." *Los Angeles Times*, 1 January 2006.

Schwarcz, J. "Take It With a Grain of Salt." *Canadian Chemical News*, April 2002.

Schwerthöffer, D., and J. Bäuml. "'Junk-Food' Intervention in Poisoning Delusion." *Psychiatrische Praxis*, Vol. 34, 2007, pp. 400–402.

Sugarman, S. "No More Business as Usual: Enticing Companies to Sharply Lower the Public Health Costs of the Products they Sell." *Public Health*, Vol. 123, 2009, pp. 275–279.

Sugarman, S. "Performance-Based Regulation: Enterprise Responsibility for Reducing Death, Injury, and Disease Caused by Consumer Products." *Journal of Health Politics, Policy and Law*, Vol. 34, 2009, pp. 1035–1077.

Tyre, P. "Fighting 'Big Fat.'" *Newsweek*, 5 August 2002.

Watson, R. "Food Industry is Under Pressure to Drop Junk Food Advertisements." *British Medical Journal*, Vol. 330, 2005, p. 215.

Wiles, N. J., et al. "'Junk Food Diet' and Childhood Behavioural Problems: Results from the ALSPAC Cohort." *European Journal of Clinical Nutrition*, Vol. 63, 2009, pp. 491–498.

GLOSSARY

"When I use a word," Humpty Dumpty said, "it means just what I choose it to mean—neither more nor less."

—Lewis Carroll, *Alice's Adventures in Wonderland* (1865)

acesulfame potassium or **acesulfame K**: An artificial sweetener.

acetaminophen: A drug used to relieve pain and fever; found in Tylenol and other brand-name products.

acetylsalicylic acid (ASA): Aspirin; a drug used to relieve pain, fever, and inflammation.

acne: Pimples.

acoustic neuroma: A benign tumor of the acoustic (hearing) nerve.

acute infection: An infection with a sudden onset, sharp rise, and relatively short course.

addiction: Physical or psychological dependence on a substance, often with physiological symptoms on withdrawal.

additives: Substances added to food to improve color, texture, flavor, or keeping qualities.

adjuvant: A substance added to a vaccine to increase its effectiveness.

adult-onset diabetes: See type 2 diabetes.

aerosol: Tiny particles (droplet nuclei, dust, spores, etc.) suspended in air.

aflatoxin: Cancer-causing toxin produced by the fungus *Aspergillus flavus*.

agroterrorism: Terrorism involving the destruction of crops or livestock.

AHB: Africanized honeybee.

AIDS: Acquired immune deficiency syndrome; a T-cell deficiency disease caused by infection with the human immunodeficiency virus (HIV).

airborne transmission: Transmission (of an infectious agent) to a susceptible host by inhalation of an aerosol.

Alar: A brand name for daminozide, a plant growth regulator.

algae: A group of variously defined unicellular and multicellular photosynthetic organisms.

alimentary canal: The digestive system; a tube extending from the mouth to the anus.

alitame: An artificial sweetener.

alkaloid: Any of a diverse group of plant chemicals with pharmacological activity.

allergen: A substance to which an individual is hypersensitive.

allergy: An adverse reaction to a chemical, resulting from previous sensitization to that chemical or a similar one; examples are hay fever or contact dermatitis.

alpha particle: A positively charged nuclear particle that is ejected at high speed in certain radioactive transformations.

Alzheimer's disease: A progressive form of presenile or senile dementia.

amaranth: A red chemical dye.

Amblyomma: A genus of hard ticks that serve as vectors for Lyme and other diseases.

ameba or **amoeba**: Any of a group of widely distributed protozoans with pseudopodia (temporary protrusions used in locomotion or feeding).

amebiasis or **amoebiasis**: Infection with an ameba.

amebic or **amoebic dysentery**: Dysentery caused by infection with an ameba.

aminotriazole: A chemical weed killer.

amnesic shellfish poisoning: An illness caused by consumption of seafood contaminated with domoic acid.

anaerobic: Occurring in the absence of oxygen.

anaphylactic shock: Severe, sometimes fatal shock symptoms resulting from exposure to an antigen to which an individual is hypersensitive (allergic).

anaphylaxis: A severe allergic reaction.

anemia: A deficiency of red blood cells, hemoglobin, or total blood volume.

anencephaly: A birth defect in which all or part of the brain is missing.

antagonism (in toxicology): The situation in which two chemicals administered together interfere with each other's actions.

anthrax: An infectious disease caused by the bacterium *Bacillus anthracis*.

antibacterial: Capable of destroying or inhibiting the growth of bacteria.

antibiotic: Any of a number of organic compounds, either produced by microorganisms or synthesized in the laboratory, that can kill or inhibit the growth of other microorganisms.

antibiotic resistance: The ability of certain microorganisms to resist antibiotics.

antibody: A protein that acts against a specific antigen in the body.

antigen: Any substance (usually a protein) that provokes an immune response.

antihistamine: Any of various chemical compounds that counteract histamine in the body; used to treat allergic reactions and symptoms of the common cold.

antimicrobial: Capable of destroying or inhibiting the growth of microorganisms.

antioxidant: A substance that inhibits oxidation reactions.

antitoxin: An antibody that is capable of neutralizing a specific toxin in the body, or a serum containing such antibodies.

arenavirus: Any of a group of RNA viruses that cause hemorrhagic fevers and other diseases transmitted from rodents to humans.

argyria: Discoloration of the skin and mucous membranes caused by exposure to silver.

arthritis: Inflammation of joints.

arthropod: Any of a group of invertebrate animals with a segmented body and jointed appendages; includes insects, spiders, mites, and others.

ascorbic acid: Vitamin C.

Asian or Asiatic flu: The 1957 influenza A pandemic.

aspartame: An artificial sweetener.

aspirin: Acetylsalicylic acid, a drug used to relieve pain, fever, and inflammation.

asthma: A condition characterized by labored breathing, wheezing, coughing, and a sense of constriction in the chest.

attenuated: Reduced in virulence; weakened.

autism: A controversial disorder of brain development that begins in early childhood and is characterized by impaired communication and social skills.

autoimmune: Of, relating to, or caused by antibodies or lymphocytes that attack the organism producing them.

avian influenza: An infectious disease of birds, caused by an avian strain of influenza A virus; some strains are transmissible to humans.

babesiosis: A tickborne parasitic disease of livestock and humans.

bacillary dysentery: Shigellosis.

Bacillus anthracis: A gram-positive bacterium that causes anthrax.

bacteria (singular, **bacterium**): Microscopic, single-celled organisms that lack a nucleus.

bacterial meningitis: Meningitis caused by a bacterial infection.

bacterial pneumonia: Pneumonia caused by a bacterial infection.

bacteriophage: A virus that infects bacteria.

benzoate: A food preservative.

BH: Biological hazard.

BHA: Butylated hydroxyanisole, a food preservative.

BHT: Butylated hydroxytoluene, an antioxidant food preservative.

Big Drug: A collective term (often derogatory) for the pharmaceutical industry.

Big Food: A collective term (often derogatory) for large companies that manufacture highly processed or unhealthy foods.

binge: A short period of overindulgence; usually refers to food or drink.

biological hazard or **biohazard**: Anything of biological origin that can harm human beings, either directly or indirectly.

biological warfare: Warfare in which the weapons are living organisms or biological toxins.

biological weapon: An organism (usually microscopic) or biological toxin used as an instrument of warfare or terrorism.

bioterrorism: Terrorist activity involving the use of biological weapons.

bird flu: Avian influenza.

bisphenol A (BPA): An organic compound used in the manufacture of certain plastics.

botulin: A neurotoxin produced by the bacterium *Clostridium botulinum*.

botulism: An acute paralytic foodborne or waterborne disease caused by botulin.

bovine growth hormone (BGH): A pituitary hormone of cattle.

bovine somatotropin (BST): Bovine growth hormone.

bovine spongiform encephalopathy (BSE): Mad cow disease; an infectious foodborne prion disease of cattle.

bovine tuberculosis: A chronic bacterial disease of cattle that can also infect humans.

BPA: Bisphenol A.

breakthrough infection: An infectious disease acquired after vaccination for that disease.

brucellosis: An infectious disease of livestock and humans, caused by the bacterium *Brucella abortus*.

BSE: Bovine spongiform encephalopathy.

BST: Bovine somatotropin.

bush meat: Meat of terrestrial wild animals.

cable mites: Tiny fictitious creatures said to live on cables in offices.

caffeine: An alkaloid found in certain plants (such as coffee) and used as a stimulant.

campylobacteriosis: Infection with bacteria in the genus *Campylobacter*.

cancer: Any of numerous diseases caused by abnormal changes in cells that lead to the growth of invasive tumors in the body.

Canderel: An artificial sweetener that contains aspartame.

carbon dioxide (CO_2): A colorless gas formed by respiration and by the combustion or decay of organic matter.

carcinogen: A chemical, virus, or other agent that causes cancer.

carmine: A red dye made from insects.

carrier: An individual infected with a disease but showing no symptoms.

case: An individual animal or person with a a specific disease.

case-control study: A study design in which the investigators compare two groups of subjects, one group with a given disease (cases) and the other without the disease (controls).

CBW: Chemical and biological warfare.

CDC: The U.S. Centers for Disease Control and Prevention.

chickenpox: An infectious disease caused by the varicella-zoster virus (HHV-3).

chlorination: Treatment with chlorine or a chlorine compound.

cholera: An infectious waterborne or foodborne disease caused by the bacterium *Vibrio cholerae*.

chronic infection: An infection of long duration and slow progress.

ciprofloxacin: A synthetic antibiotic that blocks bacterial DNA replication.

CJD: Creutzfeldt-Jakob disease.

cocaine: An alkaloid derived from leaves of the coca plant (*Erythroxylon coca*).

coffee: A beverage made from the seeds of the coffee plant (*Coffea arabica* and relatives).

colloidal: Consisting of small particles dispersed throughout another substance.

colonic irrigation or **colon hydrotherapy**: Exactly what it sounds like.

Colorado tick fever: One of several viral diseases transmitted by ticks.

colostrum: The first milk secreted by the mammary glands at the end of pregnancy, containing antibodies that give the infant temporary passive immunity to some diseases.

communicable disease: A disease that can be transmitted from one host to another (either directly or indirectly) by an infectious agent, such as a bacterium or virus.

community-acquired: Refers to a disease or infection in a person who has not recently been in a hospital or other medical institution.

comparative risk assessment: Systematic evaluation of the actual or potential effects of modifying exposure to one or more risk factors.

contact: (1) Association with an infected person or animal or with a contaminated environment. (2) A person or animal that has been in such association.

contagious disease: A highly communicable disease that is transmitted directly from one host to another.

contamination: The presence of an infectious agent or other unwanted material.

contraception: Birth control.

control: (1) The process of limiting the spread of an infectious disease by measures such as vaccination, treatment, quarantine, and disinfection. (2) In an experiment, a person or animal that does not have the condition being studied.

cowpox: A mild viral disease of cattle that can also infect humans.

crack: A solid, smokable form of cocaine.

Creutzfeldt-Jakob disease (CJD): A human transmissible spongiform encephalopathy.

cryptosporidiosis: A waterborne or foodborne infectious disease caused by the protozoan parasite *Cryptosporidium parvum*.

cyanide: Any chemical compound that contains the cyano group (a carbon atom triple-bonded to a nitrogen atom).

cyclamate: An artificial sweetener.

cyclosporosis: A waterborne or foodborne infectious disease caused by protozoan parasites in the genus *Cyclospora*.

daminozide: A plant growth regulator.

DDVP: Dimethyl 2,2-dichlorovinylphosphate, an organophosphate pesticide.

Delaney Clause: 1958 amendment to the 1938 U.S. Federal Food, Drug, and Cosmetic Act; prohibits FDA approval of food additives that cause cancer in laboratory animals.

delusional or **delusory parasitosis**: The false belief that one is infested with external or internal parasites.

deoxyribonucleic acid (DNA): One type of chemical that encodes genetic information.

dermatitis: Inflammation of the skin.

DES: Diethylstilbestrol.

diabetes: Any of a group of diseases characterized by inadequate production or utilization of insulin, with high levels of sugar in the blood and urine.

diarrhea: Abnormally frequent bowel movements with more or less liquid stool.

dichlorvos: DDVP.

diethylstilbestrol (DES): A nonsteroidal synthetic form of estrogen.

diminished capacity: A legal defense by which defendants argue that they are not responsible for their actions because their mental functions were impaired at the time.

dinoflagellate: Any of a group of single-celled, mostly marine planktonic organisms.

direct transmission: Transmission (of an infectious agent) directly from an infected person or animal to a susceptible host.

disaster: A sudden event bringing great damage, loss, or destruction.

disease: A condition of a living organism that impairs normal functioning.

disinfectant: A chemical that destroys harmful microorganisms.

DNA: Deoxyribonucleic acid.

domoic acid: A toxin produced by certain marine diatoms.

dose: A measured quantity of a therapeutic agent or toxin.

dose-response relationship: A graph or equation describing the response of an individual or population of a given species to varying doses of a given chemical.

DPT or **DTP**: A vaccine that protects against diphtheria, pertussis, and tetanus.

droplet nuclei: Residues released into the air when fluid from an infected host evaporates.

dust mite: Any of several closely related mite species that feed on shed human skin cells.

dysentery: Severe diarrhea with passage of mucus and blood.

E. coli: The bacterium *Escherichia coli*.

Ebola hemorrhagic fever: An infectious disease caused by a filovirus.

ehrlichiosis: Any of a number of tickborne bacterial diseases.

ELF: Extremely low frequency.

emerging disease: An infectious disease that has recently appeared in a human population, or one that has shown a rapid increase in incidence or geographic range.

EMF: Electromagnetic field or fields.

emulsifier: An agent that disperses a substance as droplets or particles within a liquid.

encephalitis: Inflammation of the brain.

encephalomyelitis: Inflammation of the brain and spinal cord.

encephalopathy: A disease of the brain, especially one that involves changes in brain structure.

endemic: Present in a given geographic area.

endometriosis: The presence of endometrial cells in places other than the uterine lining.

enriched food: Food (such as flour) to which nutrients lost in processing have been restored.

entamoeba: Any of a group of protozoan parasites (genus *Entamoeba*) that cause dysentery and other diseases.

enzyme: A protein that catalyzes a biological reaction.

epidemic: The occurrence of a higher-than-expected number of cases of a given disease, often derived from a common source.

epidemiology: The science that deals with the incidence, distribution, and control of disease in a population.

epigenetics: The study of changes in gene expression that occur without changes in the DNA.

Equal: An artificial sweetener that contains aspartame.

eradication: Reduction of the prevalence of a disease to zero.

Escherichia coli (**E. coli**): A bacterium that normally lives in the gastrointestinal tract. Some strains can also cause serious infections.

estrogen: Any of several female steroid sex hormones that produce estrus.

excitotoxicity: The process by which glutamate and related substances damage nerve cells.

excitotoxin: Chemicals that bind to glutamate receptors.

exotic: Foreign; not native to the place where found.

exposure: An opportunity to contract a disease or absorb a toxin.

false negative: A negative test result when the subject actually has the attribute that the test is designed to detect.

false positive: A positive test result when the subject does not actually have the attribute that the test is designed to detect.

famine: A widespread shortage of food.

fascioliasis or **fasciolosis**: Infestation with flatworms called liver flukes (genus *Fasciola*).

fatality rate: The percentage of persons with a given illness who die as a result of that illness.

fecal-oral route: A route of disease transmission in which fecal contamination is transferred to the mouth, as, for example, by a food preparer with inadequately washed hands.

fever: (1) An above-normal body temperature. (2) Any of a number of diseases in which fever is a prominent symptom.

fibromyalgia: A chronic disorder that causes widespread pain and tenderness in the muscles and tendons.

filovirus: Any of a group of RNA viruses that can cause severe hemorrhagic fevers in humans and nonhuman primates.

flesh-eating bacteria: Any bacteria that can cause necrotizing fasciitis.

flu: Influenza.

fluoridation: The controlled addition of fluoride to a public water supply for the purpose of reducing tooth decay.

follicle mite: A mite (*Demodex folliculorum* or *D. brevis*) that lives in human hair follicles and sebaceous glands.

foodborne disease: A disease caused by an infectious agent ingested with food.

food poisoning: (1) Gastrointestinal illness caused by toxins produced by foodborne bacteria. (2) Any gastrointestinal illness caused by a foodborne infectious agent.

fortified food: Food (such as dairy products) to which nutrients have been added.

Fournier gangrene: Necrotizing fasciitis of the male genitalia.

Frankenfood (slang): Food derived from genetically modified organisms.

fructose: A sugar found in fruit juices and honey.

fungicide: Any chemical used for the destruction of fungi.

fungus: Any of a group of organisms including yeasts, molds, and mushrooms.

gangrene: Local tissue death due to loss of blood supply.

gastrointestinal (GI) tract: (1) The stomach and intestines. (2) The entire alimentary canal.

genetically modified organism (GMO): An animal, plant, or microbe whose genetic material has been altered using genetic engineering techniques.

germ warfare: Biological warfare.

giardiasis: A waterborne disease caused by the protozoan *Giardia lamblia*.

glucose: A sugar that serves as the principal source of energy for man and many other organisms.

glucose intolerance: A condition in which glucose is not properly absorbed into cells.

glutamic acid: One of the amino acids.

glycoprotein: A type of protein with a carbohydrate component.

GMF: Genetically modified food.

GMO: Genetically modified organism.

gonorrhea: A sexually transmitted disease caused by the bacterium *Neisseria gonorrhoeae*.

GPA: Growth-promoting antibiotics.

GRAS: Generally recognized as safe.

greenhouse gas: Any of a number of atmospheric gases that contribute to global warming by absorbing and emitting radiation in the thermal infrared range.

group A streptococci: Any of a group of *Streptococcus* bacteria that cause diseases such as endocarditis, strep throat, impetigo, and necrotizing fasciitis.

group B streptococci: Any of a group of *Streptococcus* bacteria that cause diseases such as pneumonia, encephalitis, and meningitis.

growth-promoting antibiotics (GPA): Antibiotics added to animal feed to promote more rapid growth by improving feed conversion.

Guillain-Barré syndrome: Paralysis or muscular weakness that may occur after certain viral infections or vaccinations.

HAB: Harmful algal bloom.

hazard: A potential source of harm or loss.

HDL: High-density lipoprotein cholesterol ("good" cholesterol).

health scare: A highly publicized health threat, either real or bogus.

Helicobacter pylori: A bacterium that causes duodenal and gastric ulcers.

hemagglutinin: A type of glycoprotein found on the surface of a virus.

hemorrhagic fever: A syndrome of high fever with severe internal and/or external bleeding.

hepatitis: Any of several diseases marked by inflammation of the liver.

hepatitis A virus (HAV): A foodborne or waterborne RNA virus that can cause acute or subacute hepatitis, with recovery usual.

hepatitis B virus (HBV): A DNA virus that can cause acute or chronic hepatitis; transmitted by blood products or other fluid exchange.

herbicide: Any chemical used for the destruction of plants.

herd immunity: Immunity (to a given disease) in a high enough percentage of a population that spread of the disease is unlikely.

heroin: An addictive narcotic drug derived from morphine.

herpes simplex: An infectious disease caused by the herpes simplex viruses HSV-1 or HSV-2.

histamine: A compound released by the body during allergic reactions, causing dilatation of capillaries and contraction of smooth muscle.

HIV: Human immunodeficiency virus, a retrovirus that causes AIDS.

HMO: Health maintenance organization.

hospital-acquired: Refers to an infection that is contracted by a hospitalized patient.

host: A person or animal used by an infectious agent for subsistence or lodgment.

household transmission: Transmission (of an infectious agent) by inapparent exposure to body fluids of household members who are not sex partners.

HRT: Hormone replacement therapy.

hydrargyria: Mercury poisoning.

hydrotherapy: The use of water in any therapeutic procedure.

hyperactivity: The state of being abnormally excitable or impulsive.

hypersensitivity: Allergy.

hypoglycemia: An abnormally low level of sugar in the blood.

hypospadias: The presence of abnormal openings in the wall of the urethra.

Ig: Immunoglobulin.

immune: Having protective antibodies or cellular immunity to a given disease as a result of prior exposure or immunization.

immunity: Resistance to an infectious agent, usually associated with possession of antibodies.

immunization: Vaccination.

immunoglobulin: Any of a class of proteins that function as antibodies.

inapparent infection: An infection that produces no noticeable symptoms.

incidence rate: The number of cases of a disease diagnosed or reported during a given time period, divided by the total number of persons or animals in the affected population.

incubation period: The time interval between exposure to an infectious agent and the appearance of the first sign or symptom of the disease.

infantile paralysis: An old name for polio.

infection: The entry and development or multiplication of an infectious agent in the body.

infectious agent: An organism that is capable of producing infection or infectious disease.

infectious disease: A disease resulting either from an infection or from overgrowth of a host's normal microbes.

infestation: (1) The development and reproduction of arthropods on the body surface or in clothing. (2) The presence of any parasite in or on a host.

influenza: An acute, highly contagious respiratory disease caused by any of several influenza viruses.

insecticide: Any chemical used to kill insects or other arthropods.

insulin: A pancreatic hormone that is essential in carbohydrate metabolism.

insulin resistance: Glucose intolerance.

intoxication: (1) An abnormal physiological state induced by a toxin or other poison. (2) The state of being incapacitated by alcohol or drugs.

isotope: Any of two or more chemicals with the same atomic number but different mass.

isotretinoin: A drug used to treat acne.

krypton: An inert gas with a radioactive isotope that is released during the reprocessing of fuel rods from nuclear reactors.

late blight of potato: A plant disease caused by *Phytophthora infestans*.

latrodectism: Envenomation by the black widow spider.

LD$_{50}$: The dose of a given substance required to kill 50 percent of exposed subjects.

LDL: Low-density lipoprotein cholesterol ("bad" cholesterol).

leishmaniasis: An infectious disease caused by protozoa in the genus *Leishmania*.

leptospirosis: An infectious disease caused by the bacterium *Leptospira interrogans*.

lesion: A wound, injury, or pathological change in a tissue.

lichen planus: A skin disease that causes itching and spots on the arms or legs.

listeriosis: An infectious disease caused by the bacterium *Listeria monocytogenes*.

liver fluke: A parasitic flatworm.

love apple: An old name for the tomato.

loxoscelism: Envenomation by one of the recluse or violin spiders.

lupus erythematosus: A chronic inflammatory disease of connective tissue.

lycopene: A chemical found in tomatoes and other red fruits and vegetables.

Lyme disease: An infectious disease caused by the spirochete *Borrelia burgdorferi* and transmitted by ticks.

lymphocyte: Any of several types of white blood cell involved in immune reactions.

mad cow disease: Bovine spongiform encephalopathy.

malaria: Any of four mosquitoborne diseases caused by protozoa in the genus *Plasmodium*.

margarine: A butter substitute made from vegetable oil.

marijuana: The dried leaves and flowering tops of the female hemp plant (*Cannabis sativa*).

measles: An infectious viral disease that causes a high fever and rash.

meltdown: (1) Severe overheating of a nuclear reactor core, resulting in the escape of radiation. (2) Any major physical, emotional, or economic breakdown.

meningitis: Inflammation of the meninges (membranes surrounding the brain and spinal cord).

meningoencephalitis: Inflammation of the meninges and brain.

mercurialism: Mercury poisoning.

methicillin: An antibiotic related to penicillin.

microbe: Microorganism.

microorganism: An organism that is too small to observe in detail without a microscope, such as the bacteria and single-celled algae.

mildew: A whitish growth or discoloration on organic matter, caused by various fungi.

mitochondria (singular, **mitochondrion**): Structures that produce energy in living cells.

MMR: A vaccine that protects against measles, mumps, and rubella.

mold: A furry-looking fungal growth on the surface of damp organic matter.

monkeypox: An acute infectious disease that is similar to smallpox and caused by a related poxvirus.

monosodium glutamate (MSG): A food additive used as a flavor enhancer.

mortality rate: The number of deaths occurring in a population during a given time period, divided by the total number of persons or animals in the affected population.

MRSA: Methicillin-resistant *Staphylococcus aureus*.

MSG: Monosodium glutamate.

multiple sclerosis: A chronic, progressive disorder that involves the loss of the protective myelin sheath from certain nerve fibers.

mumps: An infectious viral disease that causes inflammation of the salivary glands.

mutagen: Any agent that causes mutations (changes in DNA).

myasthenia gravis: A chronic disease that causes muscular weakness and fatigue.

mycotoxin: Any of a number of toxins produced by fungi.

myocarditis: Inflammation of the heart muscle.

nanny state: A government that is seen as restricting its citizens' options to an extent that interferes with the public good.

natural flavor: A substance extracted, distilled, or otherwise derived from plant or animal matter, either directly from the matter itself or after it has been roasted, heated or fermented.

necrotizing fasciitis: A severe invasive disease caused by group A streptococci or certain other bacteria.

neural tube defect: Any of a number of birth defects involving the brain or spinal cord.

neuraminidase: A type of enzyme found on the surface of a virus.

neurotoxic: Toxic to the nervous system.

neurotoxin: A poisonous substance (usually a protein) that acts on the nervous system.

New variant Creutzfeldt-Jakob disease (nvCJD): A transmissible spongiform encephalopathy in humans, linked to BSE in cattle.

nicotine: A poisonous alkaloid found in tobacco and other plants.

nitrate: A salt or ester of nitric acid.

nitrite: A salt or ester of nitrous acid.

nm: Nanometer; a unit of measurement equal to one billionth of a meter.

notifiable disease: A disease that must be brought to the attention of a health agency (such as the CDC), once detected or suspected.

NSAID: Nonsteroidal anti-inflammatory drug.

NTD: Neural tube defect.

NutraSweet: A brand name for aspartame.

obesogen: A substance or action that promotes weight gain by increasing fat storage.

oleomargarine: An old word for margarine.

onanism: An old word for masturbation.

Oömycetes: A class of microscopic organisms that resemble fungi, but are more closely related to certain algae.

opportunistic infection: An infection caused by pathogens that usually do not cause disease in a healthy immune system.

organophosphate: Any of a group of organic compounds that contain phosphorus; often used as pesticides or chemical weapons.

ORS: Oral rehydration salts.

outbreak: A sudden rise in the incidence of a disease or the numbers of a harmful organism within a given area; usually smaller or more localized than an epidemic.

ozone: A highly reactive gas composed of three atoms of oxygen (O_3).

ozone layer: An atmospheric layer with high ozone content.

pandemic: A major outbreak of a disease over a wide geographic area.

panflu: Pandemic influenza.

paper lice: (1) Cable mites. (2) Book lice (tiny insects that live on stored paper).

parasite: Any organism that lives in or on the body of a larger organism of a different species, called the host, on which the parasite depends for food.

parasitic disease: A disease caused by infestation with a parasite.

paratyphoid fever: An infectious disease caused by any of several species of bacteria in the genus *Salmonella*.

passive immunity: Short-term immunity that results from maternal transfer or inoculation with antibodies.

pasteurization: Partial sterilization of a substance (such as milk) by heat or radiation.

pathogen: A bacterium, virus, or other agent that causes disease.

pathogenicity: The capability of an infectious agent to cause disease in a susceptible host.

PEAS: Possible estuary-associated syndrome.

penicillin: Any of a class of antibiotics discovered in 1928.

peptide: A molecule consisting of two or more amino acids; a component of a protein.

personal beliefs exemption: A policy in some states that enables parents to refuse to have their children vaccinated against childhood infectious diseases.

pertussis: Whooping cough.

pest: (1) Any organism that causes economic harm to humans by damaging crops, livestock, or their stored products. (2) An old name for plague.

pesticide: Any chemical used to kill unwanted lower organisms.

Pfiesteria: A dinoflagellate (*Pfiesteria piscicida*) that may cause fish kills and human illness.

Phytophthora infestans: The oömycete that causes late blight of potato and tomato.

pinworm: A small parasitic nematode worm.

placebo effect: Beneficial effects from an inert substance as a result of belief or expectation.

placental transfer: Transfer (of an infectious agent, toxin, or other entity) from a female mammal to a fetus via the placenta.

plague: (1) An infectious disease caused by the bacterium *Yersinia pestis*. (2) Any major disease epidemic.

pneumonia: A disease of the lungs with inflammation and consolidation, caused by any of a variety of bacteria, fungi, viruses, or chemicals.

poison: Any chemical agent that kills or harms an organism.

poisonous: Having the properties or effects of a poison.

poliomyelitis or **polio**: An infectious disease caused by a poliovirus.

polyarthritis: Arthritis involving five or more joints.

polyvinyl chloride: A polymer that is widely used in construction materials.

possible estuary-associated syndrome (PEAS): Controversial human illness attributed to Pfiesteria.

poxvirus: Any of a group of DNA viruses that cause diseases such as smallpox and cowpox.

precautionary principle: A risk management policy often used in circumstances with a high degree of scientific uncertainty, reflecting the need to take action for a potentially serious risk without awaiting the results of scientific research.

preservatives: Food additives used to prevent spoilage.

prevalence or **prevalence rate**: The percentage of persons or animals in a population having a certain disease or condition at a given time.

primary host: A host species in which a parasite passes the adult or reproductive stage in its life cycle.

prion: A nonliving, self-replicating infectious particle composed entirely of protein.

prophylaxis: The prevention of disease.

ptomaine: An old term for poisonous substances (such as toxic amines) formed during bacterial decomposition of protein.

pustule: A small elevation of the skin that contains pus.

pyrethrum: An insecticide made from chrysanthemum flowers.

Q fever: An infectious disease caused by the rickettsia *Coxiella burneti*.

quarantine: A state of enforced isolation, usually to prevent the spread of a disease.

radioactive decay: The spontaneous disintegration of a radioactive substance with the emission of ionizing radiation.

raw milk: Milk that has not been pasteurized.

red tide: A proliferation of certain types of ocean plankton that produce toxins.

reportable disease: Notifiable disease.

reservoir host: An animal species that carries and maintains an infectious agent and serves as a source of infection for other species.

resistance: (1) The ability of the body to resist the invasion or multiplication of infectious agents or damage by their toxic products. (2) The ability of a microorganism or vector to survive exposure to an antibiotic or other drug.

Reye's syndrome: An acute, potentially fatal metabolic disease seen primarily in children, often following an infectious disease such as chickenpox.

rheumatic fever: A group A streptococcal infection that may damage the heart valves.

rhinitis: Inflammation of the mucous membrane of the nose.

ribonucleic acid (RNA): One type of chemical that encodes genetic information.

rickets: A deficiency disease that results from inadequate vitamin D or sunlight.

rickettsia: Any of a group of small bacteria-like organisms that can live only as parasites inside cells.

ring vaccination: The process of vaccinating all susceptible persons who have been in close contact with an infected patient.

risk: A measure of the probability of exposure to a given hazard, combined with the probability of being harmed by that exposure.

risk assessment: The process of identifying hazards and measuring and prioritizing their associated risks.

risk compression: The human tendency to overestimate rare risks and to underestimate common ones.

risk management: A structured approach to reducing risk associated with a threat.

risk society: A human society that is preoccupied with risks, particularly those resulting from modernization.

RNA: Ribonucleic acid.

Rocky Mountain spotted fever: A tickborne disease caused by *Rickettsia rickettsi*.

rosacea: A skin disease that causes reddened areas on the nose, forehead and cheeks.

rubella: German measles; a usually mild infectious viral disease that can cause birth defects if contracted by a pregnant woman.

rubeola: Measles. Not the same as rubella.

Russian flu: The influenza pandemic of 1889.

Sabin polio vaccine: An oral polio vaccine developed from live attenuated poliovirus.

saccharin: An artificial sweetener.

Salk polio vaccine: An injected polio vaccine developed from inactivated (dead) poliovirus.

salmonellosis: Infection with bacteria of the genus *Salmonella* (other than *S. typhi*).

SARS: Severe acute respiratory syndrome.

scarlet fever: A group A streptococcal disease characterized by a skin rash and high fever.

screen: To test for the presence of a disease or other characteristic.

seasonal influenza: The normal annual outbreak of respiratory illness caused by influenza A, usually in winter in temperate climates.

secondary infection: An infection that occurs during or after treatment of another, already existing infection.

sensitivity (of a diagnostic test): A measure of how many cases of a given disease the test can find. A highly sensitive test may yield many false positives.

sensitization: The process of becoming sensitized (allergic) to an antigen.

septicemia: Invasion of the bloodstream by virulent microorganisms.

seroconversion: The appearance of an antibody in the blood.

seroprevalence: The percentage of a population whose blood tests positive for a specific disease.

serotype or **serovar**: A group of closely related microorganisms with a common set of antigens.

shigellosis: An infectious disease caused by bacteria in the genus *Shigella*.

sick building syndrome: A situation in which a building's occupants report symptoms such as fatigue, headaches, or difficulty in concentrating.

silver nitrate: A silver compound used as a disinfectant.

smallpox: An infectious disease caused by the variola poxvirus.

sodium benzoate: A chemical preservative.

sodium cyclamate: An artificial sweetener.

solanine: A toxic chemical found in green or blighted potatoes.

source (of infection): The person, animal, object, or substance from which an infectious agent passes directly to a susceptible host.

specificity (of a diagnostic test): A measure of how accurately the test diagnoses a given disease. A highly specific test may yield many false negatives.

spina bifida: A birth defect in which the spinal column is imperfectly closed.

spirochete: Any of a group of bacteria with a spiral shape.

Splenda: A brand name for sucralose.

spoilage: Any disagreeable change in a food that can be detected with the senses.

sporadic: Occurring singly rather than in groups.

spore: A small reproductive body produced by some plants, fungi, bacteria, and protozoa.

Stachybotrys: A toxigenic black fungus (*Stachybotrys chartarum*) that grows in buildings, often in water-damaged areas.

staph infection: An infection caused by bacteria in the genus *Staphylococcus*.

staphylococci: Bacteria of the genus *Staphylococcus*.

Staphylococcus aureus: A widely distributed, gram-positive bacterium that causes infections ranging from acne to wound infections and pneumonia.

STARI: Southern tick-associated rash illness.

stevia: A sweetener made from plants in the genus *Stevia*.

strep infection: An infection caused by bacteria in the genus *Streptococcus*.

strep throat: An acute sore throat caused by group A streptococci.

Streptococcus pneumoniae: An aerobic, gram-positive bacterium that is a common cause of pneumonia, meningitis, middle-ear infections, and other diseases.

strontium-90: A radioactive strontium isotope produced by the fission of uranium.

sucralose: An artificial sweetener

sulfite: A salt or ester of sulfurous acid.

sunblock: A lotion that prevents UVB light from reaching the skin.

sunscreen: A lotion that reduces the amount of UVA and UVB light reaching the skin.

susceptible: Capable of contracting a given disease if exposed.

Sweet'N Low: An artificial sweetener that contains saccharin.

swine flu: Any influenza A virus related to strains found in swine, such as H1N1 or H3N2.

Tamiflu: A trade name for oseltamivir, an antiviral drug used to treat influenza.

tapeworm: Any of a class of parasitic flatworms.

TAPOS: Tick-associated polyorganic syndrome.

TB: Tuberculosis.

teratogen: Any agent that causes birth defects.

thimerosal or **thiomersal**: An organomercury compound (trade name Merthiolate) used as an antiseptic and also as a preservative in some vaccines.

threat: (1) A hazard. (2) A major hazard, or one that involves evildoers.

Tiger River disease: Another name for listeriosis.

tolerance: A state of decreased responsiveness to a toxic effect of a chemical, resulting from prior exposure.

tomatine: A toxic chemical found in tomatoes (mainly in foliage and green fruit).

toxic: Poisonous; having the properties or effects of a toxin.

toxicology: The study of the nature, effects, and detection of poisons in living organisms.

toxic shock syndrome (TSS): A severe, invasive infection caused by *Staphylococcus aureus*, Group A streptococci, and other bacteria.

toxigenic: Producing a toxin or toxins.

toxin: A poison derived from a plant, animal, fungus, or microorganism.

toxoplasmosis: An infectious disease caused by the protozoan parasite *Toxoplasma gondii*.

trachoma: An infectious eye disease caused by the bacterium *Chlamydia trachomatis*.

trans fat: An unsaturated (liquid) fat that has been partially hydrogenated.

transgenic: Having chromosomes into which one or more genes from an unrelated species have been incorporated.

transmission (of an infectious agent): Any mechanism that exposes a susceptible host to an infectious agent.

tuberculosis: A chronic infectious disease caused by *Mycobacterium tuberculosis* in humans and by *M. bovis* in livestock.

tularemia: An infectious disease caused by the bacterium *Francisella tularensis*.

type 1 diabetes: A form of diabetes mellitus that usually starts in childhood and results from diminished production of insulin.

type 2 diabetes: A form of diabetes mellitus that usually starts in adulthood and results from resistance to the effects of insulin.

typhoid fever: An infectious disease caused by the bacterium *Salmonella typhi*.

UDMH: Unsymmetrical dimethylhydrazine, a breakdown product of daminozide.

ulcer: A persistent sore on the skin or a mucous membrane.

ulcer disease: Ulcers in the stomach or duodenum, caused by the bacterium *Helicobacter pylori*.

ultraviolet (UV) light: Radiation with a wavelength shorter than visible light and longer than X-rays.

umami: Savoriness; one of the basic tastes (other than bitter, sour, salty, and sweet).

USDA: United States Department of Agriculture.

UVA: Ultraviolet light with wavelengths of 315 to 400 nm.

UVB: Ultraviolet light with wavelengths of 280 to 315 nm.

UVC: Ultraviolet light with wavelengths of 100 to 280 nm.

vaccination: The act of administering a vaccine.

vaccine: A preparation of a weakened or killed pathogen, or a portion of the pathogen's structure, which when administered stimulates antibody production or cellular immunity.

vaccinia: The poxvirus that causes cowpox.

variola: Smallpox.

variolation: An early form of smallpox vaccination.

vasculitis: Inflammation of a blood vessel.

vCJD or nvCJD: New variant Creutzfeldt-Jakob disease.

vector: An insect or other organism that transmits a pathogen from one host to another.

virulence: The ability of an agent to cause disease in a given host.

virus: An extremely small organism that can reproduce only as a parasite inside a living cell; sometimes classified as nonliving.

waterborne disease: A disease caused by an infectious agent that is present in water.

West Nile encephalitis: A form of encephalitis caused by a virus and transmitted primarily by mosquitoes.

WHO: World Health Organization.

whooping cough: An infectious disease caused by the bacterium *Bordetella pertussis*.

WNV: West Nile virus.

wolf peach: An old name for the tomato.

xenophobia: Fear of foreigners or strangers.

yellow fats: Butter, margarine, and other spreads.

yellow journalism: Journalism that distorts or exaggerates the news to attract readers.

zoonosis: Plural, zoonoses. An infection or infectious disease that is transmissible under natural conditions from vertebrate animals to human beings.

INDEX

ABOUT THE AUTHOR

JOAN R. CALLAHAN is the award-winning author of numerous biological journal papers, environmental reports, and science books. She received her PhD from the University of Arizona and has worked as a consultant and researcher for over 30 years, most recently as an epidemiologist for the Naval Health Research Center and as a contractor for the National Institute of Standards and Technology. Her latest books include *Biological Hazards* (Oryx Press, 2002) and *Emerging Biological Threats* (Greenwood Press, 2009).